Culinary Solutions
FOR MIGRAINE SUFFERERS

Cat Browne, Founder, Culinary Solutions
& Laurie Hartford, MS, RD

Photography by Sarah Morrel Lowder

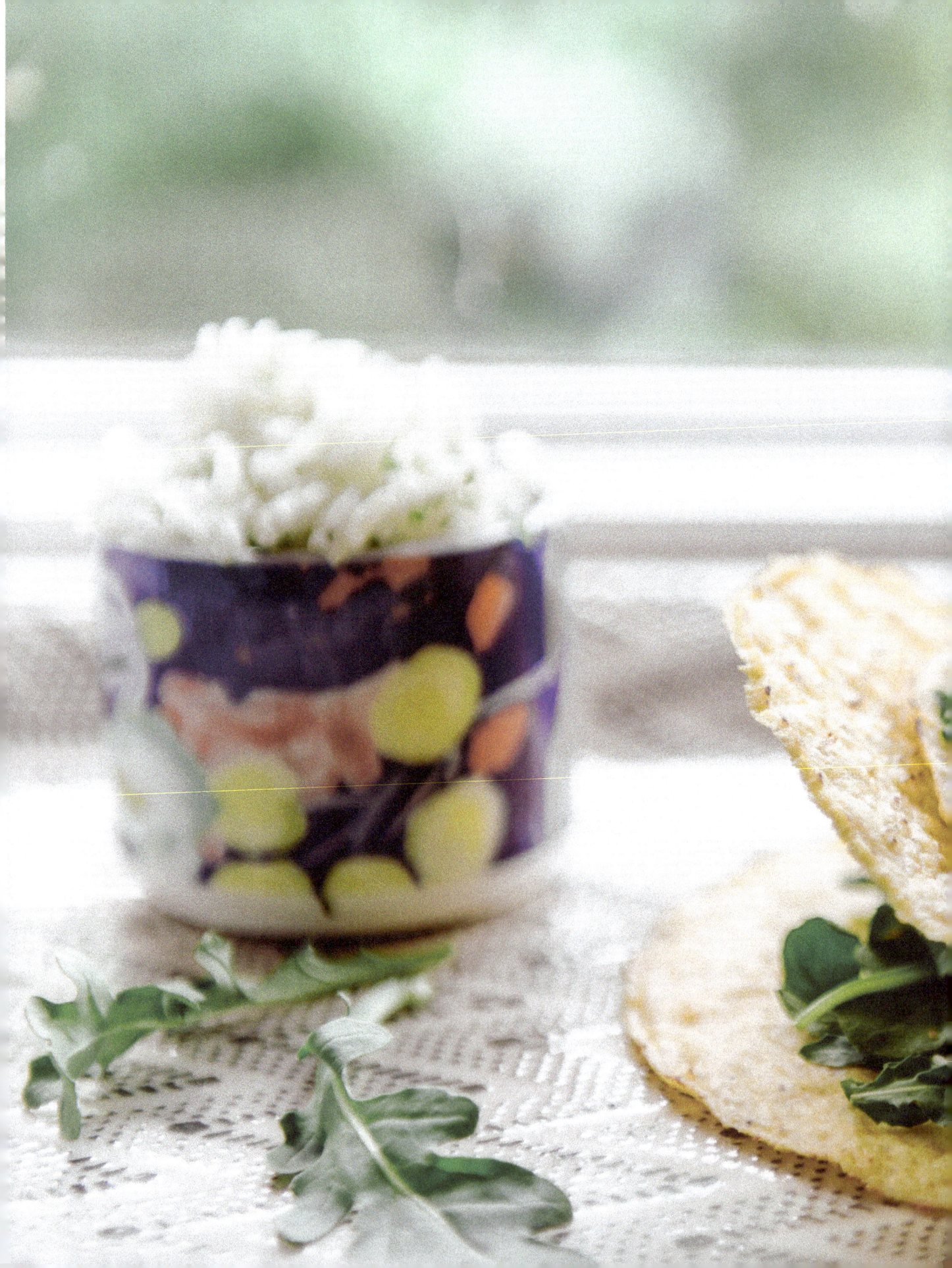

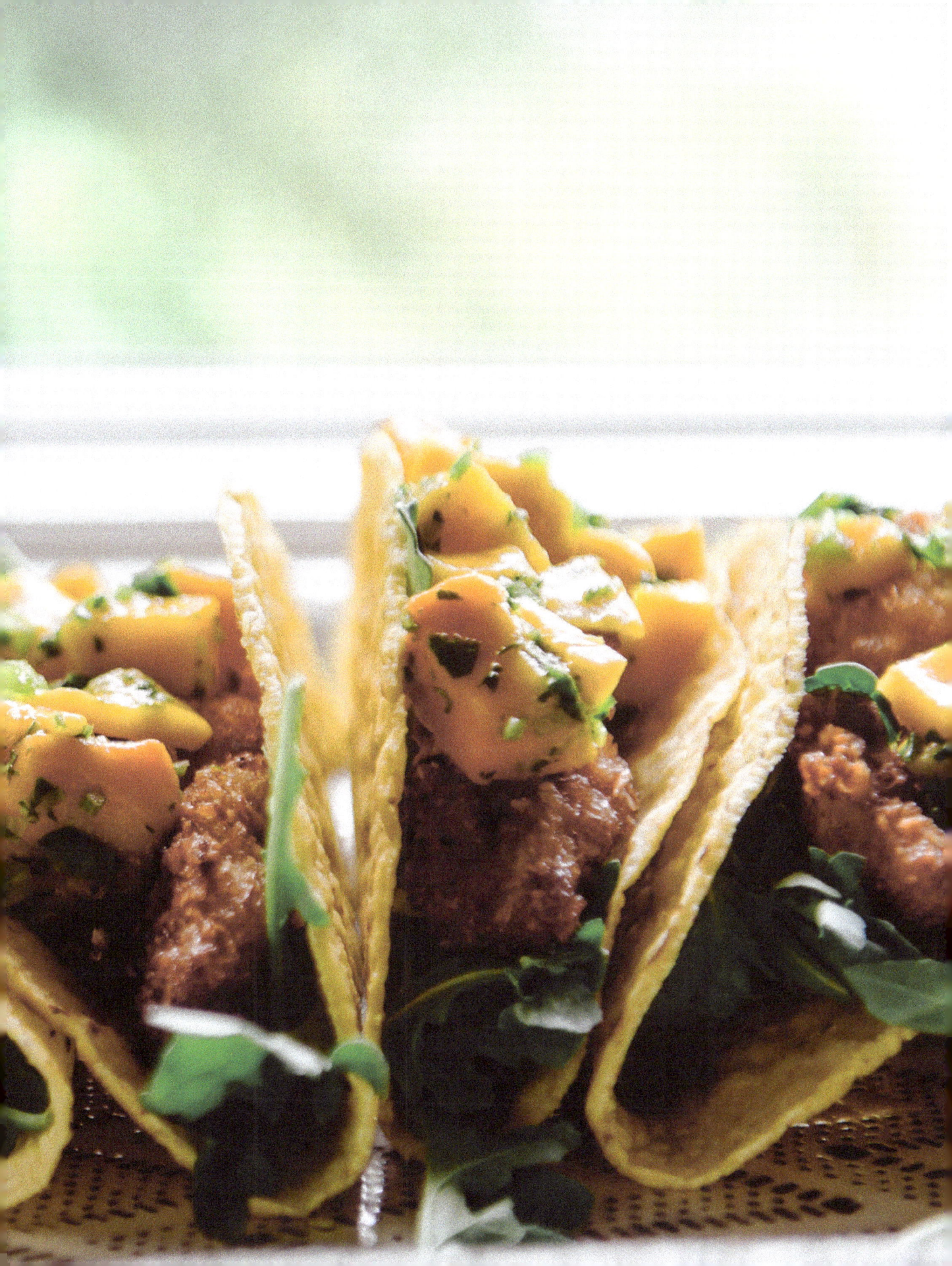

COPYRIGHT

ISBN: 979-8-9990672-0-3 (hardcover)
ISBN: 979-8-9990672-1-0 (softcover)

Photography: Sarah Morrel Lowder
Design and Layout: Vicky Vaughn Shea, Ponderosa Pine Design
Editing: Patricia Davis
Copy Editing and Proofreading: Debra Kaczynski Perry

DISCLAIMER

The information contained in this book is not designed to make or replace any form of medical or professional advice. It is in no way to suggest a cure for headaches. The material has been researched from reasonable sources and has been provided for educational and entertainment purposes. Medical treatment for headaches must be derived from licensed professional and medical practitioners.

DEDICATION/ACKNOWLEDGMENTS

Patti Davis, you helped me get this cookbook off the ground. I sincerely appreciate your work on formatting the recipes alone. Your invaluable guidance helped to shape this cookbook into what it is today.

Debra Perry, who kept everyone on track and moving forward in the final stages of editing this book.

Our talented book designer, Vicky Shea, whose professional experience and creativity brought this book to life. Thank you for creating a captivating book cover that showcases what the book has to offer.

Photographer and friend, Sarah Lowder, for seeing my colorful vision for this book. I truly enjoyed our long sessions together and appreciate all your flexibility. Your joy and love of life are contagious.

Thank you to all of my professors, chefs, colleagues, and friends at College of Charleston and The Culinary Institute of America. Your guidance and knowledge are irreplaceable, and I feel privileged to have spent chapters of my life at these wonderful schools.

A huge shout-out to all friends, family, and colleagues at Whisk and at Home for Entertaining, who tested recipes, gave input, and never stopped asking "How's the cookbook coming?" I could not ask for a more supportive group.

My grandmother, Marjorie Parker. Grandma, thank you for inspiring several recipes in this book and for the wonderful childhood memories in the kitchen. Your biscuits and cobbler will always be some of my favorites.

My brother, John Parker. Thank you for reminding me early on that recipes don't always have to be followed, and ingredients don't always have to be measured. It's now my favorite way to cook.

My dad, Chuck Parker. Dad, I will forever love our time together in the kitchen as a kid and as an adult. Thank you for all your guidance in business, recipe testing, and life in general.

Betty Parker, my mom and best friend. Mom, thank you for sending me the cooking magazines, articles, and encouraging notes when I wasn't close to home. I appreciate all the time you spent with the kids while I worked on this book and for the numerous roles you play in helping me throughout the ups and downs of life.

Dad and Mom, thank you both for your endless support and for allowing me to follow my dreams. I owe my love of cooking to you, among countless other things in this life. You are my rocks.

My little sous-chefs, Johnny and Parker: I can't imagine life without you, and I cherish our time together in the kitchen. You bring me endless joy, and I love you more than you'll ever know.

And most importantly, to Jim and Laurie Hartford, for being inspired to create this cookbook and trusting me to write the recipes. Without you this book wouldn't exist, and it has been a joy collaborating with you.

—Cat Browne

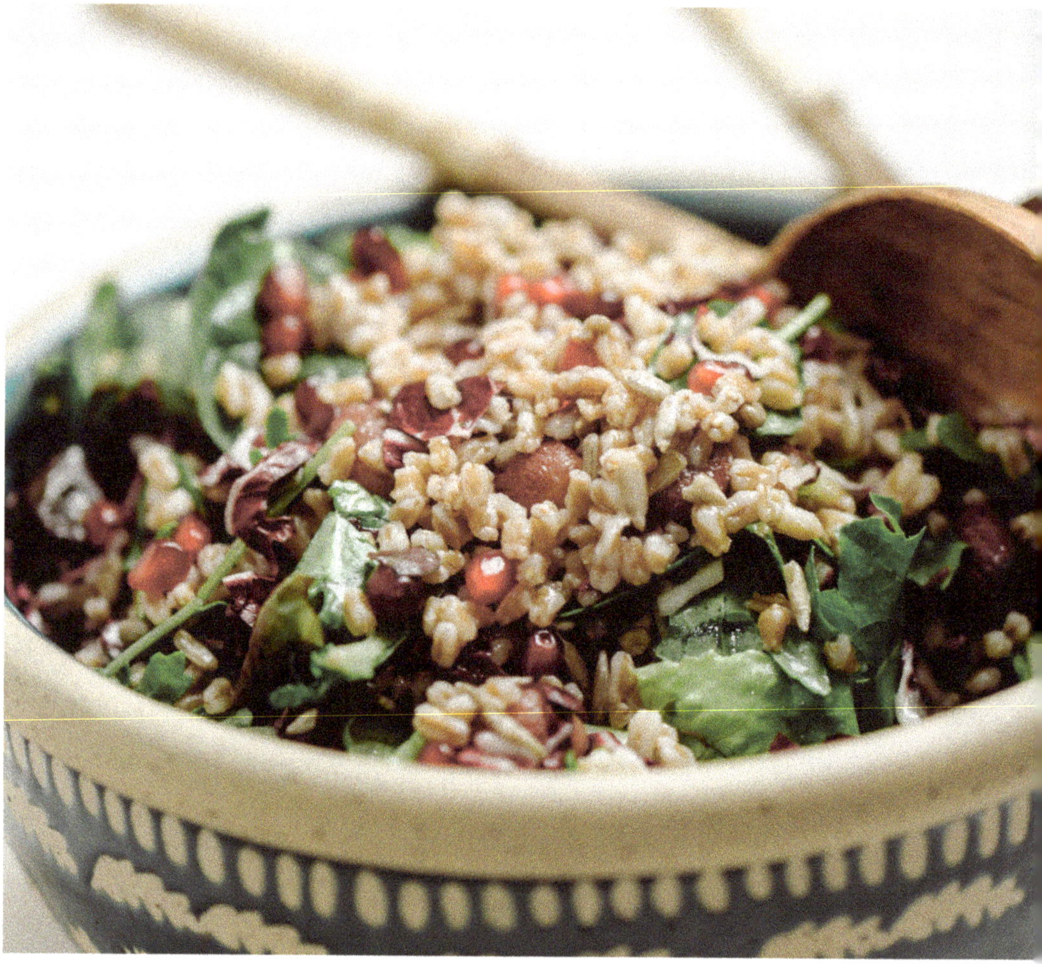

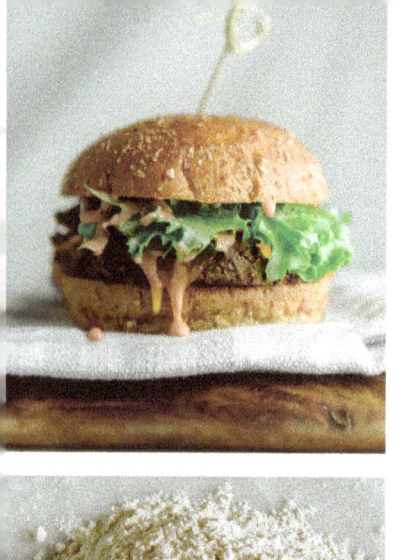
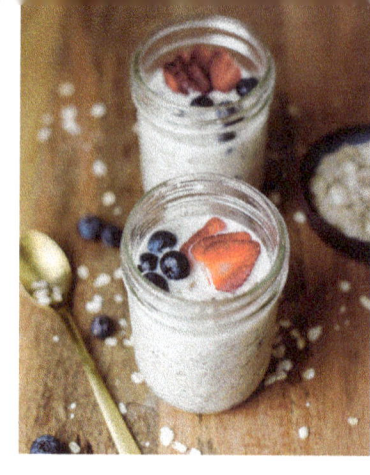
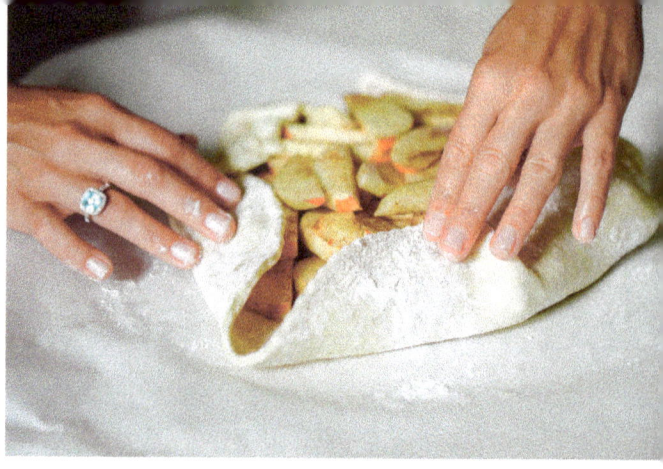
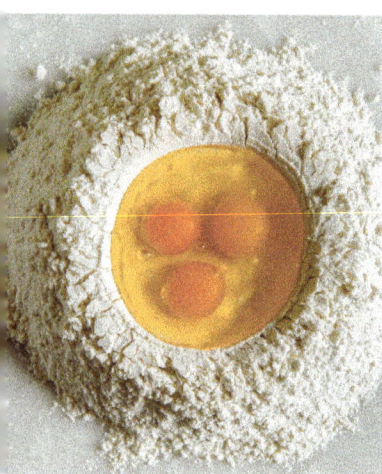
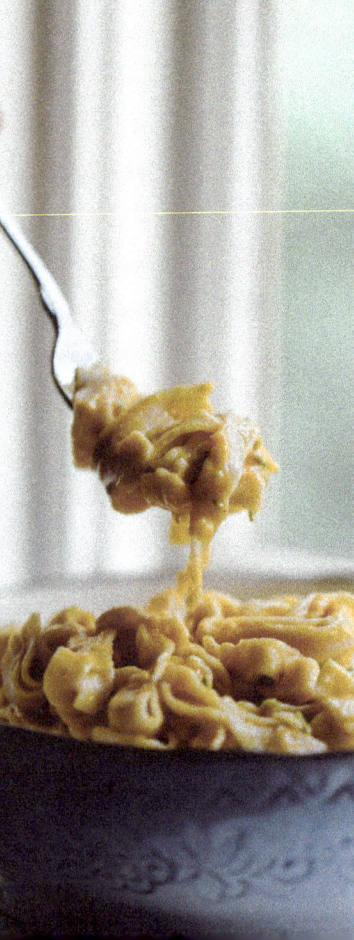
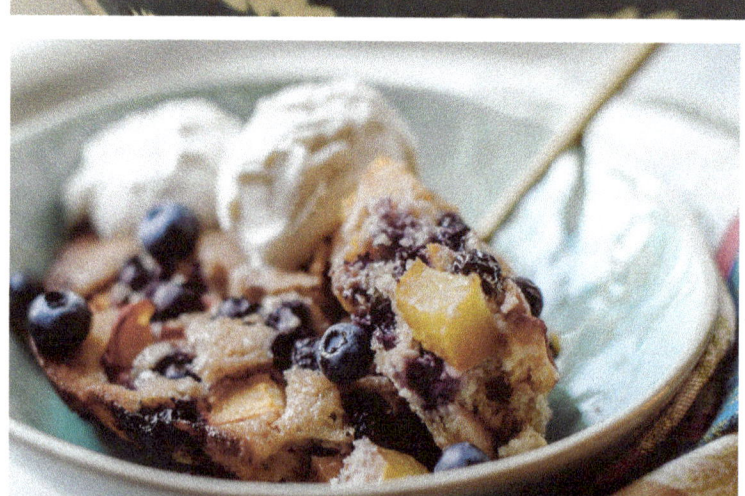
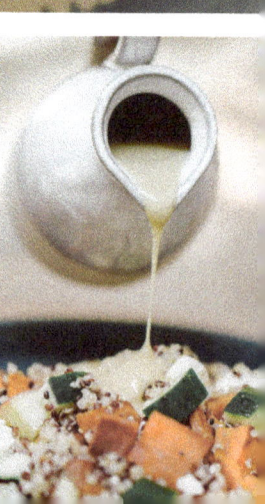

Contents

Introduction 8

Tools to Help You 11

Pantry Staples 13

Fridge and Freezer Staples 15

Smoothies and Bowls 17

Breakfast 33

Snacks 61

Stocks, Soups, Stews, and Salads 83

Vegetarian Mains 111

Meaty Mains 129

Pasta 165

Seafood 185

Sides 197

Sauces and Dips 223

Sweets 247

Index 266

About the Authors 272

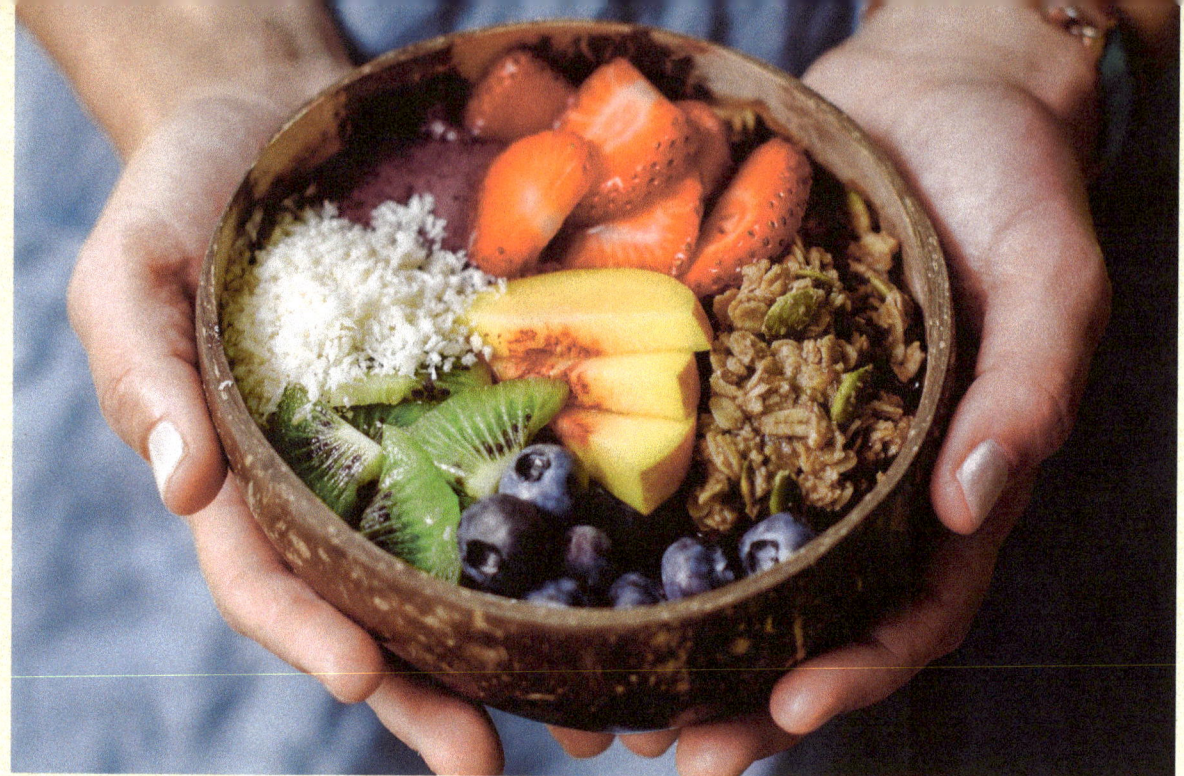

Introduction

Migraines occur in about 12% of the people aged 12 and older in the United States (about 7% women and 6% men). I have suffered from migraines for most of my adult life. I came to realize there are many things that can trigger or worsen a migraine. Some of these triggers are out of one's control: weather, environment (bright lights, strong odors, and loud noises), and hormonal fluctuations, to name a few. Many triggers, however, can be controlled: too much or too little sleep, stress, and diet.

Being a dietitian, I was most interested in diet as a trigger. I reviewed countless "lists" of foods that can be considered triggers. Ultimately, I discovered an easy-to-understand list provided by Dr. David Buchholz in his book *Heal Your Headache* (see right). In general, I found that eliminating the foods suggested by Dr. Buchholz made a significant difference in my migraines. At right is an easy-to-use chart of foods that are considered dietary triggers, which Chef Cat Browne and I try to avoid using in our recipes. Other dietary triggers include histamine and tyramine, two naturally occurring compounds in food. In developing a migraine diet, avoidance of both compounds is beneficial in the reduction of dietary headache triggers.

The goal of this book is to provide inspiring recipes that abide by the foundations of a headache diet that can be served to migraine sufferers as well as their friends and family.

—Laurie Hartford

DIETARY TRIGGERS	
Caffeine	Coffee, tea, iced tea, and cola. Even decaf coffee and tea (which contain additional chemical triggers) may be a problem. Also beware of coffee substitutes. Try caffeine-free herbal tea (without citrus and other trigger flavors).
Chocolate	White chocolate (no cocoa is OK; carob is questionable).
Monosodium Glutamate	Chinese (and other) restaurant food; soups and bouillons; Accent and seasoned salt; flavored, salty snacks; croutons and breadcrumbs; gravies; ready-to-eat meals; cheap buffets; low-fat, low-calorie foods. Watch out for hidden MSG!
Processed Meats and Fish	Aged, canned, cured, fermented, marinated, smoked, tenderized—or preserved with nitrites or nitrates. Hot dogs, sausage, salami, pepperoni, bologna (and other lunchmeats with nitrates); liverwurst, beef jerky, certain hams, bacon, pâtés, smoked or pickled fish, caviar, and anchovies. Also, fresh beef liver and chicken livers, and wild game (which contain tyramine).
Cheese and Other Dairy Products	The more aged the cheese, the worse. (Permissible cheeses include cottage cheese, ricotta, cream cheese, and good-quality American cheese). Beware of foods containing cheese, including pizza. Yogurt (including frozen yogurt), sour cream, and buttermilk are also triggers.
Nuts	Avoid all kinds, as well as nut butters. Seeds are OK.
Alcohol and Vinegar	Especially red wine. Champagne and dark or heavy drinks. Vodka is best tolerated. Clear (ideally, distilled) vinegar is *allowable*. Don't overdo condiments (ketchup, mustard, and mayonnaise) made with vinegar.
Certain Fruits and Juices	Citrus fruits (oranges, grapefruits, lemons, limes, tangerines, clementines, and pineapples) and their juices—as well as bananas. Also avoid raisins (and other dried fruits if preserved with sulfites), raspberries, red plums, papayas, passion fruit, figs, dates, and avocados.
Certain Vegetables, Especially Onions	Plus sauerkraut, pea pods, and certain beans (broad Italian, lima, fava, navy, and lentils). *Allowed*: leeks, scallions, shallots, spring onions, garlic.
Fresh Yeast-Risen Baked Goods	Less than one-day-old homemade (or restaurant-baked) breads, especially sourdough, as well as bagels, doughnuts, pizza dough, soft pretzels and coffee cake.
Aspartame	Saccharin (Sweet'n Low) may also be a trigger for some. Sucralose (Splenda) may not be a trigger.
Others	Perhaps soy products, especially if cultured (miso), fermented (tempeh) or otherwise highly processed (e.g., soy protein isolate/concentrate). Watch out for soy sauce containing MSG. Less risky are unflavored tofu and soy milk and flour. Soy oil is safe. Possibly tomatoes (and tomato-based sauces), mushrooms... whatever gives *you* a headache.

Chart from *Heal Your Headache: The 1-2-3 Program for Taking Charge of Your Pain*, by David Buchholz, MD, pages 74–75. Workman Publishing, New York, NY. Copyright © 2002. Reprinted with permission Workman Publishing an imprint of Hachette Book Group, Inc.

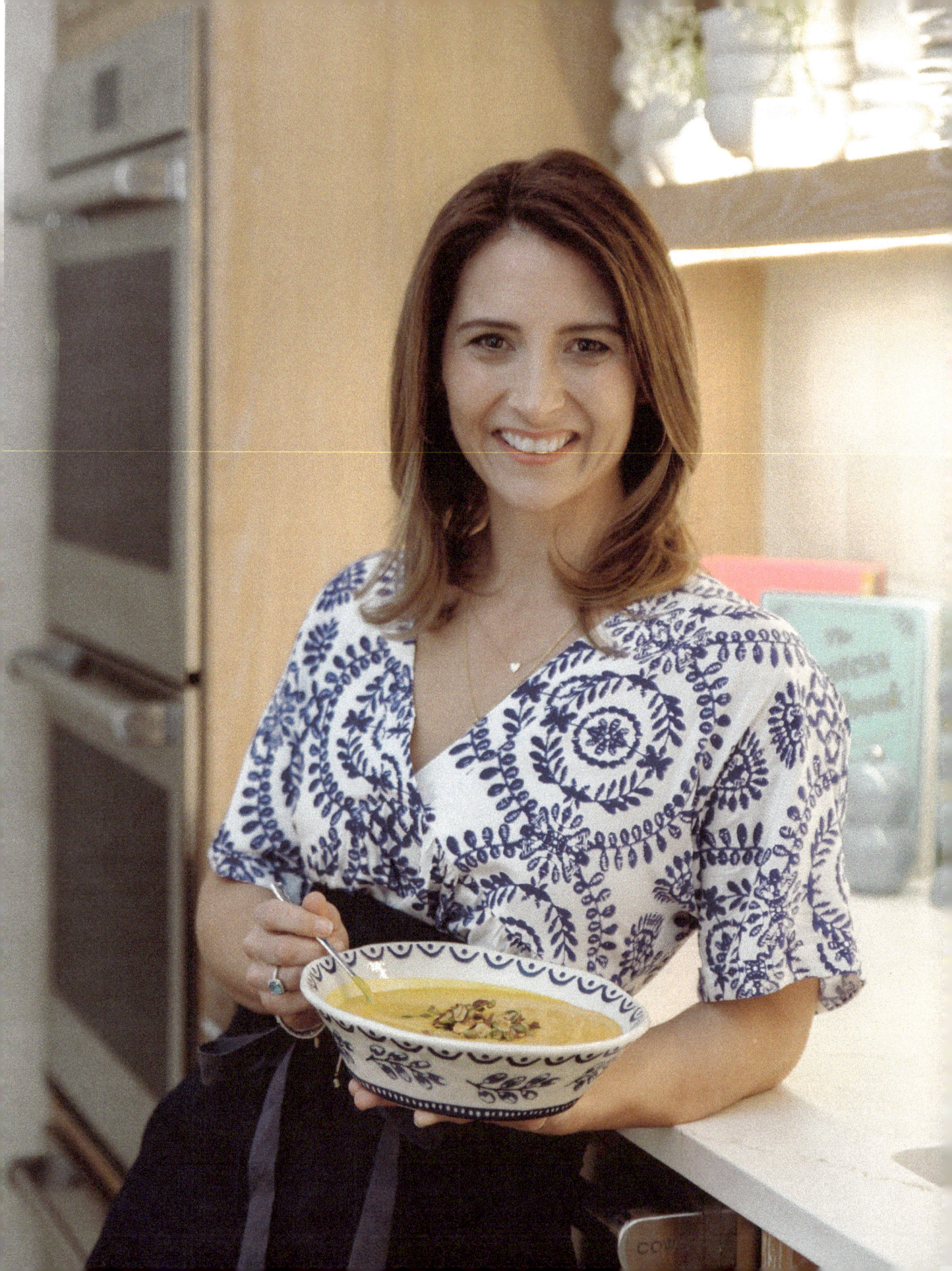

Tools to Help You

SHARP KNIFE

This is by far the most important tool in your kitchen. A dull knife can make your entire kitchen experience frustrating, especially if you have a lot of prep to do before you begin cooking. I recommend having your knives professionally sharpened about once a year. If you are thinking about purchasing a knife but don't necessarily want to buy an entire set, start with a chef's knife. An 8-inch (or similar) chef's knife can go a long way in the kitchen.

FOOD PROCESSOR

A quality food processor is one of the best kitchen tools to have. It reduces prep work if you need to rough-chop or mince many vegetables. I use it for Grandma Parker's Pasta Bolognese (page 169) and other soups and stews as well as Strawberry Coconut Bites (page 69).

VITAMIX OR OTHER HIGH-SPEED BLENDER

This is one of my favorite pieces of kitchen equipment, one that I use daily. Whether it's blending up a smoothie, creating a pesto, or even making baby food purées, a high-speed blender can be a game-changer in the kitchen. The Vitamix can be a bit pricey, but my refurbished (half-price) one has been going strong for over eight years now.

MASHER OR PASTRY BLENDER

A pastry blender or masher is a great tool to have when making biscuits and pie crusts. It helps cut the butter into small pieces while keeping it cold. It is also great for potatoes or mashing avocado for guacamole (if avocados are not a trigger).

BENCH SCRAPER

This tool makes pasta making (and working with dough in general) much more enjoyable. It not only can be used to cut your dough (or butter) but also helps to clean the flour off your countertops. A bench scraper also makes transporting a pile of chopped vegetables a breeze.

RICER OR FOOD MILL

A ricer is helpful if you are working with potatoes for dishes like gnocchi. It breaks down boiled potatoes into thin, rice-like pieces that are then incorporated into recipes. However, if you plan to do larger batches or want to break down foods like roasted beets and tomatoes, a food mill might be the better choice.

INSTANT-READ THERMOMETER

An instant-read thermometer is extremely important to have on hand to confirm the internal temperatures of fish and meats. It is best to avoid cutting into meat to check for doneness. Slicing into the meat releases all the juices and flavor before the meat has time to rest.

IMMERSION BLENDER

This tool is a simple but effective one. It is a handheld blender that makes puréed soups and half-blended stews a breeze. You can also make big batches of homemade mayonnaise as well as blend jams and applesauce with it.

INSTANT POT (OR OTHER PRESSURE COOKER)

The love I have for my Instant Pot was not immediate. I enjoyed the long, slow process of cooking stews all day on the stove. (This was obviously before kids!) When I received an Instant Pot as a gift, it sat on the counter for a while, since like most new pieces of kitchen equipment, it takes time to familiarize yourself with your new item. When I finally decided to get to know my Instant Pot, it took several tries to get it right. I am still not exactly sure what I was doing wrong and, once again, I didn't understand why they were so popular. Then it clicked! Maybe I just needed to read one more tutorial or I hadn't gotten the venting right, but once it worked, I was hooked. It's hard to imagine my kitchen without it now. As a personal chef I can now offer clients short ribs and stews that would otherwise take too long. If it's solely pressurized cooking you want, there are many good-quality pressure cookers out there. But if you like a combo pressure cooker and slow cooker all in one, the Instant Pot might be for you.

SILPAT AND OTHER SILICONE BAKING MATS

You can always line a baking sheet with parchment paper, but to reduce waste, a Silpat (or other brand) silicone baking mat is the way to go. The mats are made of durable, food-grade silicone, don't absorb food odors, and are a snap to clean in the sink or dishwasher. Best of all, they distribute heat evenly and can be rolled up for easy storage.

—Cat Browne

Pantry Staples

KOSHER SALT

If you ask a chef what's the most important ingredient when cooking, chances are they will say salt. Just a small pinch of salt can bring food to life!

In this book Morton's kosher salt was used in testing all of the recipes. Kosher salt enhances flavors without adding chemical taste that table salt can have.

Kosher salt is widely available, inexpensive, and a great choice for any cook. Even different types of kosher salt vary slightly by brand, so I suggest picking one and sticking to it.

You will notice throughout the book that in some recipes I give specific amounts of salt (for items like muffins, that you might not taste as you go) and, in others I say salt to taste. I encourage you to taste as you go, when possible, and add salt to match your preference.

HIGH-QUALITY OILS: OLIVE OIL AND EXTRA VIRGIN OLIVE OIL

I always have a nice extra virgin olive oil for drizzling on salads and pastas or in pesto and other recipes that don't require heat. Then I use regular olive oil for most cooking. It's less expensive, more mellow in flavor, and has a higher smoke point.

You don't want to go overboard when using any oil, since it's extremely high in fat and processed. Oils can also easily overpower a dish if you add too much.

For a higher-heat oil I use avocado oil or ghee (clarified butter).

Try to avoid using a lot of refined vegetable oil, such as corn, canola, and soybean.

OATS AND OAT FLOUR

Oats are one of my favorite foods! They are a great source of fiber and protein and can help lower cholesterol and blood sugar levels. They are widely available, affordable, and can be used in so many ways. Of all the different types of oats, I usually use rolled oats, which are oat groats that have been steamed and pressed/flattened. They are less processed than quick-cooking oats and are great for making oat flour. Steel-cut oats are even less processed than rolled oats, but they take longer to cook.

To make oat flour, just blend rolled or quick-cooking oats in a high-speed blender until you have a fine consistency. I make several cups at once and store in an airtight container in the pantry.

SEEDS

Seeds are a nutrient-dense powerhouse. They have lots of vitamins and minerals, protein, fiber, and healthy fats.

QUINOA

Quinoa is a fantastic plant protein for those who don't eat a lot of meat (and for those who do!). Quinoa is considered a complete protein and can be used when making pancakes or veggie burgers and can be added to soups to give them some texture and more protein.

BEANS

Migraine-friendly beans are great sources of protein, fiber, and antioxidants. Black beans provide the body with lots of iron and potassium, while chickpeas (aka garbanzo beans) offer more magnesium and folate. While canned beans provide convenience for the busy cook, I try to use dry whenever possible. Just make sure you soak them overnight and rinse before cooking.

VANILLA

Most of the recipes in this book call for vanilla extract, which most people have in their pantry. Just ensure it is high-quality, pure vanilla extract and not imitation vanilla. Imitation vanilla has artificial flavorings usually made from by-products and can be diluted with water and alcohol. You will pay a little more for the quality vanilla, but it's worth it. When you really want the vanilla in a recipe to shine (as in Coconut Caramel Sauce, page 259), opt for vanilla bean paste, which includes the seeds as well. Check the label to ensure the ratio is 1:1 to vanilla extract.

OTHER PANTRY STAPLES TO NOTE

Local (real) honey

Look for local honey or "pure" honey. Some of the large industrial honey producers add fillers, such as corn syrup, to reduce costs. A local farmers market or health-food store is a good place to look for quality honey.

Coconut sugar

This is a good option if you are looking for a natural sweetener. It comes from dehydrating the sap of the coconut palm and is minimally processed.

Chia seeds

These tiny little seeds pack a lot of nutrition. They are full of fiber, protein, and omega-3 fatty acids. We call them "sprinkles" in our house, and the kids enjoy putting them on their oats, açaí bowls, avocado toast, and more.

—Cat Browne

Fridge and Freezer Staples

TAHINI

Made from sesame seeds, tahini adds a great depth of flavor to many dishes. It is a wonderful nut-free option that I find myself using frequently in sauces, dressings, and, of course, hummus.

COCONUT WATER

We keep coconut water on hand and use as a base for a lot of smoothies. It is packed with natural electrolytes that refuel the body. Find a brand without added sugars, preservatives, or flavorings.

PURE MAPLE SYRUP

A good-quality maple syrup is my go-to sweetener. It is less processed and includes more minerals and antioxidants compared to standard cane sugar. While it is lower on the glycemic index, it is still sugar, so don't go too crazy. Be sure to read the label to confirm there are no added ingredients.

QUALITY ANIMAL PRODUCTS
(Beef, pork, poultry, eggs, milk, butter, etc.)

I cannot stress enough the importance of high-quality animal proteins. Whether it's 100% grass-fed, pasture-raised beef, wild- and sustainable-caught fish, or eggs from pasture-raised poultry, it's important to know where your food comes from. Not only are there more nutrients in top-quality animal proteins, but they leave out all the unnecessary additives.

HOMEMADE STOCKS

Homemade stocks are usually better in flavor and nutrition than store-bought and free from preservatives and additives. If you do purchase stock, check the label for unnecessary MSG, sugar, and preservatives, and buy organic when possible.

FRUITS, IDEALLY LOCAL OR ORGANIC

Sometimes local farmers don't want to go through the trouble or pay additional costs to label their foods "organic," but that doesn't mean they don't use organic practices. Ask the farmers at the market if they use chemical pesticides or synthetic fertilizers (or other products) on their produce. When the local farmers market has seasonal fruits, I stock up and freeze some to enjoy when they are out of season. Whether you buy local or conventional produce, give your fruits, vegetables, and herbs a good rinse before enjoying.

—Cat Browne

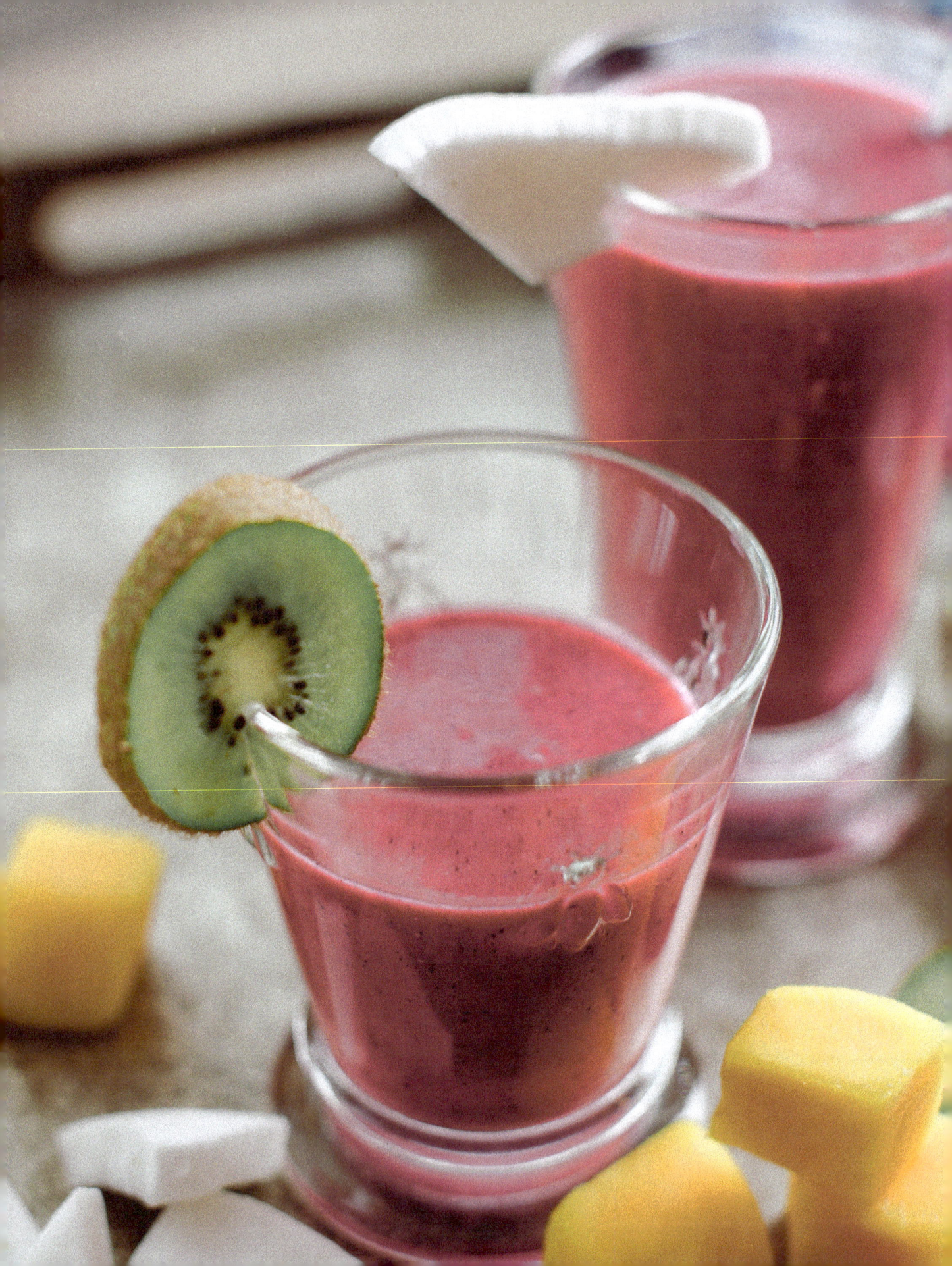

Smoothies and Bowls

Minty Mango Kale Smoothie...18

Strawberry Mint Refresher...19

Sweet Potato Pie Smoothie...20

Herby Glow Smoothie 21

Strawberry Rhubarb Smoothie..22

Roasted Blueberry Smoothie 23

Mixed Berry and Beet Smoothie...24

SB&J Smoothie 25

Pink Dragon Smoothie 26

Hidden Veggie Smoothie 27

Peach Pie Smoothie (or Bowl) 28

Açaí Berry Bowl...31

Minty Mango Kale Smoothie

This refreshing, spa-like smoothie is one of my favorite recipes in this book. Come springtime, we make this smoothie several times a week when our garden is overflowing with mint. And bonus: It is just as tasty the next day!

YIELD: 2 SERVINGS

INGREDIENTS

1 cup kale, packed

1½ cups coconut water

½ cup canned coconut milk

1-inch knob fresh ginger, peeled

Juice of ½ lime

¼ cup mint leaves

Small pinch salt

½ cup frozen sliced peaches

2 cups frozen diced mango

INSTRUCTIONS

Place all ingredients in a high-speed blender in the order listed then blend until smooth.

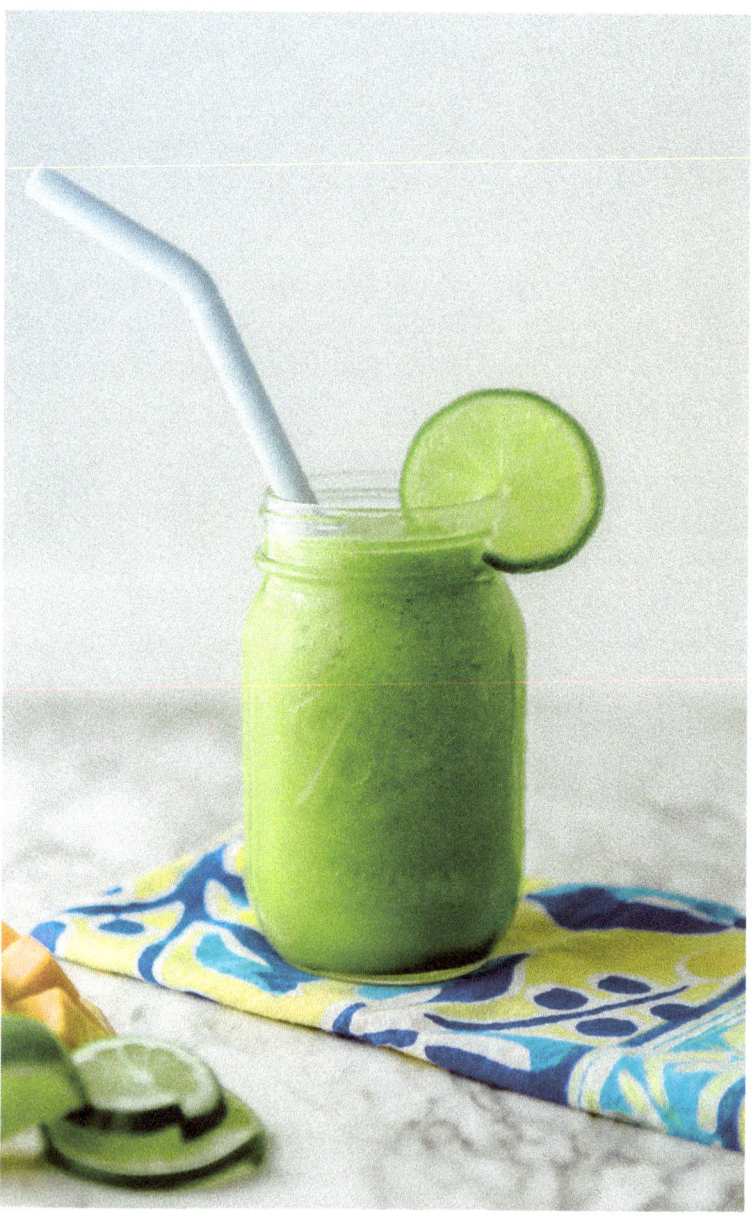

Strawberry Mint Refresher

Staying hydrated is one of the most important things you can do for your body, and food is here to help. Both strawberries and cucumbers are over 90% water and have plenty of benefits to keep your body thriving. I love this drink as a late afternoon snack on a warm spring day.

YIELD: 2 SERVINGS

INGREDIENTS

¼ cup fresh mint leaves, packed

1 cup cucumber, peeled and cubed

1¼ cups coconut water

2 teaspoons honey

3 cups strawberries, preferably frozen

Small pinch salt

2 teaspoons chia seeds

INSTRUCTIONS

1. Blend the first 6 ingredients in a high-speed blender until smooth.
2. Pour into a couple of glasses and stir in the chia seeds.
3. Wait a few minutes until the chia seeds plump up, stir again, and enjoy.

NOTE: You can also blend the chia seeds right into the smoothie if you prefer a smoother consistency.

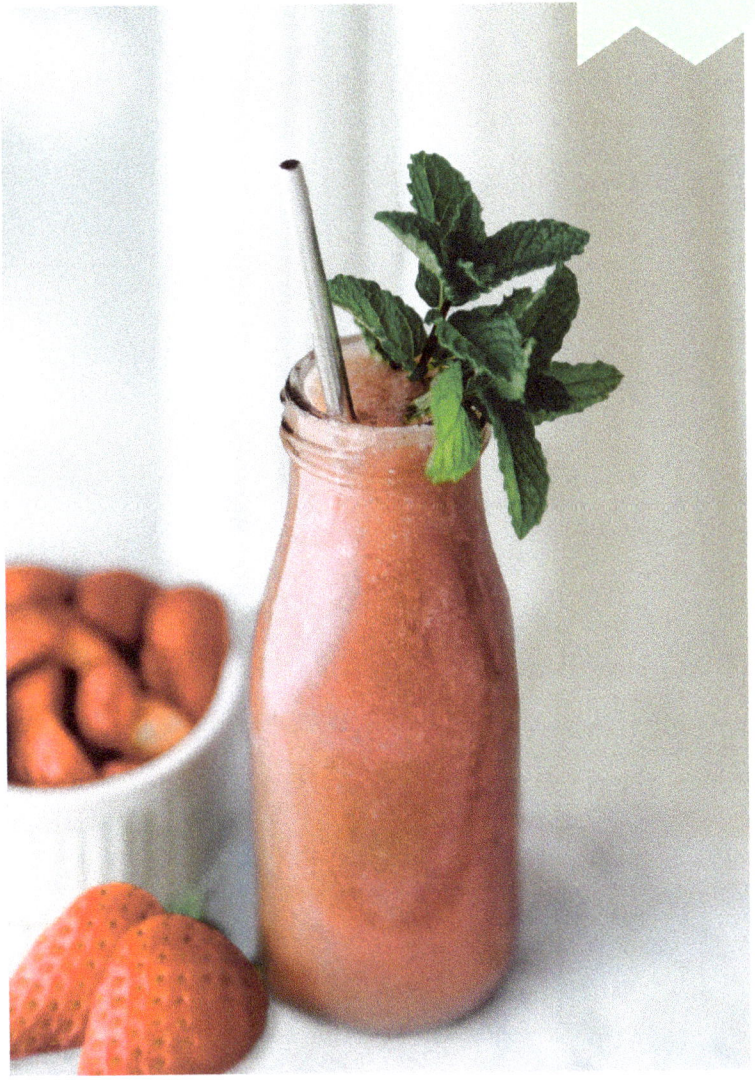

Sweet Potato Pie Smoothie

Sweet potatoes contain lots of potassium (more than bananas!), magnesium, and vitamins A, B6, and C. When digested they help balance electrolytes in the body. When I cook sweet potatoes, I always cook a couple extra and freeze them in small amounts for future smoothies.

YIELD: 2 SERVINGS

INGREDIENTS

1½ cups milk of choice

1 cup coconut water

½ teaspoon ground cinnamon

½ teaspoon pumpkin pie spice

¼ cup rolled oats

2 tablespoons sunflower seed butter

1 teaspoon pure vanilla extract

2 tablespoons maple syrup

Small pinch salt

1 cup cooked sweet potato, preferably chilled or frozen in cubes

1 handful ice if the sweet potato isn't frozen

INSTRUCTIONS

Place all ingredients in a high-speed blender in the order listed then blend until smooth.

TIP: To speed things up, you can use canned sweet potato purée. Extra purée can be frozen and used for future smoothies.

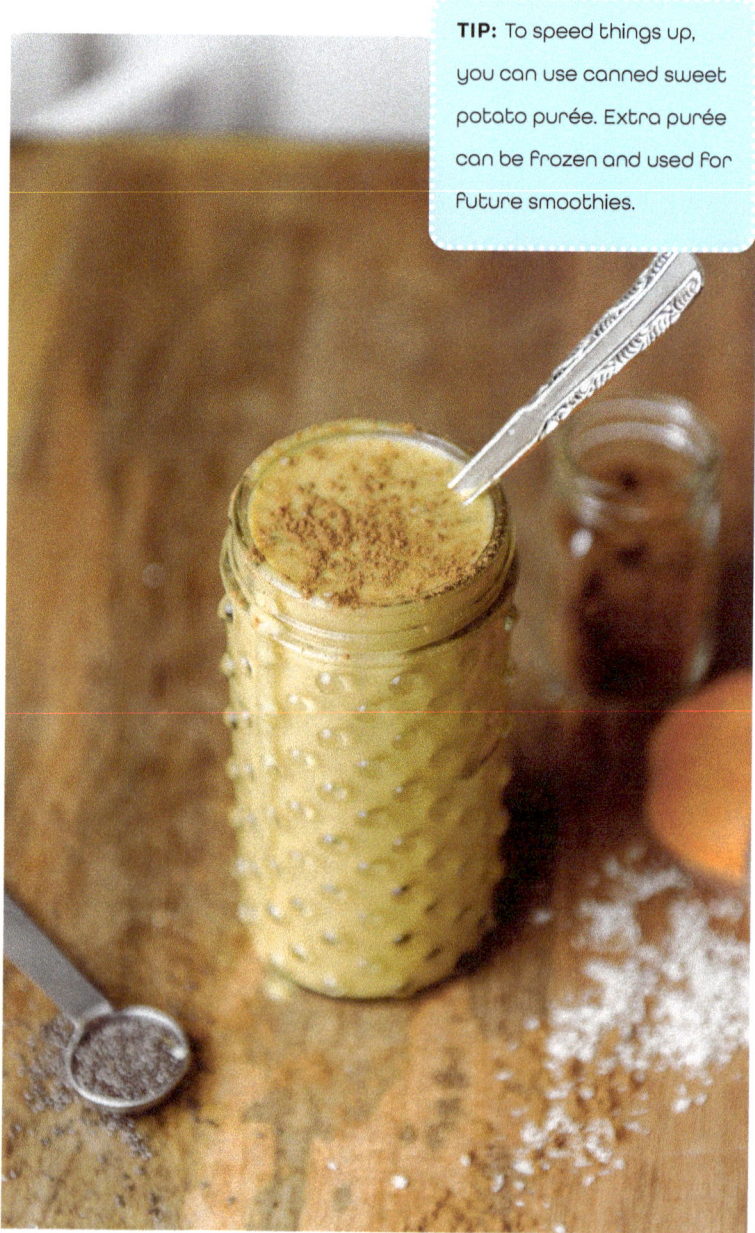

Herby Glow Smoothie

This is a nice "green" smoothie, as my kids call it. Feel free to add honey if you prefer a sweeter smoothie.

YIELD: 2 SERVINGS

INGREDIENTS

½ cup fresh parsley, some stems are OK

¼ cup fresh cilantro, some stems are OK

½ large apple, such as Granny Smith or Honeycrisp, cored and chopped

1 cup spinach

1½ cups coconut water

½ cup canned coconut milk

1 (10 oz) bag diced frozen mango, or about 2 cups

Small pinch salt

1–2 teaspoons honey (optional)

INSTRUCTIONS

Place all ingredients in a high-speed blender in the order listed then blend until smooth.

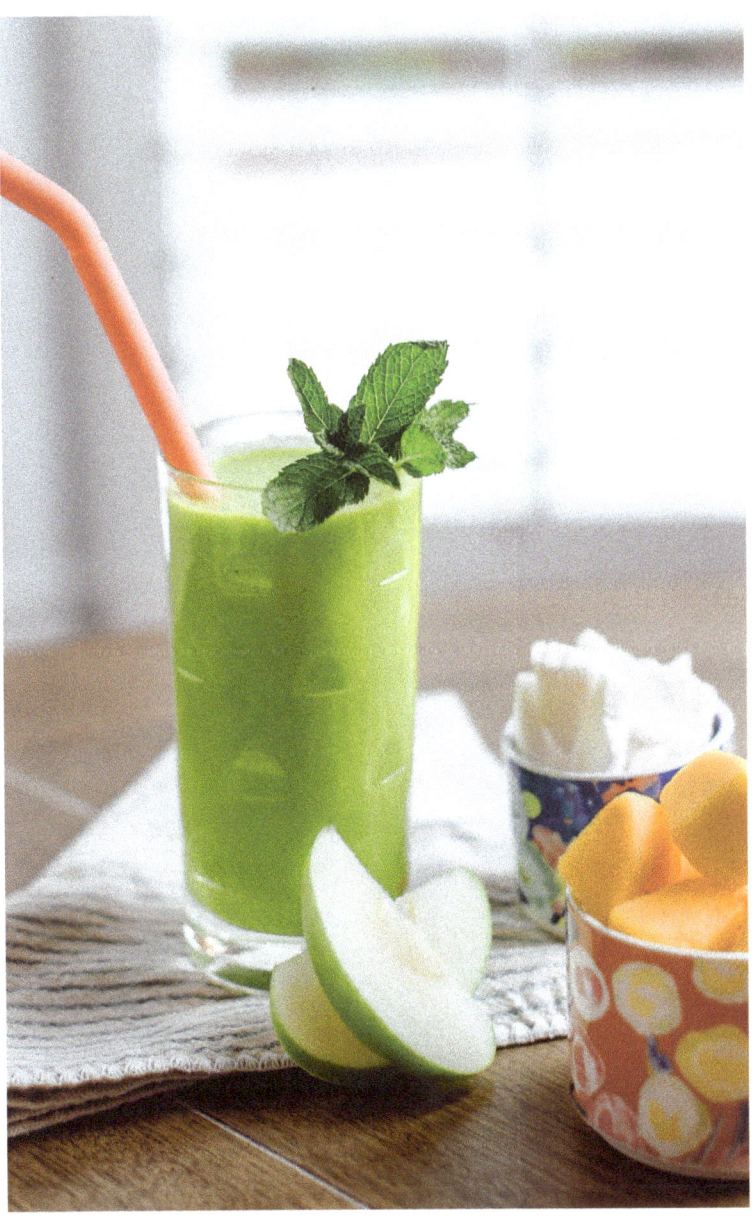

Strawberry Rhubarb Smoothie

Rhubarb is somewhat bitter when it's raw. You can heat it along with ½ cup water in a small saucepot over medium heat until most of the water evaporates. Allow it to cool slightly while carrying on making the smoothie.

YIELD: 2 SERVINGS

INGREDIENTS

2 stalks rhubarb, trimmed and chopped

½ cup canned coconut milk or other milk of choice

1 cup coconut water

½ cup pomegranate juice

1 tablespoon hemp hearts

1–3 teaspoons honey, or to taste

2 cups frozen strawberries

Small pinch salt

INSTRUCTIONS

Place all ingredients in a high-speed blender in the order listed then blend until smooth.

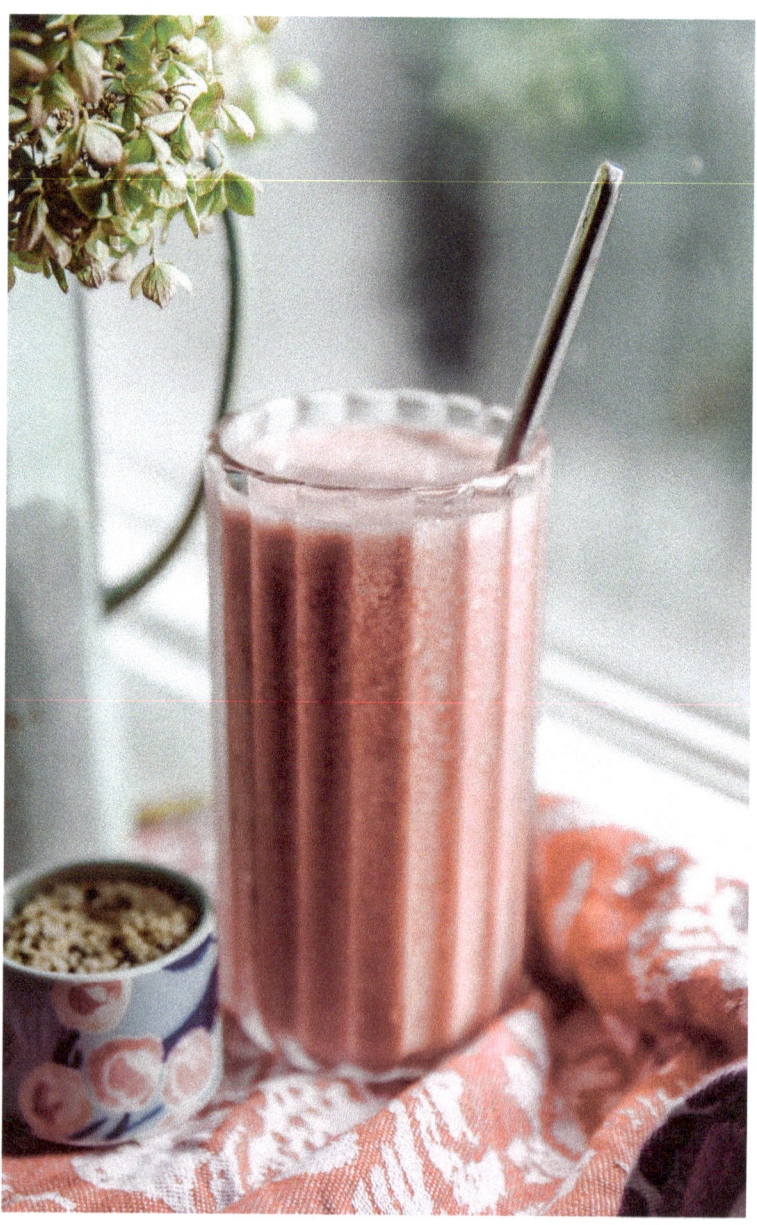

Roasted Blueberry Smoothie

While this smoothie can be made without roasting the blueberries, I don't recommend skipping that step. Roasting fruit concentrates the flavor and therefore brings out even more of the natural sweetness.

YIELD: 2 SERVINGS

INGREDIENTS

2 cups fresh blueberries, roasted (see Instructions)

¾ cup canned coconut milk or other milk of choice

¾ cup pomegranate juice

1 handful fresh spinach or kale (optional)

1 cup frozen cubed mango

1 handful ice

Small pinch salt

TIP: This smoothie is best enjoyed right away.

INSTRUCTIONS

1. To roast blueberries, place them on a parchment or Silpat mat-lined baking sheet and roast at 425°F for about 8 minutes or until one or two have burst open.

2. Once the blueberries cool, combine everything in a high-speed blender in the order listed then blend until smooth.

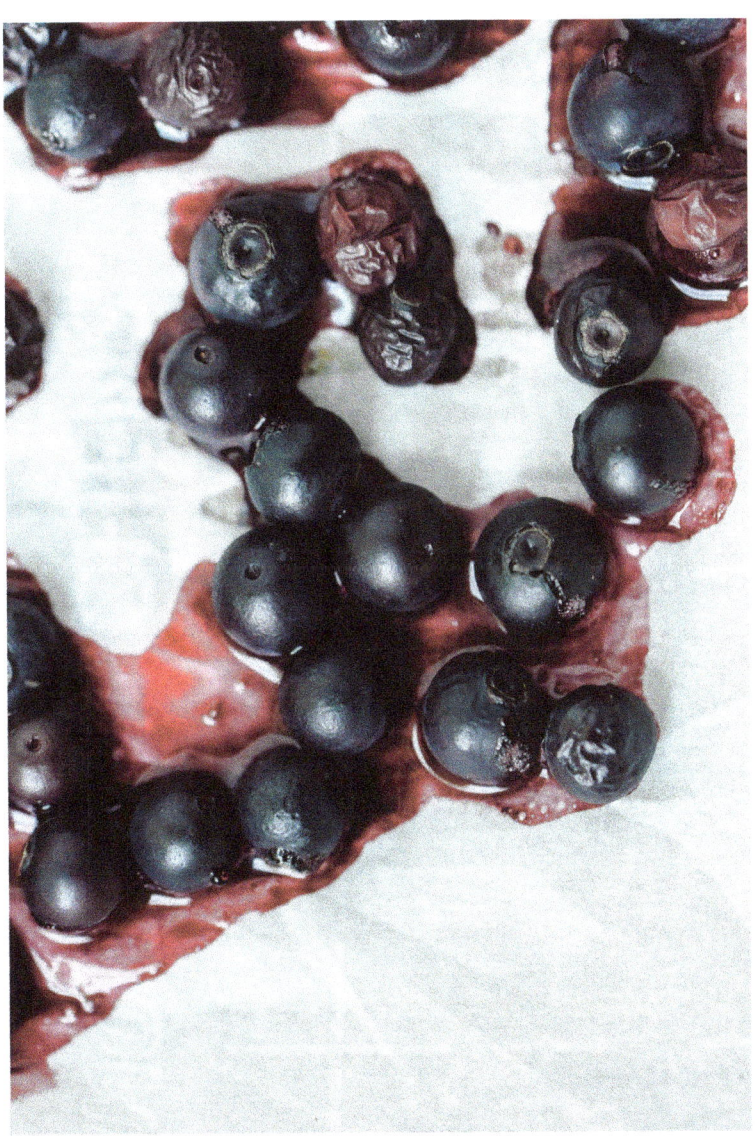

Mixed Berry and Beet Smoothie

My kids love beets. They just don't know it! If I give them pieces of cooked beets, they won't touch them. However, if I hand them a smoothie that has beets in it, they can't drink it fast enough.

YIELD: 2 SERVINGS

INGREDIENTS

1 small–medium beet, cooked and peeled

1¼ cups frozen mixed berries

¾ cup milk of choice

1 cup coconut water

½-inch knob ginger, peeled

Small pinch salt

INSTRUCTIONS

1. To roast beets, preheat oven to 400°F. Rinse beets then place them in a baking dish such as a large loaf or 8" x 8" pan along with 1 cup water. Cover with foil and bake for 45 minutes—1½ hours depending on beet size. They are done when you can pierce them with a fork easily.

2. Remove foil and let beets cool slightly before peeling. (I roast several beets at once and freeze the extra ones for future smoothies.) Blend all ingredients in a high-speed blender in the order listed until smooth.

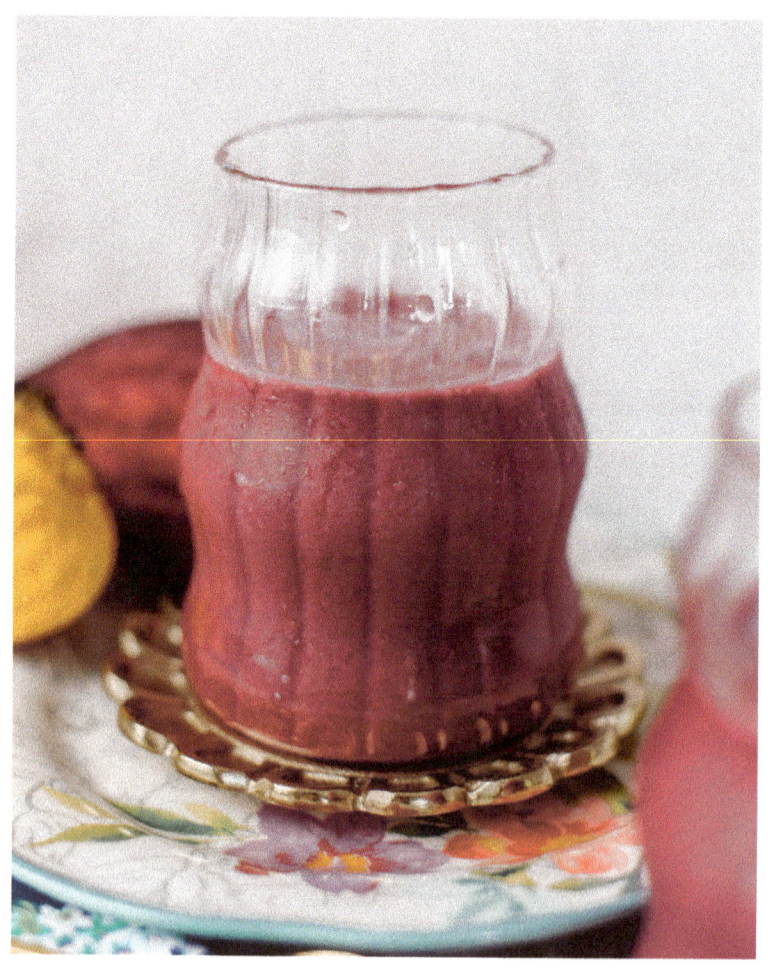

SB&J Smoothie

Whether it's on a sandwich or in a smoothie, this nut-free combo has become very popular. Sunflower seed butter is a great alternative to peanut butter, whether you suffer from migraines or are looking for a nut-free alternative to send in your child's lunch box. Like peanut butter, there are sweetened and unsweetened options. Be sure to read the label.

YIELD: 2 SERVINGS

INGREDIENTS

½ apple, such as Pink Lady or Honeycrisp, cored and chopped

1½ cups milk of choice

1 cup grapes

3 tablespoons sunflower seed butter*

2 cups frozen mixed berries

INSTRUCTIONS

Place all ingredients in a high-speed blender in the order listed then blend until smooth.

*NOTE: If peanuts are not a trigger for you, feel free to substitute peanut butter for the sunflower seed butter for a true PB&J smoothie.

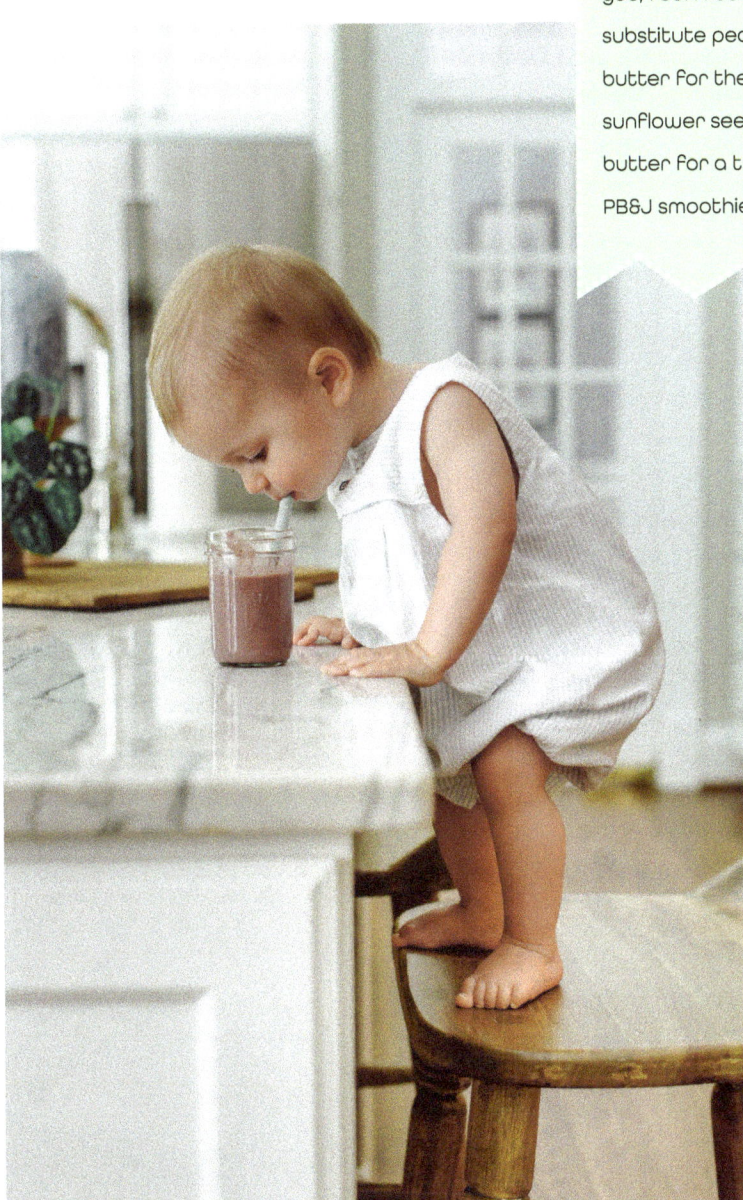

Pink Dragon Smoothie

Dragon fruit is also known as strawberry pear or cactus fruit. You can find frozen packets of its pulp in most health-food stores and some grocery stores. This tropical fruit has great iron content, lots of vitamin C, and plenty of antioxidants.

YIELD: 2 SERVINGS

INGREDIENTS

1 (3.5 oz) packet of frozen dragon fruit purée

1 cup coconut water

½ cup canned coconut milk

2 ripe kiwis*

1½ cups frozen mango chunks

1–2 teaspoons honey (optional)

Small pinch salt

*NOTE: You can peel the kiwi fruit before using, or, for an added boost of fiber and vitamins C and E, you can leave the peel on. Simply rinse the kiwi before using.

INSTRUCTIONS

1. Thaw the dragon fruit purée slightly by running warm water over the packet. It does not need to thaw completely.
2. Place all ingredients in a high-speed blender in the order listed then blend until smooth.

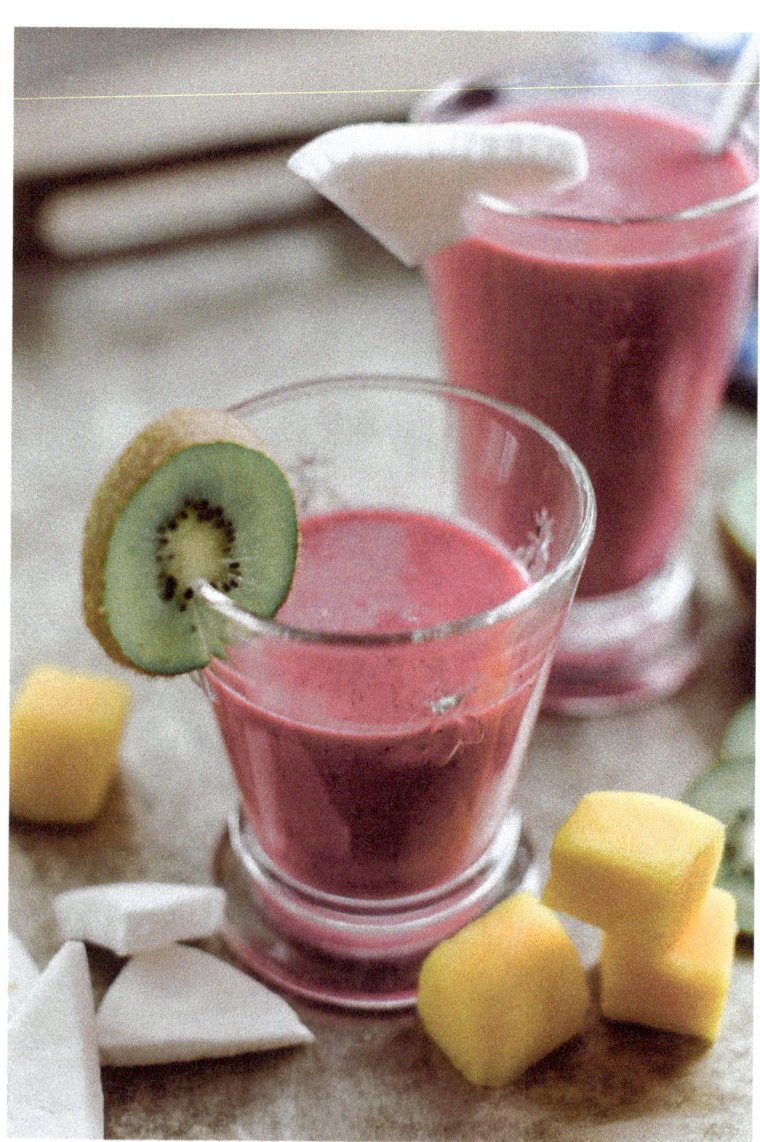

Hidden Veggie Smoothie

Smoothies are a great way to sneak an extra serving of vegetables in your kids, or yourself! Carrots and beets are some other great options to add to your smoothie. Cauliflower and spinach go almost undetected.

YIELD: 2 SERVINGS

INGREDIENTS

1½ cups pomegranate juice

1 cup fresh spinach

¾ cup milk of choice

½ cup frozen riced cauliflower

2 cups frozen sweet cherries, pitted

1 cup frozen mango chunks or frozen mixed berries

Small pinch salt

1 teaspoon chia seeds (optional)

INSTRUCTIONS

Place all ingredients in a high-speed blender in the order listed then blend until smooth.

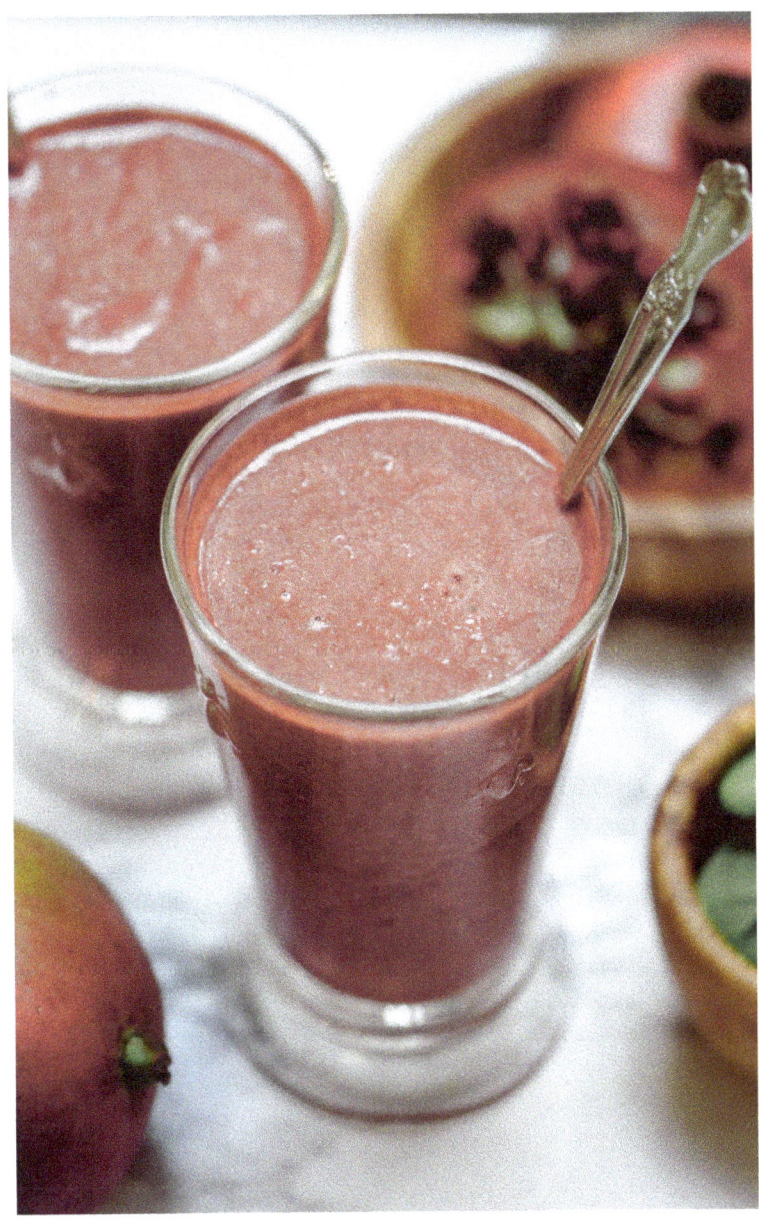

Peach Pie Smoothie (or Bowl)

If the South had a smoothie, this would be it. You can do so much with a fresh Southern peach, and don't even think about throwing away those slightly bruised ones. They are great cut up and frozen for smoothies or used in jam.

YIELD: 2 SERVINGS

INGREDIENTS

1 cup canned coconut milk

1 cup coconut water

½ teaspoon ground cinnamon

⅛ teaspoon ground ginger

Pinch nutmeg

½ teaspoon vanilla extract

Small pinch salt

1 tablespoon maple syrup

2½ cups sliced frozen peaches

½ cup strawberries

¼ cup or more riced cauliflower (optional)

INSTRUCTIONS

1. Place all ingredients in a high-speed blender in the order listed then blend until smooth.

2. Add your choice of toppings, such as toasted coconut, hemp hearts, chia seeds, granola, sliced peaches, strawberries, and blueberries.

TIP: To turn this into a smoothie bowl, reduce the amounts of coconut milk and coconut water by half. If you have trouble getting it to blend and your blender comes with a tamper, use that to push the fruit down.

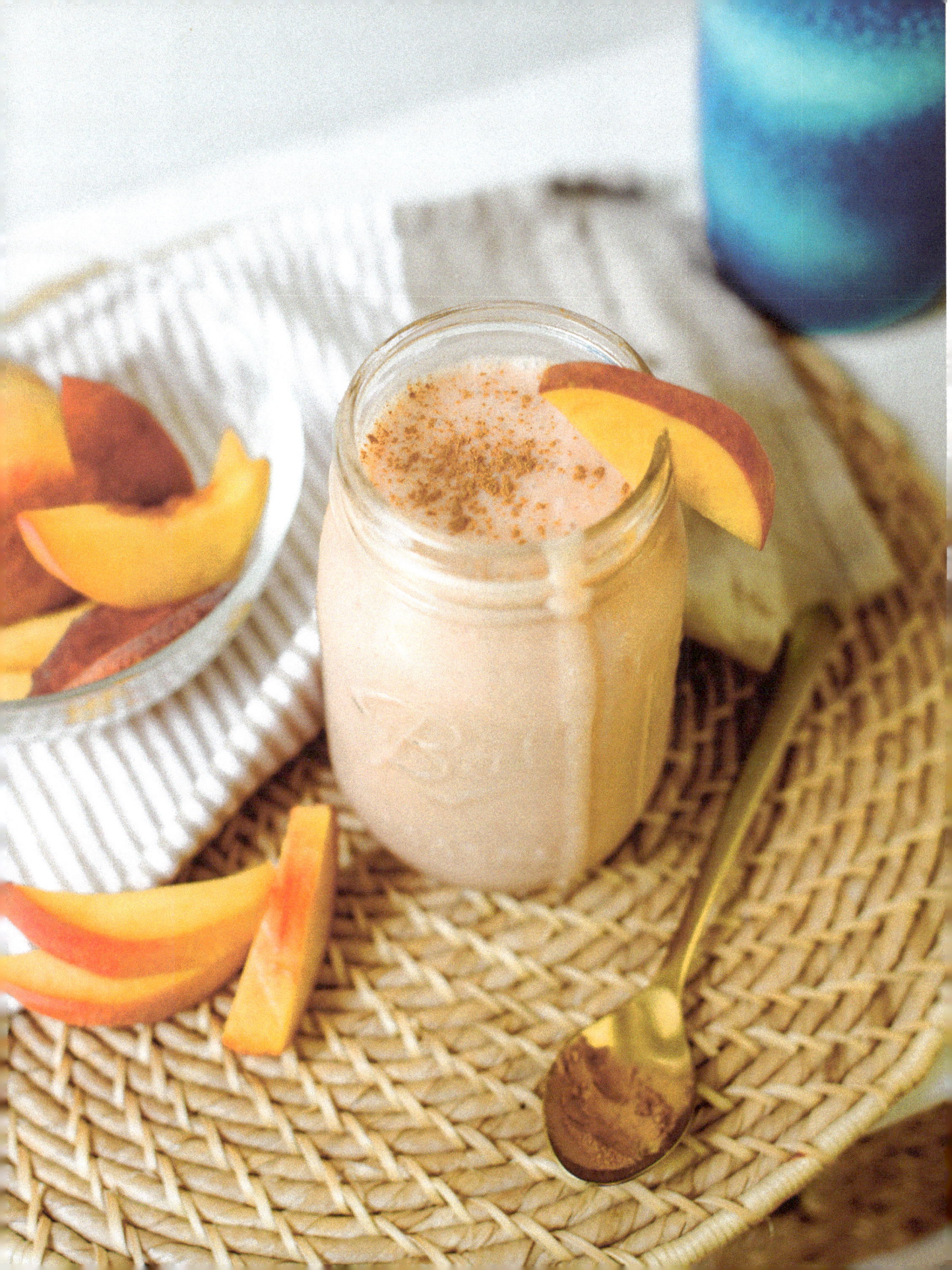

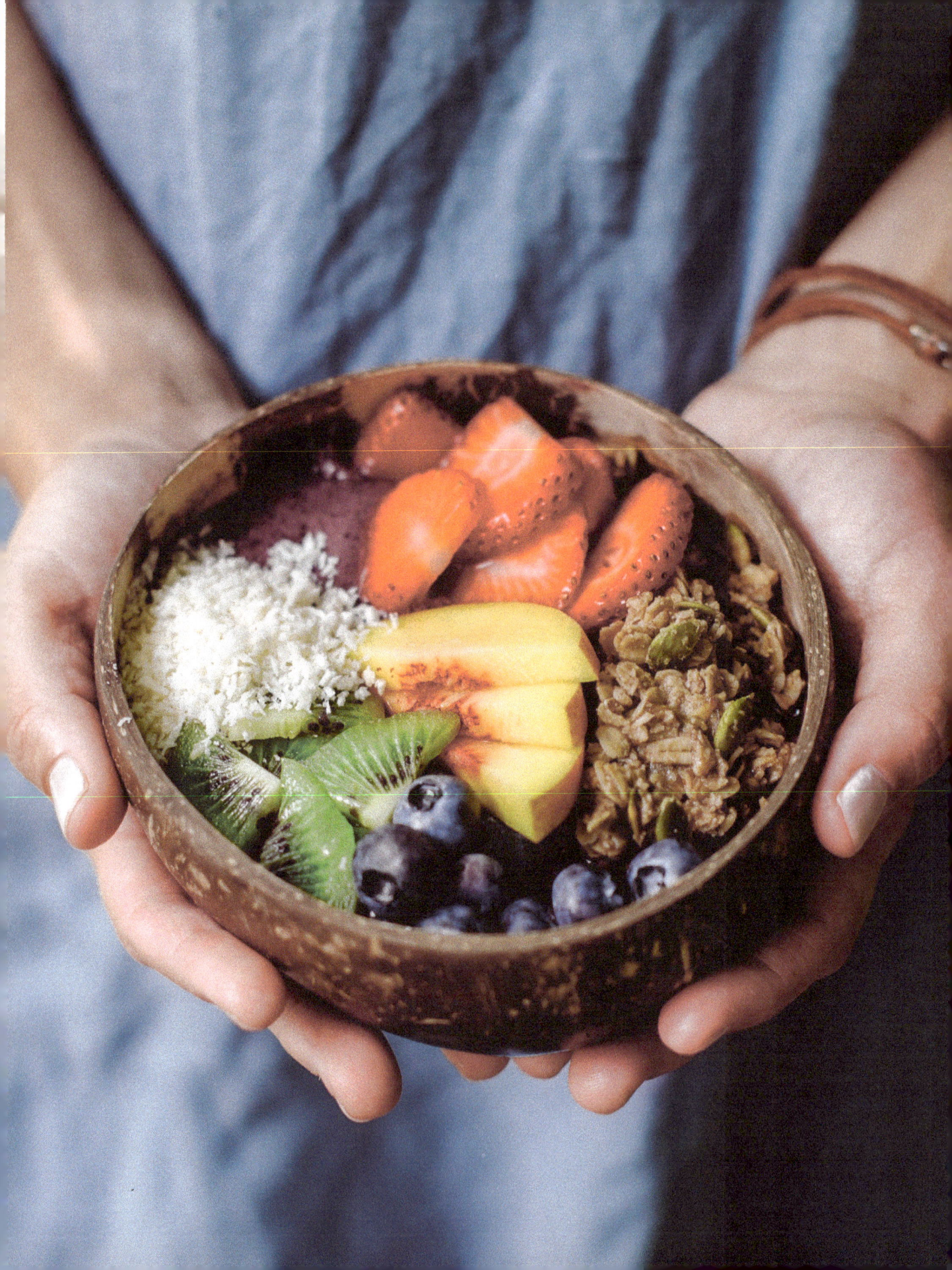

Açaí Berry Bowl

When my girlfriends and I travel together, we make a point to seek out some yummy açaí bowls wherever we are. The bowls are always a little different, but they hit the spot every time. Feel free to use dairy-free milk and maple syrup in place of honey for a vegan-friendly option.

YIELD: 2 BOWLS

INGREDIENTS

1 (3.5 oz) frozen packet açaí pulp

1½ cups frozen mixed berries

¾ cup milk of choice, I recommend canned coconut milk or grass-fed whole milk

1–3 teaspoons honey (optional)

Small pinch salt

Optional Toppings

Super Seed Granola (page 37) or another nut-free granola

Fresh blueberries, blackberries, or strawberries

Shredded coconut

Sliced peaches

Chia seeds

Hemp hearts

Bee pollen

Coconut Whipped Cream (page 259)

INSTRUCTIONS

1. Combine the first 5 ingredients in a high-speed blender then blend until smooth.

2. Pour into two bowls and add toppings of choice.

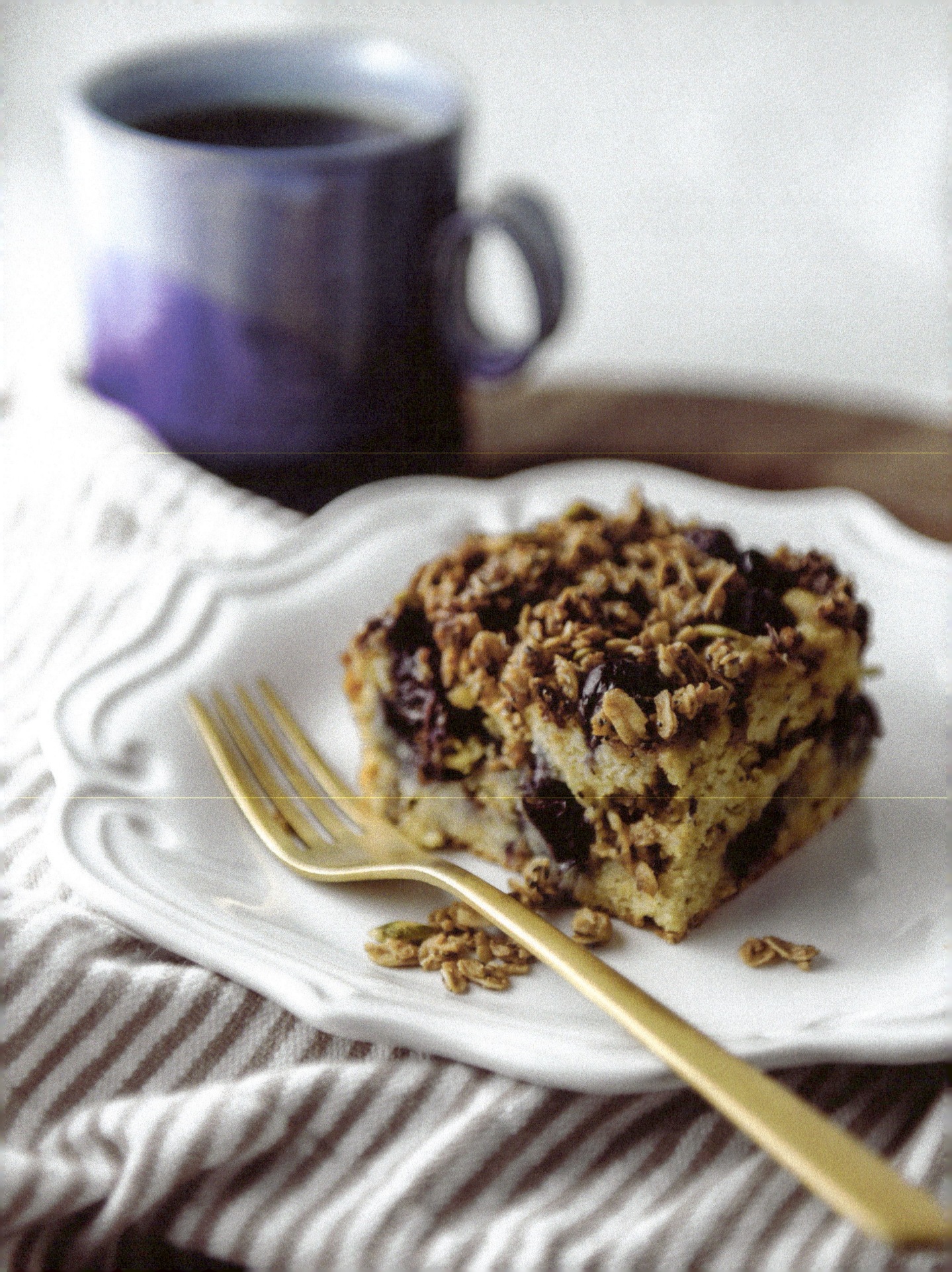

Breakfast

Apple Pancakes with Sage Leaves 34

Super Seed Granola...37

Power Blueberry Coffee Cake 38

Snickerdoodle Muffins with Streusel Topping 41

Migraine-Free Morning Glory Muffins...42

Johnny's Pumpkin Muffins 45

Egg Frittata Muffins 46

Sweet Potato Apple Breakfast Bake.. 49

Overnight Oats Three Ways 50

Make Your Own Sausage 53

Saturday Morning Breakfast Hash.. 54

Migraine-Friendly Frittata... 57

Southern Biscuits..58

Apple Pancakes with Sage Leaves

After moving to Napa for culinary school, my roommate asked if I wanted to volunteer at a farmers market event with her. When I learned we were going to be helping a chef make pancakes, I was even more excited. Of course, they weren't just regular pancakes. The batter was made with a sourdough starter, and they were topped with battered sage leaves that had been cooked on the griddle. I have created a migraine-friendly version that always reminds me of that fun event.

YIELD: 12–14 PANCAKES

INGREDIENTS

1¼ cups all-purpose or gluten-free flour (such as Bob's Red Mill)

½ cup oat flour (page 13)

Heaping ¼ teaspoon salt

1 tablespoon coconut sugar

1 teaspoon ground cinnamon

⅛ teaspoon ground nutmeg

⅛ teaspoon ground cloves

1 teaspoon baking powder

½ teaspoon baking soda

2 eggs, separated

1 cup milk, preferably whole milk

3 tablespoons unsalted butter, melted, plus more for cooking

1 teaspoon pure vanilla extract

¾ cup applesauce (page 62) or about 1 small–medium apple, finely shredded

Around 12 sage leaves*

Maple syrup for serving

INSTRUCTIONS

1. Combine the first 9 ingredients in a bowl. Stir and set aside.
2. In a separate large bowl add the egg yolks, milk, 3 tablespoons butter, and the vanilla. Mix thoroughly then add the applesauce or finely shredded apple.
3. With a stand mixer or handheld beaters, whip the egg whites with a whisk attachment until stiff peaks form. Set it aside.
4. In two batches add the dry ingredients into the wet ingredients, making sure not to overmix.
5. Gently fold in the egg whites.
6. In a large skillet or cast-iron pan, heat some butter over medium heat.
7. Pour ¼ cup batter in the skillet, fitting as many pancakes as you can in the pan while leaving room to flip. Once golden-brown, flip pancakes over and finish cooking. Repeat until there is about ¼ cup batter left.
8. Add a little more butter to the pan and dip the sage leaves in the batter. Place in the skillet and cook for about 30 seconds on each side until lightly golden.
9. To serve, top pancakes with sage leaves and maple syrup.

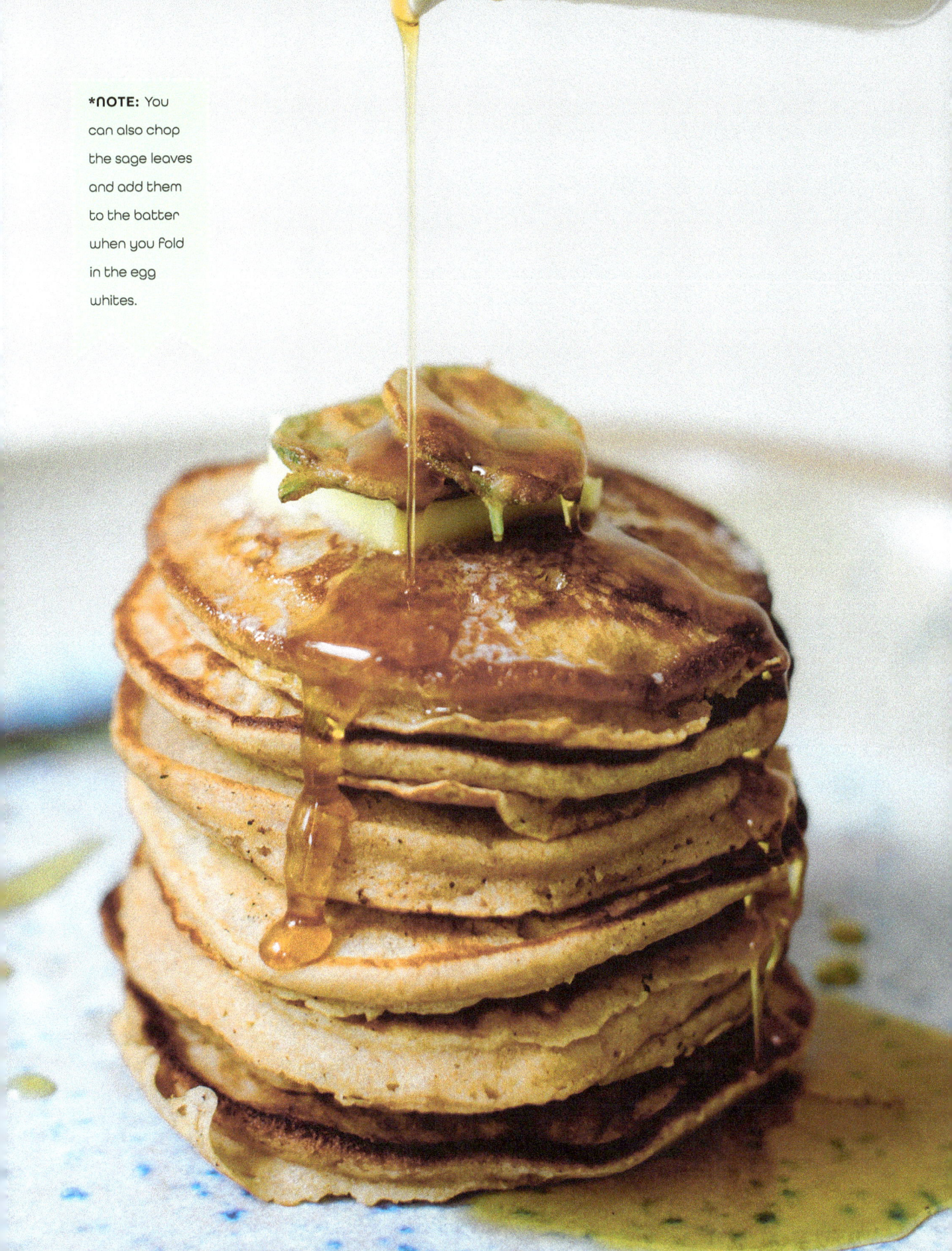

*NOTE: You can also chop the sage leaves and add them to the batter when you fold in the egg whites.

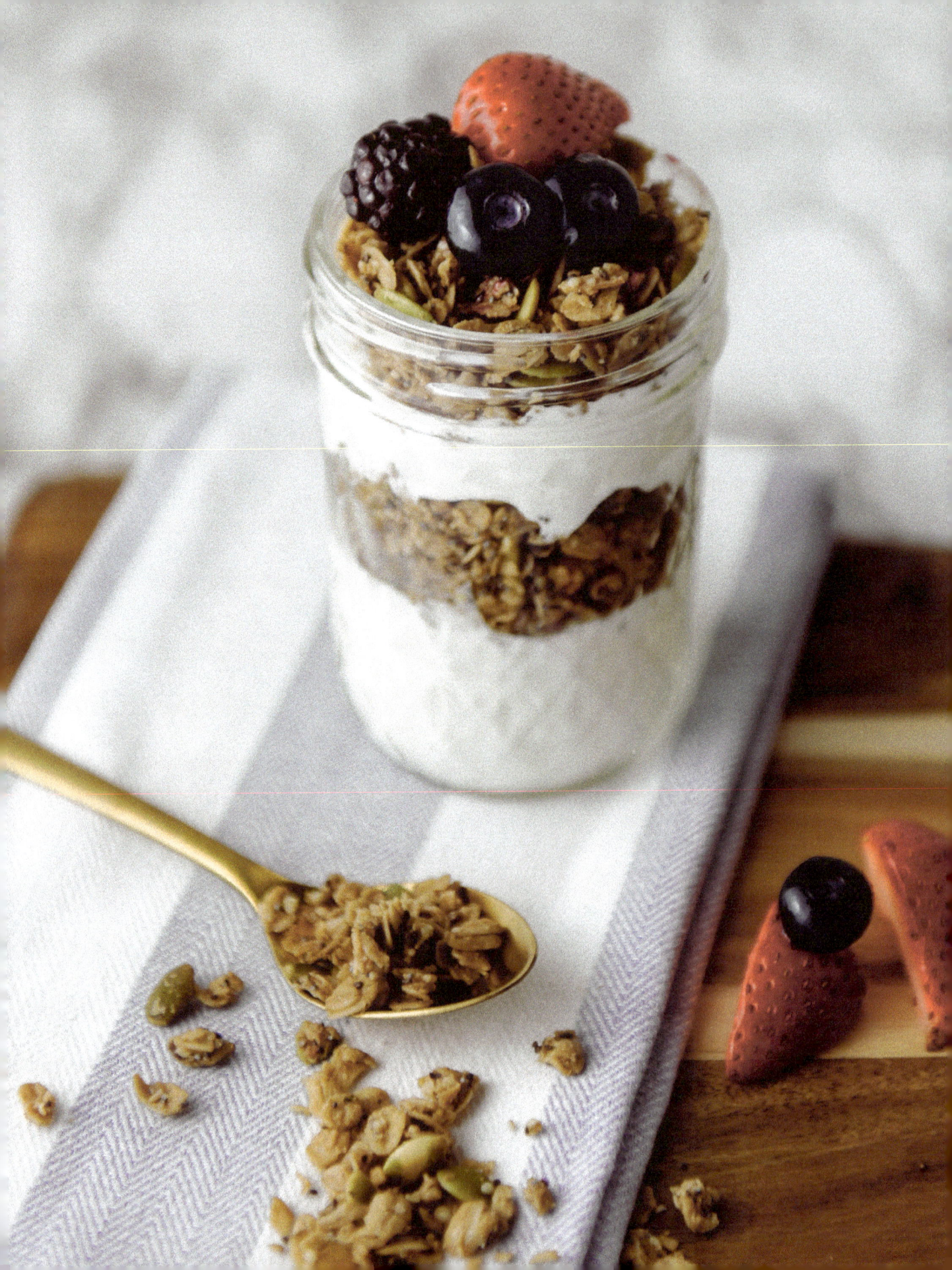

Super Seed Granola

I have been a long-time believer of making your own granola. This recipe has all the flavor without overdoing it on the sugar. It's great on top of an Açaí Berry Bowl (page 31) or in the Power Blueberry Coffee Cake (page 38).

YIELD: 8 CUPS

INGREDIENTS

3 cups rolled oats

1 recipe Super Seed Mix (page 242)

1 cup raw pumpkin seeds

1 cup shredded coconut

2 teaspoons ground cinnamon

½ teaspoon ground ginger

½ teaspoon kosher salt

¼ cup coconut oil

3 tablespoons sunflower seed butter

½ cup maple syrup

1 teaspoon pure vanilla extract

INSTRUCTIONS

1. Preheat oven to 275°F and line a baking tray with parchment paper or Silpat mat.
2. In a large bowl, combine the first 7 ingredients and stir.
3. Place the coconut oil, sunflower seed butter, and syrup in a small bowl. Heat in the microwave until everything is melted. Remove and add the vanilla.
4. Mix the wet mixture into the oats mixture until all dry ingredients are coated evenly.
5. Spread the mixture out on the baking sheet. Bake for 40 minutes, stirring the granola every 15 minutes.
6. Remove from oven and cool completely before breaking apart and storing in a sealed container at room temperature.

Granola will keep for about 2 weeks at room temperature.

Power Blueberry Coffee Cake

Come blueberry season, this recipe is made almost weekly at our house. There is nothing better than coming home from an early morning run and having this waiting for you.

INGREDIENTS

1 cup oat flour (page 13)

½ cup coconut flour

½ teaspoon kosher salt

1 teaspoon baking powder

1½ teaspoons ground cinnamon, divided

4 eggs, room temperature

¼ cup olive oil

¼ cup maple syrup, plus another 2 tablespoons

1 teaspoon pure vanilla extract

¾ cup canned coconut milk, full fat

2 cups blueberries

1 cup Super Seed Granola (page 37) or other migraine-friendly granola

3 tablespoons coconut oil

INSTRUCTIONS

1. Preheat oven to 350°F.
2. Line an 8" x 8" baking dish with parchment paper.
3. In a large bowl whisk the oat flour, coconut flour, salt, baking powder, and a ½ teaspoon of the cinnamon to combine.
4. In another bowl add the eggs, olive oil, ¼ cup maple syrup, vanilla, and coconut milk. Stir until combined.
5. Add the oat flour mixture into the wet ingredients and stir until combined into a batter.
6. In a separate bowl, stir together the granola, coconut oil, 1 teaspoon cinnamon, and 2 tablespoons maple syrup. Set it aside.
7. Place half the batter mixture in the bottom of the baking dish and top with half of the blueberries. Then top with half of the granola mixture.
8. Repeat Step 7 to create a second layer, then lightly press down the cake.
9. Bake for 55 minutes until the cake is done in the center and a toothpick comes out clean. Allow it to cool for 30 minutes before slicing.

This coffee cake is best served warm but may be stored for up to 2 days at room temperature or 5 days in the fridge. It may also be frozen. From the fridge, I recommend microwaving the coffee cake for about 15 seconds before enjoying.

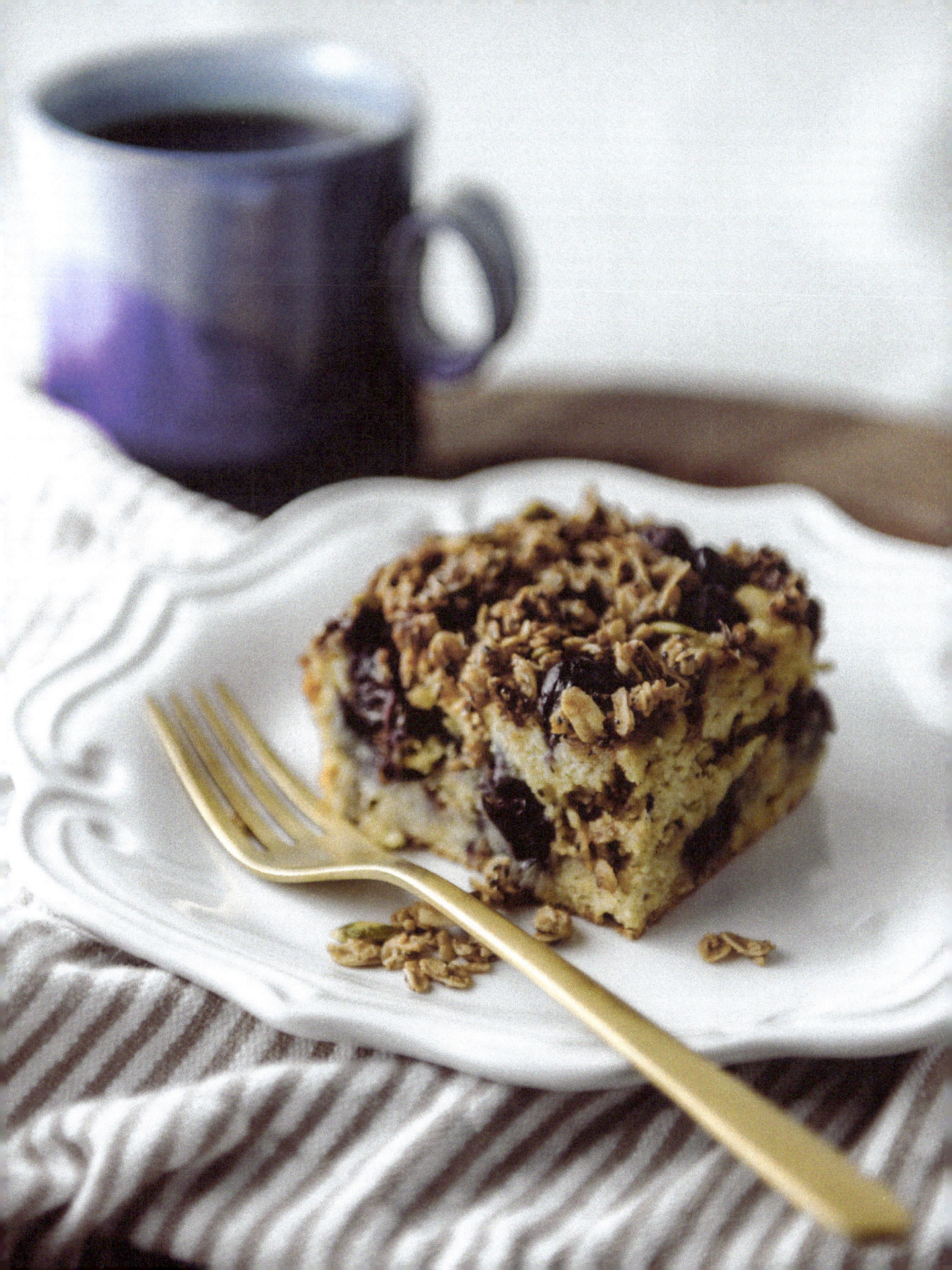

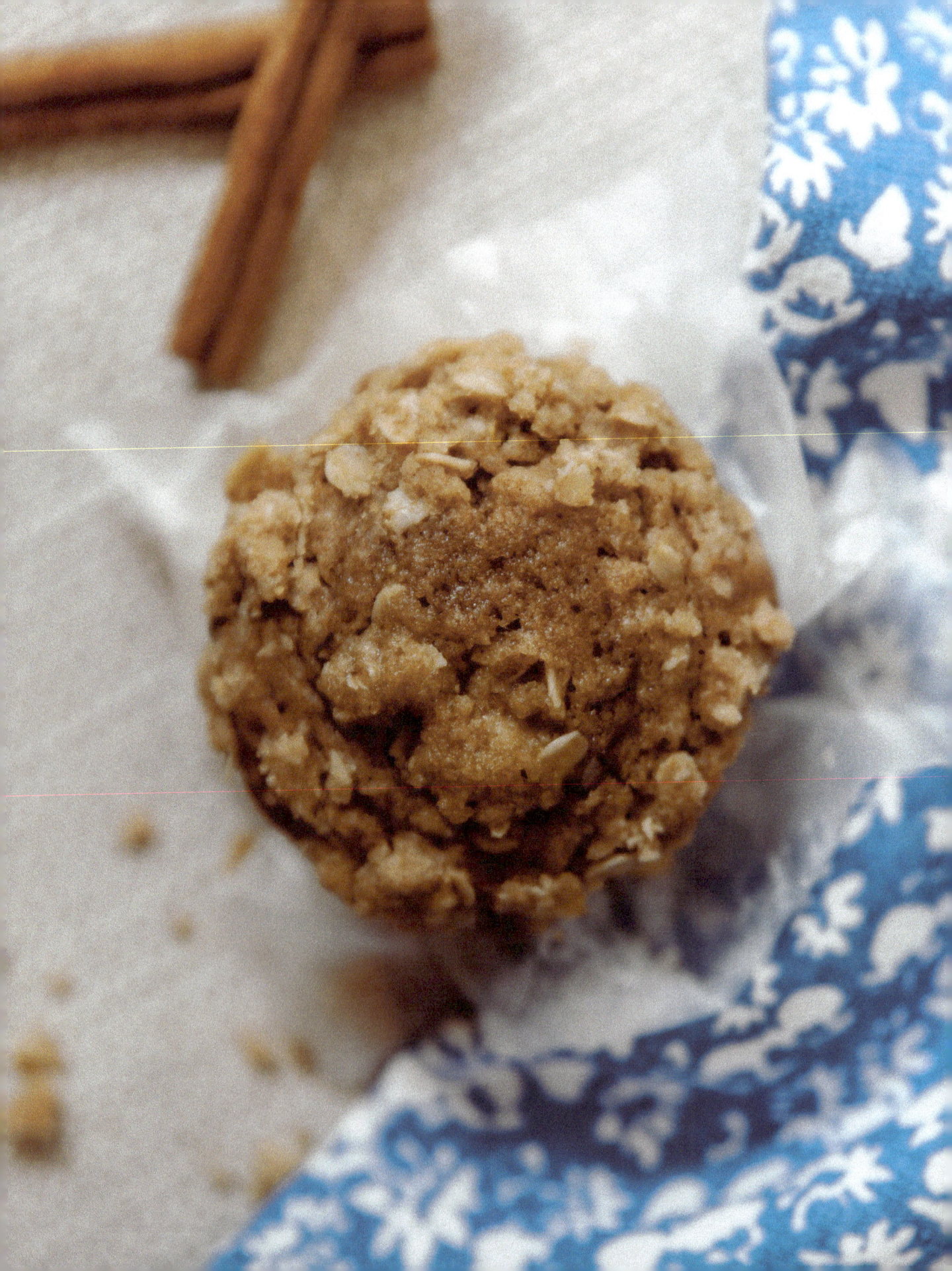

Snickerdoodle Muffins with Streusel Topping

This recipe took many, many test batches to get right (could be worse), but I am glad it made it into the book. As a kid some of my favorite muffins were cinnamon swirl muffins from a box. Sometimes on my birthday my mom would wake me up singing "Happy Birthday," holding one of these muffins with a candle in it (love you, Mom!). These muffins are a tasty, less-processed alternative to a boxed mix.

YIELD: 12 MUFFINS

INGREDIENTS

Batter

8 tablespoons unsalted butter, room temperature

⅔ cup brown sugar

2 eggs

¾ cup whole milk or canned light coconut milk

¼ cup applesauce (page 62)

1 teaspoon vanilla

1⅔ cups all-purpose flour or gluten-free flour

1½ teaspoons baking powder

½ teaspoon baking soda

½ teaspoon salt

1¾ teaspoons cinnamon

Streusel Topping

¼ cup all-purpose flour or gluten-free flour

¼ cup rolled oats

3 tablespoons brown sugar

¼ teaspoon cinnamon

Pinch of salt

4 tablespoons unsalted butter, cold and diced

INSTRUCTIONS

1. Preheat oven to 350°F. Line a 12-cup muffin tin with paper muffin cups or place reusable nonstick muffin cups on a parchment or Silpat mat-lined baking tray.

2. For the batter, by hand or using a stand mixer with paddle attachment, cream the butter and brown sugar together.

3. Add 2 eggs and continue mixing.

4. Add the milk, applesauce, and vanilla. Stir.

5. For the batter, in a separate bowl, add the flour, baking powder, baking soda, salt, and cinnamon. Whisk until combined.

6. Add the batter's dry ingredients into its wet ingredients in a large bowl in a couple of batches. Stir just enough to combine. Do not overmix.

7. Divide among muffin cups.

8. For the streusel topping, add the flour, rolled oats, brown sugar, cinnamon, and salt into a bowl and mix. Then cut the butter in with a pastry blender or your hands.

9. Distribute the streusel evenly on top of the batter-filled muffin cups.

10. Bake for 22–26 minutes or until a toothpick inserted into a muffin comes out clean.

11. Remove and allow to cool completely before storing in an airtight container.

These will keep stored at room temperature for 2 days or in the fridge for 5 days, or they can be frozen. From the fridge, I recommend microwaving them for about 15 seconds before enjoying.

Migraine-Free Morning Glory Muffins

The typical morning glory muffin contains loads of sugar and dried fruit. This recipe focuses more on apples, carrots, and coconut, which gives you long-lasting energy throughout your (migraine-free) day.

YIELD: 12 MUFFINS

INGREDIENTS

3 eggs, room temperature

⅓ cup coconut oil, melted

½ cup maple syrup

½ cup applesauce (page 62) or finely grated apple

½ cup milk of choice

1½ teaspoon pure vanilla extract

¾ cup finely grated carrots (about 2 medium carrots can be grated quickly in a food processor)

2 cups oat flour (page 13)

¼ cup coconut flour

⅔ cup rolled oats

½ teaspoon kosher salt

2½ teaspoons baking powder

2 teaspoons ground cinnamon

Topping

1 tablespoon coconut oil, melted

2 tablespoons rolled oats

2 tablespoons finely shredded coconut flakes

1 teaspoon maple syrup

INSTRUCTIONS

1. Preheat oven to 375°F. Line a 12-cup muffin tin with paper muffin cups or place reusable nonstick muffin cups on a parchment or Silpat mat-lined baking tray.

2. In a large bowl, combine the eggs, coconut oil, syrup, applesauce, milk, and vanilla. Mix thoroughly. Add the grated carrot. Note: If the coconut oil solidifies, you can place the bowl in a microwave and heat for up to 20 seconds at a time. Just don't heat it too much or you will cook the eggs.

3. In a separate bowl stir together the oat flour, coconut flour, oats, salt, baking powder, and cinnamon.

4. Add the dry ingredients to the wet and stir until just combined. Divide the mixture among 12 muffin cups.

5. Combine ingredients for topping in a small bowl and divide evenly on top of the muffins, pressing down lightly into the batter.

6. Bake for 20–25 minutes or until a toothpick inserted into a muffin comes out clean.

7. Remove and allow to cool completely before storing.

These will keep stored at room temperature for 2 days or in the fridge for 5 days, or they can be frozen. From the fridge, I recommend microwaving them for about 15 seconds before enjoying.

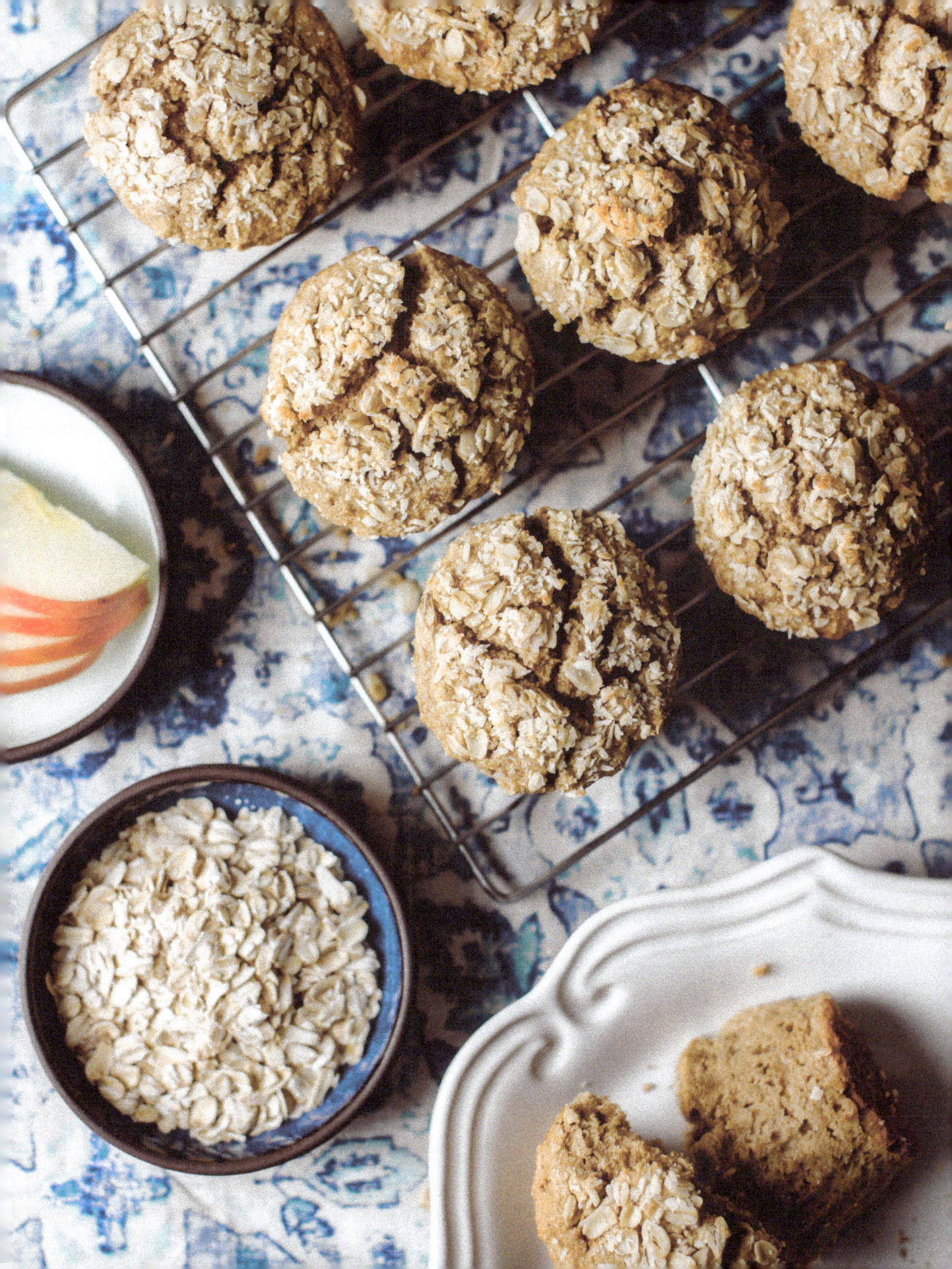

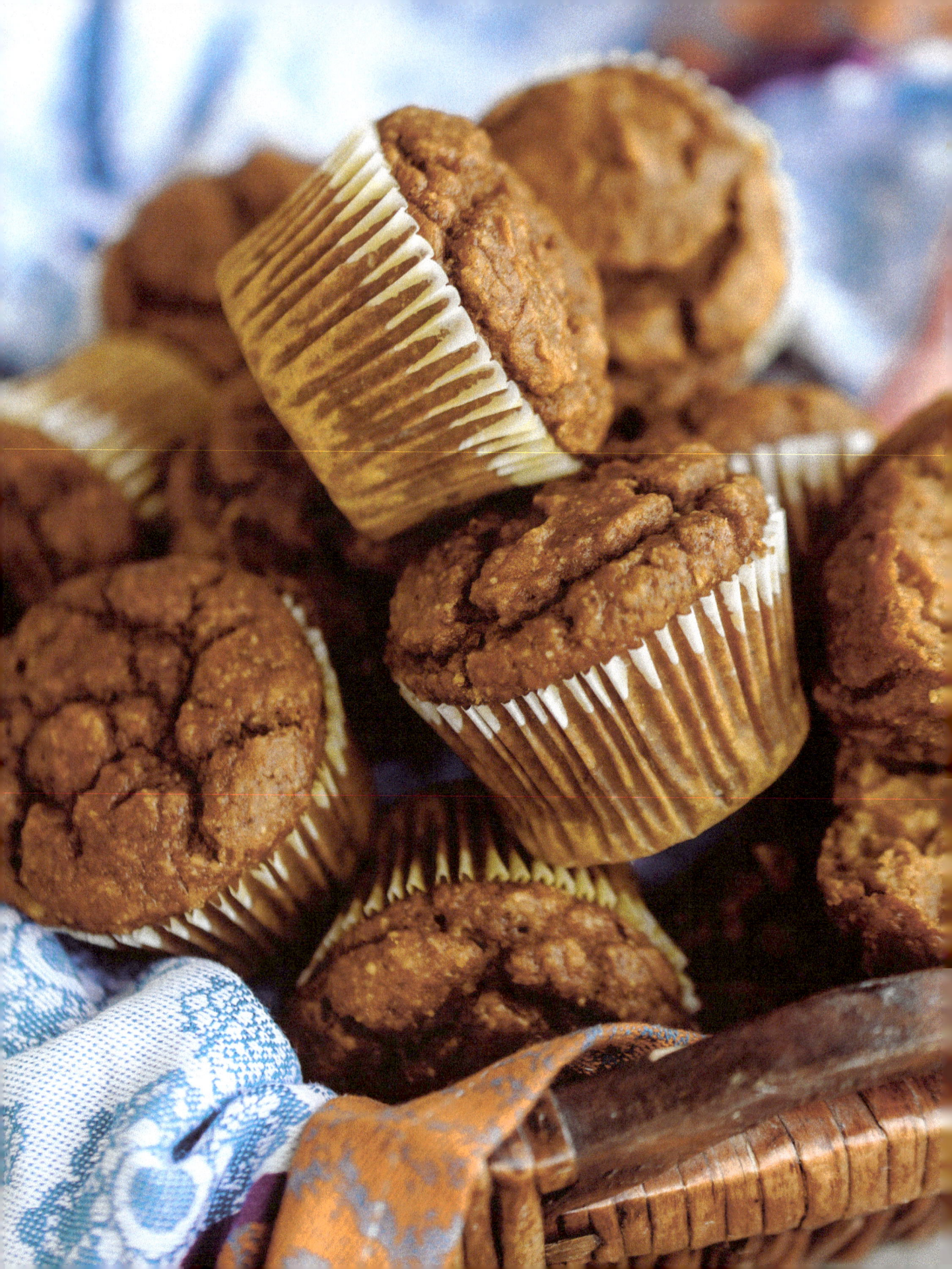

Johnny's Pumpkin Muffins

My son Johnny can't get enough of these muffins. They are great for breakfast or a snack and freeze well. To save time you can use canned pumpkin purée, just make sure it's not the canned pie filling, which has added ingredients.

YIELD: 12 MUFFINS

INGREDIENTS

1 cup pumpkin purée

½ cup maple syrup

⅓ cup coconut oil, melted

½ cup applesauce (page 62) or finely grated apple

1 teaspoon pure vanilla extract

2 eggs, room temperature

1 cup oat flour (page 13)

1¼ cups gluten-free flour (such as Bob's Red Mill) or all-purpose flour

1 teaspoon baking soda

1 tablespoon pumpkin pie spice

½ teaspoon salt

INSTRUCTIONS

1. Preheat oven to 350°F. Line a 12-cup muffin tin with paper muffin cups or place reusable nonstick muffin cups on a parchment or Silpat mat-lined baking tray.

2. Add the first 6 ingredients in a large bowl and whisk.

3. In a separate bowl combine the oat flour, gluten-free flour, baking soda, pumpkin pie spice, and salt. Whisk together.

4. Add dry ingredients to the wet and mix until combined. Divide among 12 muffin cups and bake for 20–25 minutes or until a toothpick inserted into a muffin comes out clean.

5. Allow to cool slightly before removing from muffin cups then cool completely.

These will keep stored at room temperature for 2 days or in the fridge for 5 days, or they can be frozen. From the fridge, I recommend microwaving them for about 15 seconds before enjoying.

Egg Frittata Muffins

As a personal chef, one of my goals is to create easy and healthy options for families. This protein- and vegetable-packed breakfast is just that. Make a batch at the beginning of the week and have breakfast ready all week long.

YIELD: 12–14 CUPS

INGREDIENTS

1 tablespoon olive oil

2 cups other ingredients such as broccoli, bell peppers, spinach, kale, shallots, or herbs, chopped small

12 eggs

½ cup whole milk or 2% reduced fat milk

½ teaspoon garlic granules

¾ teaspoon kosher salt

Freshly ground pepper

INSTRUCTIONS

1. Preheat oven to 375°F. Line a muffin tin with paper muffin cups or place reusable nonstick muffin cups on a parchment or Silpat mat-lined baking tray.

2. Heat the oil in a skillet. Once the oil is hot, add the vegetables, adding any greens last (hold any herbs till next step).

3. Cook a few minutes over medium heat until they begin to soften. Turn off heat and add any herbs. Set aside to cool slightly.

4. In a medium-sized bowl whisk together the eggs, milk, garlic, salt, and some pepper. Stir in the vegetable mixture.

5. Divide the mixture evenly among muffin cups. Bake until set in the middle, about 25 minutes.

6. Allow to cool slightly and remove from muffin cups.

TIP: Option to add ½ cup crumbled feta cheese in place of ½ cup of the vegetables. Just add in the cheese after you stir the vegetables into the egg mixture. If adding feta, reduce the salt to ½ teaspoon.

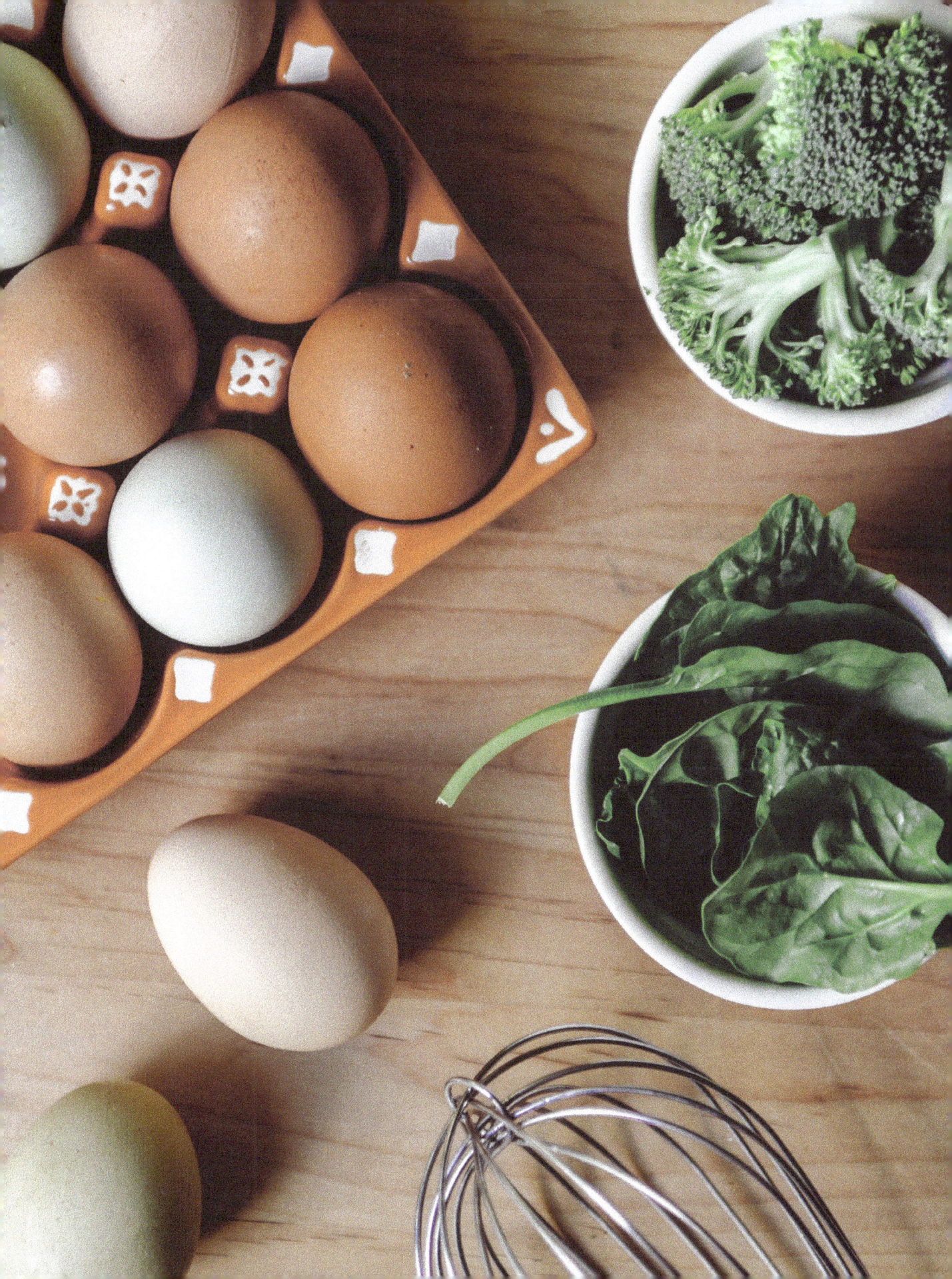

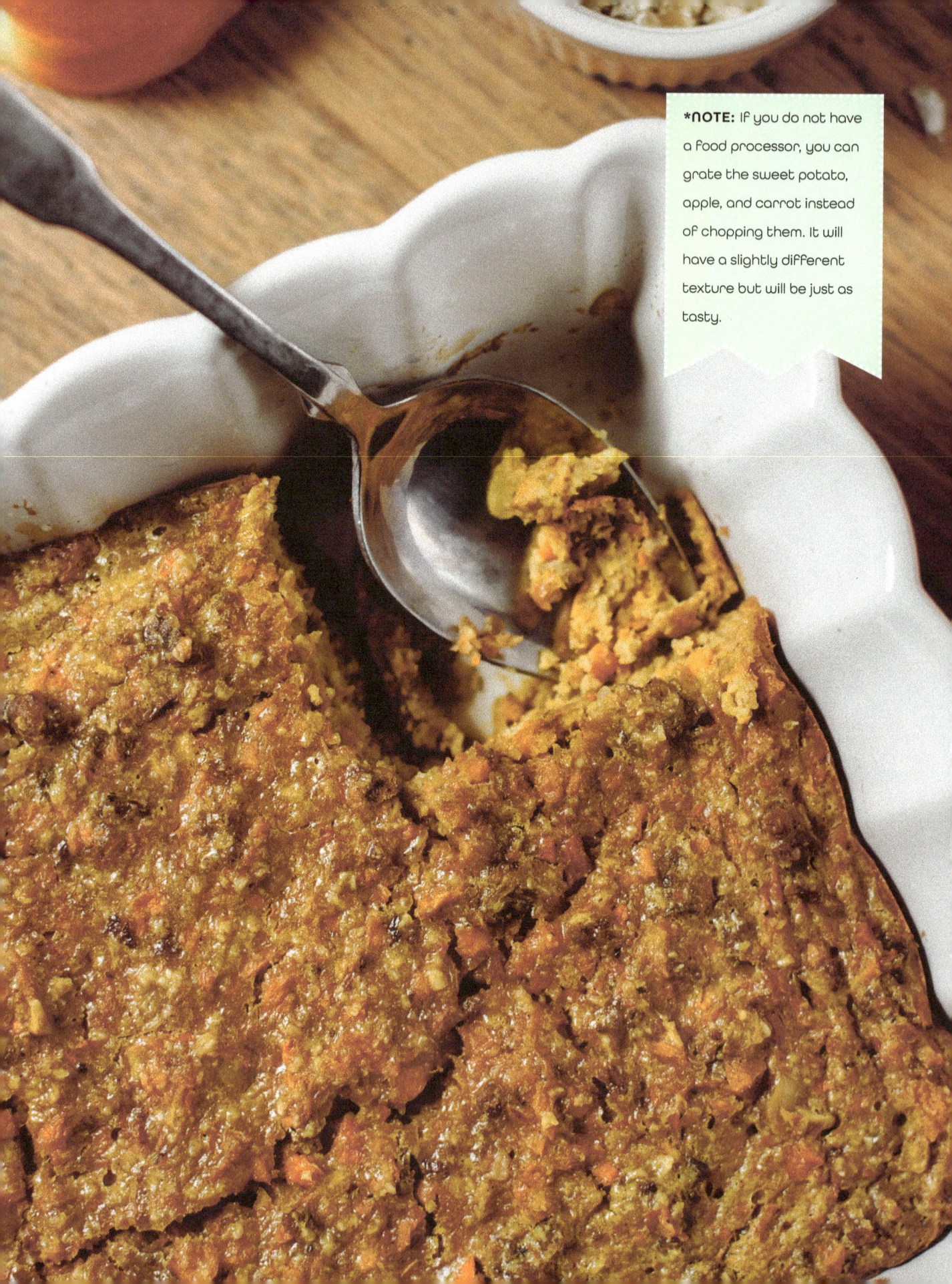

*NOTE: If you do not have a food processor, you can grate the sweet potato, apple, and carrot instead of chopping them. It will have a slightly different texture but will be just as tasty.

Sweet Potato Apple Breakfast Bake

This dish is a more nutrient-dense option compared to the heavy breakfast casseroles that can leave you feeling sluggish. I like to top mine with diced apples and a drizzle of maple syrup before serving.

YIELD: 6–8 SERVINGS

INGREDIENTS

2 tablespoons unsalted butter (can substitute coconut oil), plus extra for greasing the pan

1 medium–large sweet potato, peeled and chopped

1 apple, such as Honeycrisp or Pink Lady, cored and chopped

1 large carrot, chopped

½ recipe (or ½ pound) Make Your Own Sausage (page 53)

Kosher salt

1 teaspoon ground cinnamon

Dash of ground nutmeg

1 cup oat flour (page 13)

1 teaspoon baking powder

¾ cup canned coconut milk, full fat

3 tablespoons maple syrup

5 eggs

1½ teaspoons pure vanilla extract

Freshly ground black pepper

INSTRUCTIONS

1. Preheat oven to 375°F.
2. Lightly grease the bottom and sides of an 8" x 8" dish or similar with a little butter or coconut oil.
3. Add the sweet potato to a food processor.* Pulse until it is almost minced then remove. You should have roughly 2½ cups sweet potato. Add the apple and carrot to the food processor and process until almost minced then set aside.
4. In a large skillet cook the sausage, breaking it apart as it browns. Once cooked, remove the sausage with a slotted spoon and set aside.
5. Add the butter to the same skillet and sauté the sweet potatoes for a few minutes over medium heat. Season with ½ teaspoon salt and some pepper. If needed, you can add 1 tablespoon or more water to the bottom of the pan to prevent any burning.
6. Add the apple, carrot, and a couple big pinches of salt. Sauté another 5–7 minutes, then add the cinnamon and nutmeg. Turn off heat and allow mixture to cool slightly.
7. Meanwhile, add the oat flour, baking powder, coconut milk, syrup, eggs, vanilla, salt, and cooked sausage to a large bowl. Add the sweet potato mixture and combine.
8. Place in the greased dish. Bake for about 35 minutes or until set in the center. Remove and allow to cool before cutting.

TIP: To make this vegetarian, increase the sweet potato to 2 medium potatoes and use 1½ apples. Also increase the butter to 3 tablespoons, the cinnamon to 1½ teaspoons, and the salt to ¾–1 teaspoon.

Overnight Oats Three Ways

Overnight oats are a go-to breakfast for busy weekday mornings in our house. Oats provide your body with fiber and protein. When you are short on time in the mornings, these are a convenient and healthy option to have waiting for you in the fridge.

YIELD: 4 SERVINGS

INGREDIENTS

Base

1½ cups rolled oats

1½ cups canned light coconut milk or milk of choice

¼ cup water or additional milk of choice

1 teaspoon pure vanilla extract or vanilla bean paste*

3–4 tablespoons maple syrup or honey

¼ teaspoon kosher salt

Mango Cardamom Oats

1 teaspoon ground flax seeds

¼ teaspoon ground cardamom

1 cup diced mango

Chia Berry Oats

1 tablespoon chia seeds

1 cup blueberries or other berries such as chopped strawberries

Pumpkin Pear Oats

1 tablespoon hemp hearts

2 teaspoons pumpkin pie spice

1 cup diced pear

INSTRUCTIONS

1. Combine all the base ingredients into a medium-sized bowl and mix.
2. Add your choice of flavor ingredients and stir to combine.
3. Transfer to a container and refrigerate overnight.
4. Once ready to enjoy you can reheat in the microwave or briefly on the stovetop.

You can divide the oats into four Mason jars for a quick grab-and-go breakfast. The oats will last 4 nights in the fridge.

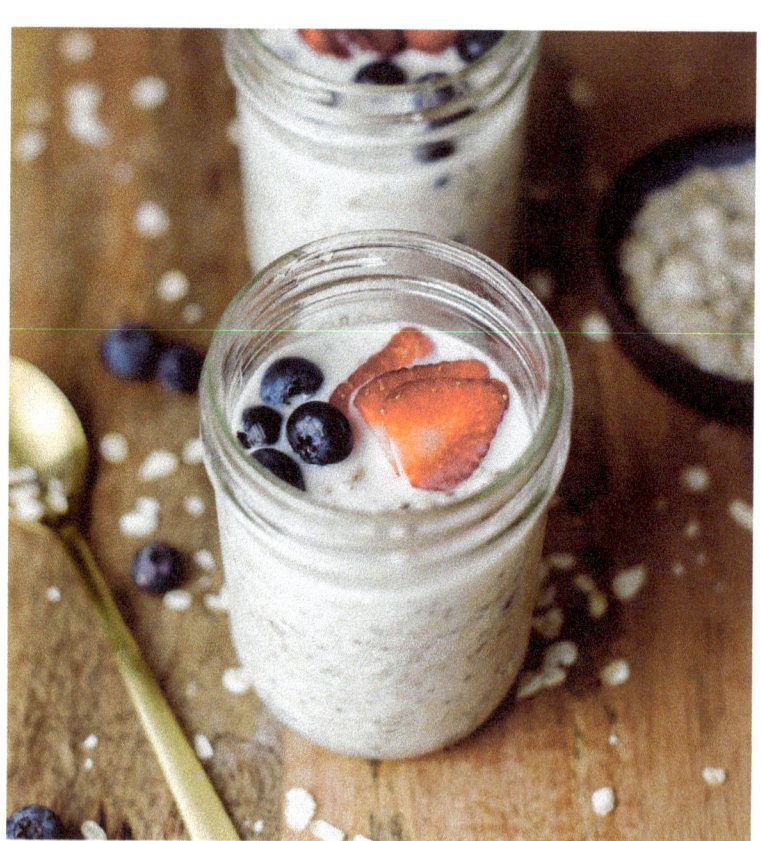

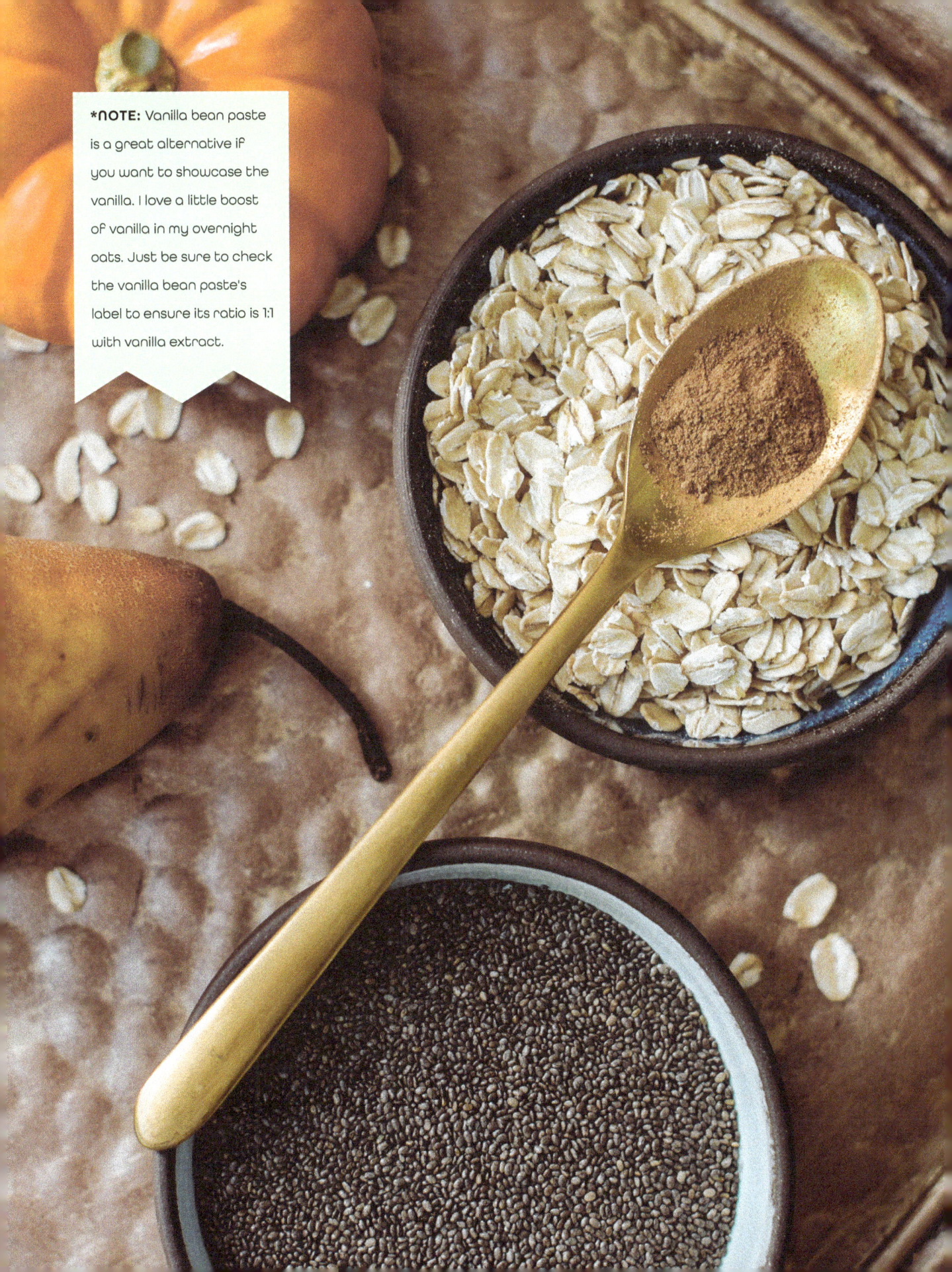

*NOTE: Vanilla bean paste is a great alternative if you want to showcase the vanilla. I love a little boost of vanilla in my overnight oats. Just be sure to check the vanilla bean paste's label to ensure its ratio is 1:1 with vanilla extract.

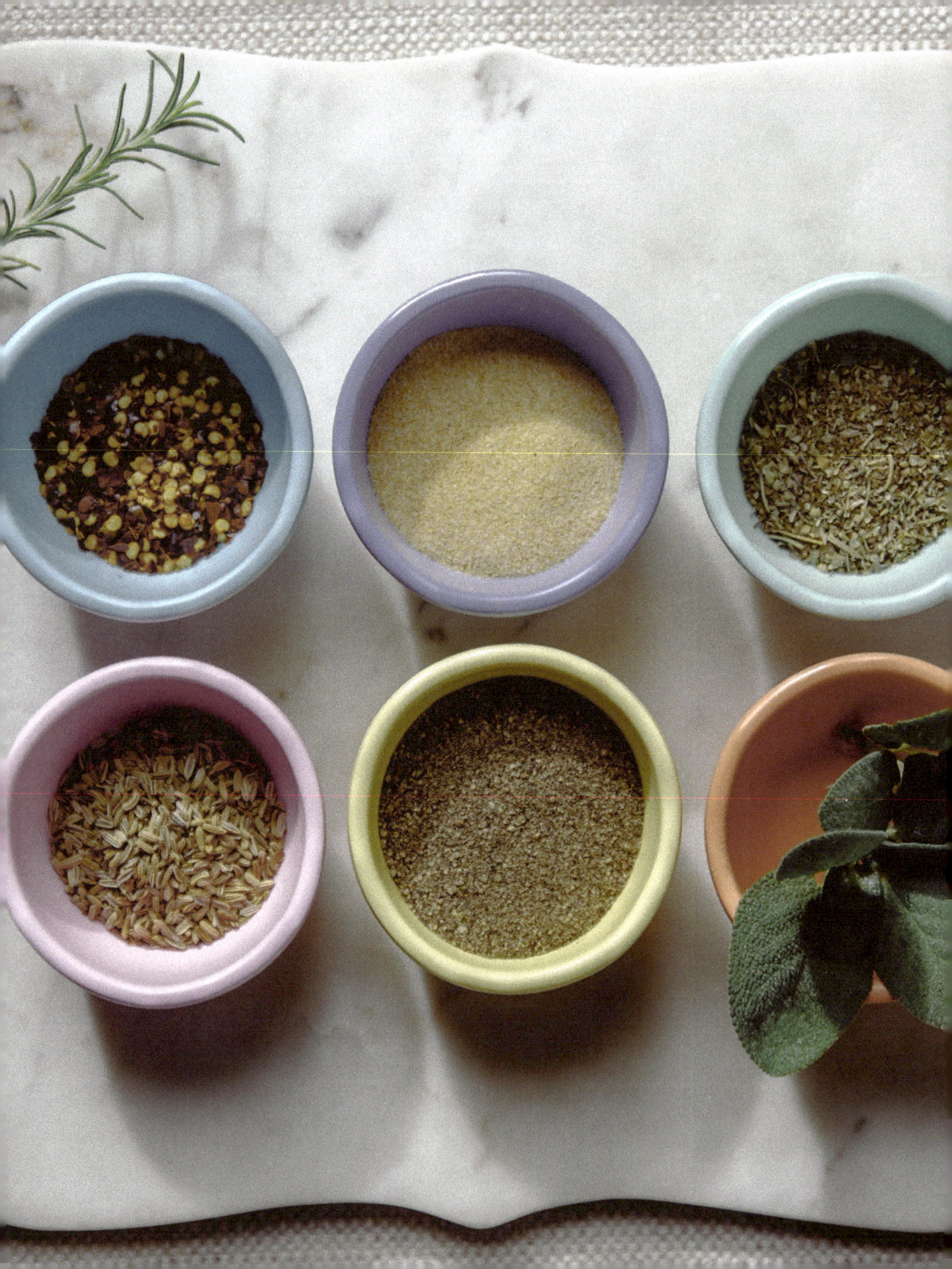

Make Your Own Sausage

Most store-bought sausages contain preservatives called nitrates, which can cause migraines. This recipe, which includes herbs, salt, and pepper, provides a much cleaner option.

YIELD: 1 POUND OF
SAUSAGE

INGREDIENTS

1 tablespoon chopped fresh sage

1 teaspoon chopped fresh rosemary

¼ teaspoon red pepper flakes

¼ teaspoon fennel seeds, lightly crushed with the side of your knife

¾–1 teaspoon kosher salt

¼ teaspoon freshly ground black pepper

½ teaspoon dried thyme

½ teaspoon garlic granules

½ teaspoon coconut sugar

1 pound ground pork, can substitute chicken or turkey,* preferably local

*NOTE: If you substitute chicken or turkey, you will want to add 1 tablespoon olive oil to the pan before cooking the meat, since it doesn't have much fat.

INSTRUCTIONS

1. Add all the ingredients except the pork to a large bowl and mix. Then add the pork and mix once more.

2. For ground sausage, cook in a large skillet over medium heat, breaking it apart as you go. Or you can form sausage patties (makes about 8 patties) or links to cook in a skillet over medium heat.

Saturday Morning Breakfast Hash

If I am roasting potatoes one night for dinner, I usually make a double batch to have on hand for a hash or frittata. Both are delicious options for a weekend brunch or savory breakfast for dinner.

YIELD: 4–6 SERVINGS

INGREDIENTS

1 recipe Make Your Own Sausage (page 53)

1 tablespoon olive oil or leftover pork fat from cooking the sausage

2 leeks, trimmed, thinly sliced and rinsed, white part only

2 bell peppers, seeded and diced (I like 1 green and 1 red)

1 jalapeño, seeded and diced

4 garlic cloves, peeled and minced or grated

1 recipe Roasted Garlic Potatoes (page 217)

Kosher salt and freshly ground pepper

TIP: Don't throw away the green parts on the leeks. They can be used for stock or soups.

INSTRUCTIONS

1. Heat the olive oil in a large sauté pan (use the same one if you just made the sausage). Once the oil is hot, add the leeks. Turn the heat to medium and cook for about 5–8 minutes or until the leeks start to soften. Add a pinch of salt.

2. Add the bell peppers and jalapeño. Cook over medium heat for another 5–10 minutes.

3. Add garlic and stir until fragrant, about 1 minute.

4. Once the peppers have softened slightly add the cooked sausage and potatoes.

5. Season to taste with salt and pepper and serve.

This hash is also delicious with a fried egg on top or scrambled eggs folded in.

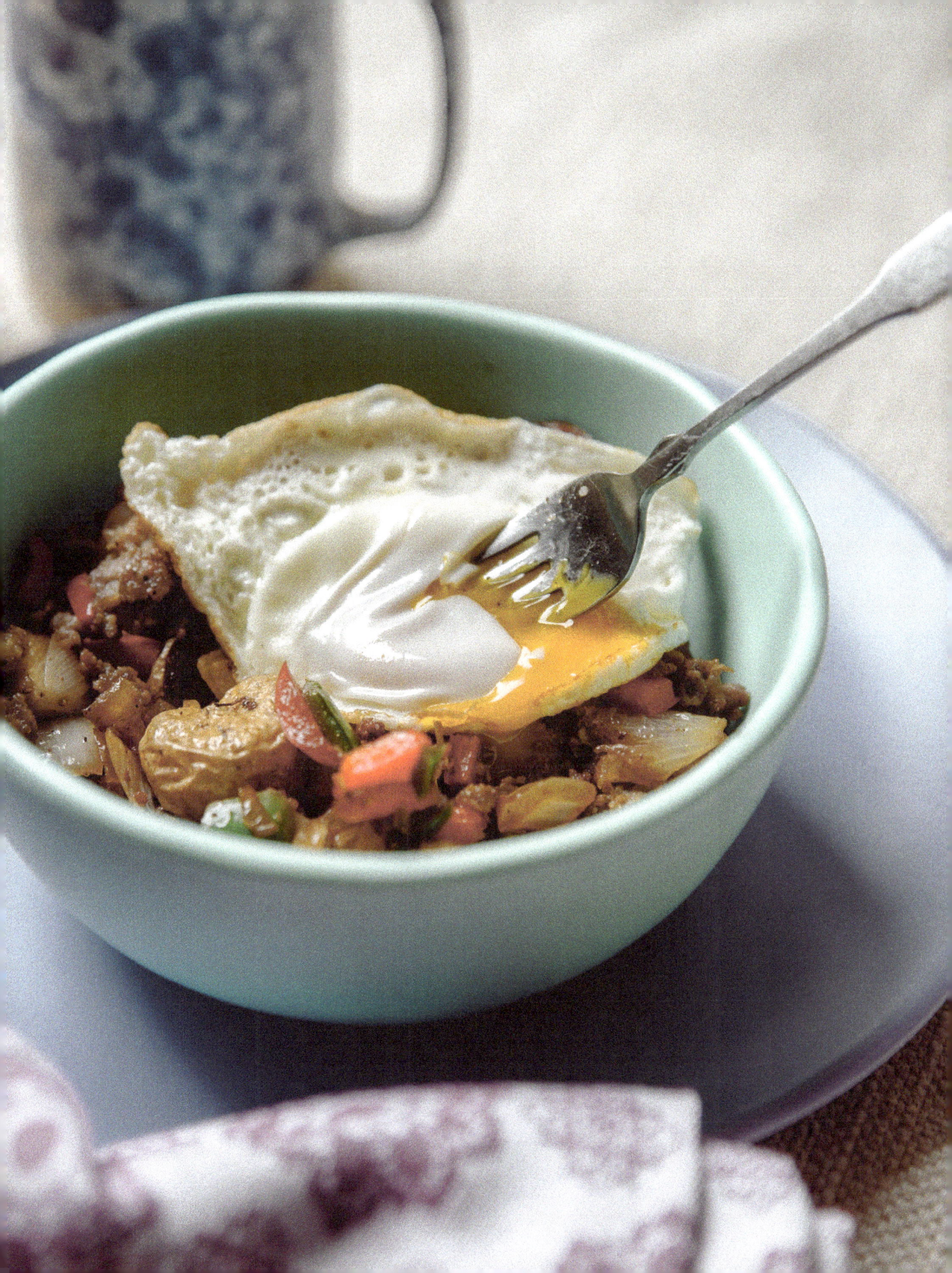

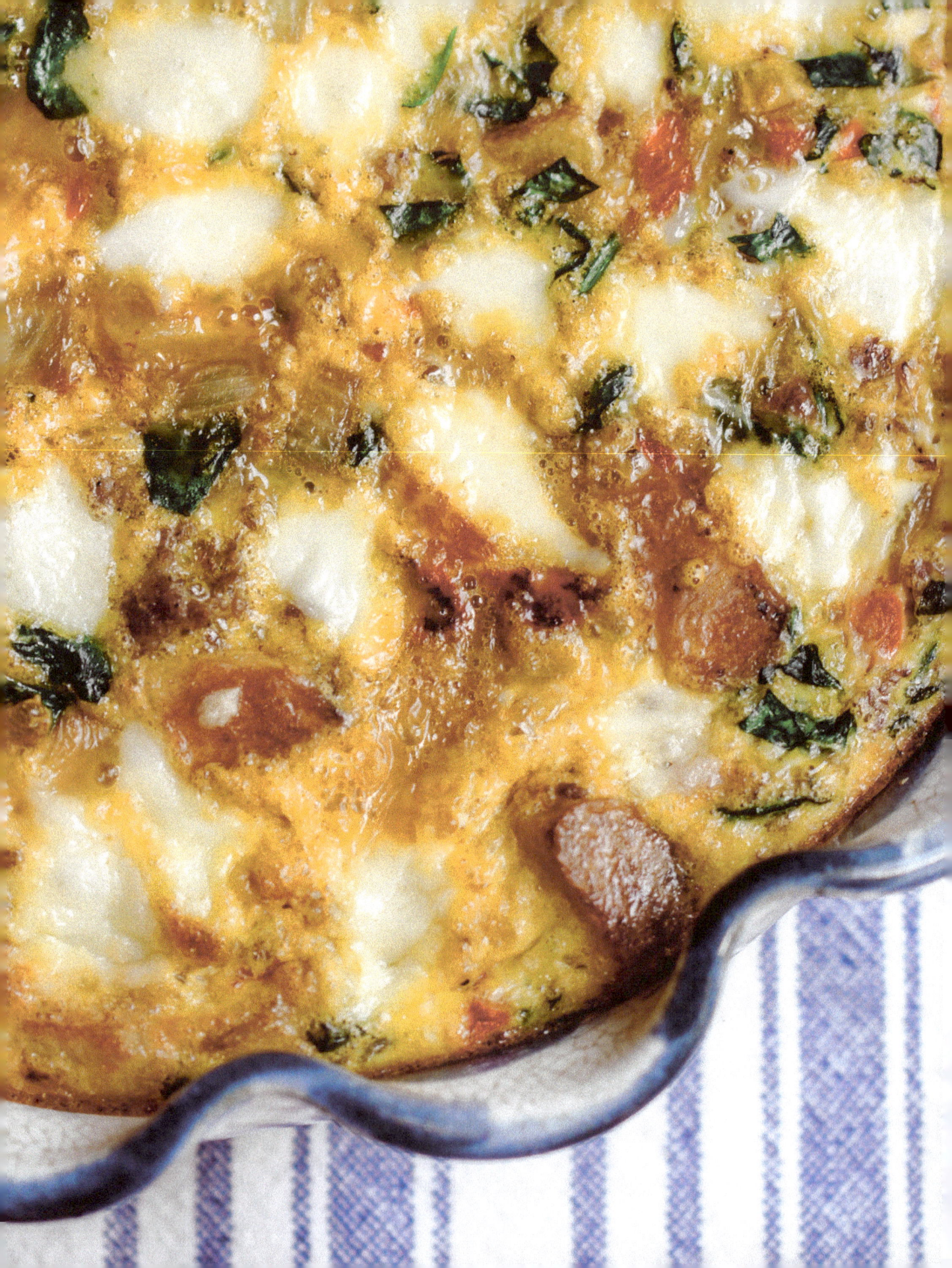

Migraine-Friendly Frittata

YIELD: 8 SERVINGS

INGREDIENTS

10 eggs

½ cup whole milk

½ teaspoon kosher salt

Freshly ground pepper

1 tablespoon olive oil or butter, plus extra for greasing the pan

2 shallots, peeled and diced

½ cup roasted red peppers, diced

2 cups spinach or kale, chopped

1½ cups (about ½ recipe) Roasted Garlic Potatoes (page 217), cooked

½ pound (½ recipe) Make Your Own Sausage (page 53) or other migraine-friendly sausage, cooked

3 oz fresh mozzarella, sliced or shredded

INSTRUCTIONS

1. Preheat oven to 375°F. Lightly grease the bottom and sides of a pie dish or dish of similar size.

2. Combine the eggs, milk, salt, and pepper in a large bowl and whisk. Set it aside.

3. Cook the sausage in a large skillet if you haven't already. Break it apart as it cooks. Once the sausage is done, remove it with a slotted spoon and set aside.

4. Heat the olive oil or butter in the same skillet and sauté the shallots over medium-high heat. Sauté for a few minutes. Once soft, add the peppers and cook another 2 minutes.

5. Next add the spinach or kale and sauté until wilted.

6. Turn off heat and add the potatoes and sausage. Spoon mixture into the greased dish.

7. Pour the egg mixture over the potatoes and gently stir, making sure the vegetables are evenly distributed. Spread the mozzarella over the top.

8. Bake for 38–45 minutes until the eggs are set. Remove and let cool slightly before serving.

Southern Biscuits

I can't tell you how many times I have made biscuits, but it's a lot! There are so many different variations of biscuits out there, from small tea biscuits to ones made with cheese and herbs. This rendition is a classic Southern biscuit with lots of flaky layers.

YIELD: 12 LARGE BISCUITS

INGREDIENTS

2½ cups cake flour (such as King Arthur)

2½ cups all-purpose flour, plus extra for rolling out the dough

1 tablespoon baking powder

½ teaspoon baking soda

Scant 2 teaspoons kosher salt

1 tablespoon sugar or coconut sugar

12 tablespoons unsalted butter, cold

About 2 cups whole milk, cold

2 tablespoons unsalted butter, melted

> **TIP:** These biscuits are great served with Sage Sausage Gravy (page 230).

INSTRUCTIONS

1. Preheat oven to 425°F. Line a sheet pan with parchment paper or a Silpat mat.

2. Combine the first 6 ingredients in a large bowl and mix thoroughly.

3. Take the butter out of the refrigerator and cut it into large chunks. Then cut the butter into the dry ingredients with a pastry blender until the butter is the size of peas. Alternatively, you can mix the dry ingredients in a food processor then add the butter and pulse a few times.

4. Starting with just under 2 cups, stir in the milk with a spatula until a loose ball forms. Do not overmix. You should still have some crumbs at the bottom of the bowl, but if the mixture looks too dry, you can add a little more milk.

5. Turn the dough onto a floured work surface and form a thick rectangle. Cut in half and stack the dough on top of each other. Repeat 4–5 times.

6. Roll into a 1½-inch thick circle. Cut with a medium-sized biscuit cutter, making 12 biscuits. You might have to reroll the dough once or twice.

7. Place each biscuit near each other, barely touching, on the sheet pan.

8. Bake for 20–25 minutes rotating the pan halfway through. Then make sure the tops started to brown and the inside is done. Brush with the melted butter and serve immediately.

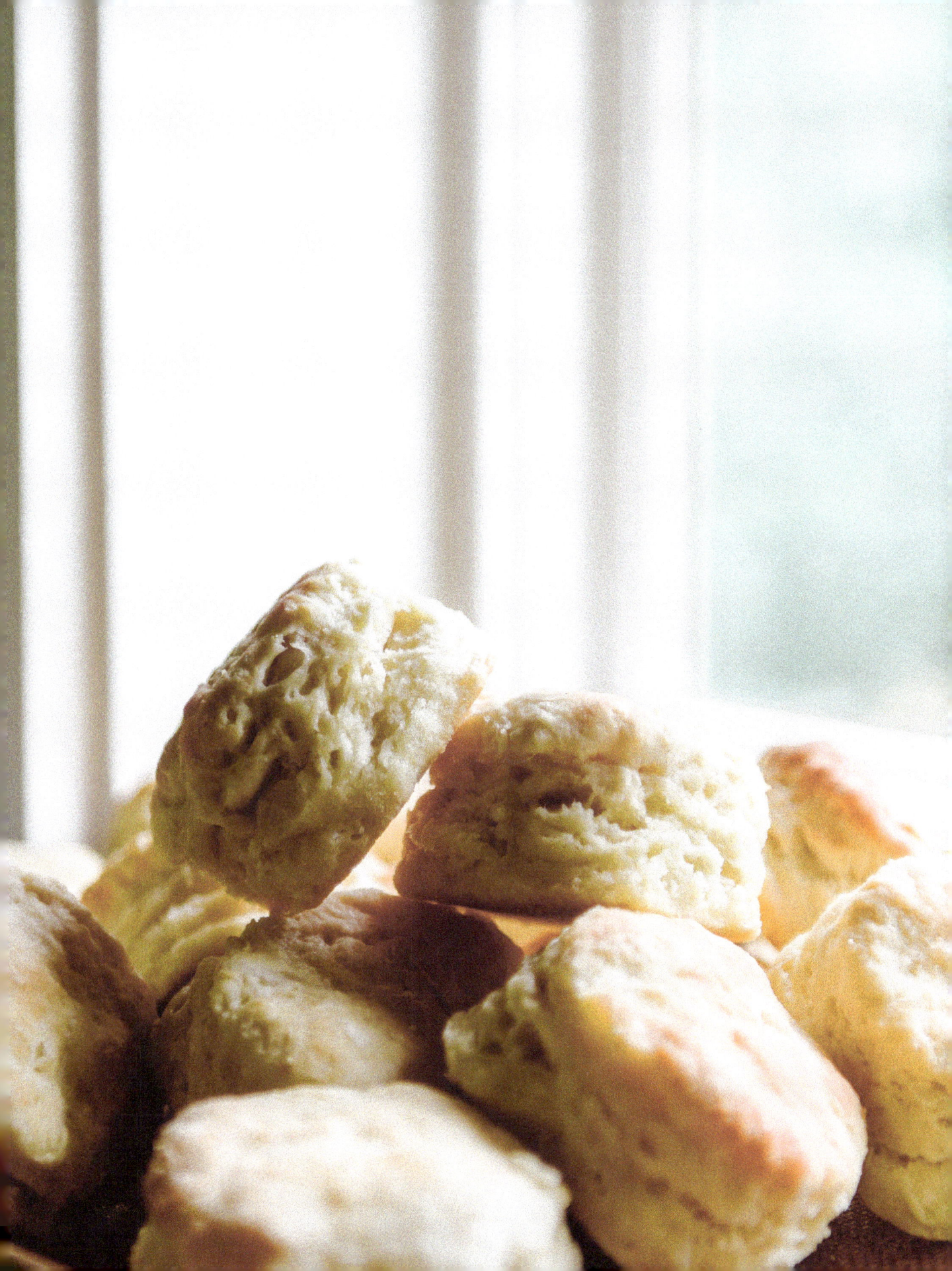

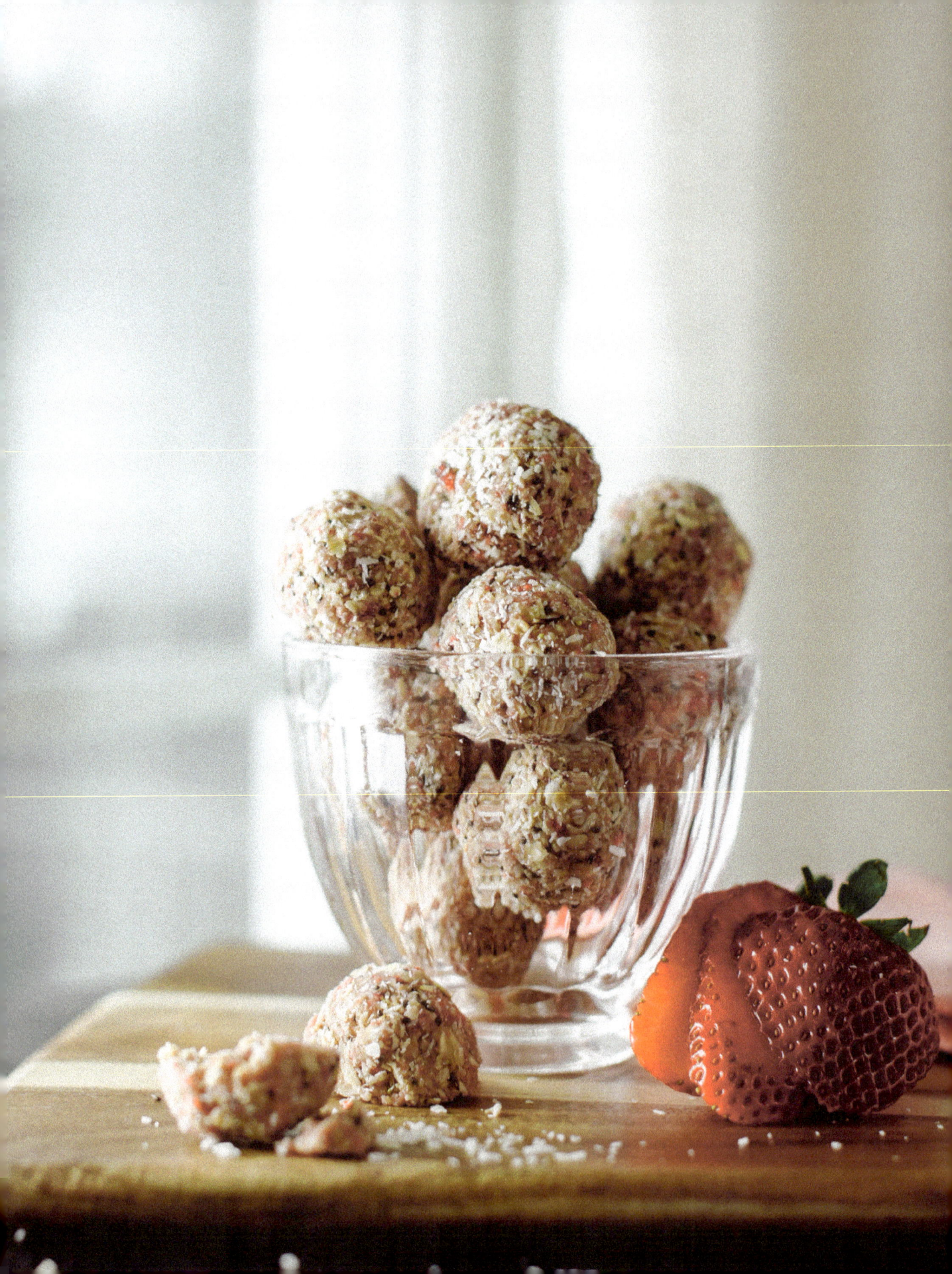

Snacks

Cinnamon Applesauce.. 62

Baba Ghanoush 65

Blueberry Bites... 66

Strawberry Coconut Bites 69

Pumpkin Seeds Two Ways 70

Herb-Roasted Garlic 73

Roasted Garlic White Bean Dip... 74

Roasted Red Pepper Hummus... 77

Sweet Pea and Basil Hummus 78

Sweet and Savory Popcorn Toppings.. 81

Cinnamon Applesauce

Come fall, we love seeking out an apple orchard and going apple picking. Between that and the nearby farmers market, we have lots and lots of apples. At least once every fall, I make a big batch of applesauce and freeze extra in 1- to 2-cup amounts. It's great for adding to yogurt and makes for a tasty, natural sweetener in muffin recipes.

YIELD: 3 CUPS

INGREDIENTS

6 medium apples (about 2½ pounds) such as Golden Delicious, Fuji, or a mixture of varieties (my favorite!)

¼ cup water

½ lemon, zested then juiced (optional)

1 teaspoon ground cinnamon

2 tablespoons (or to taste) maple syrup or honey

¼ teaspoon kosher salt

TIP: During apple season ask farmers at the farmers market if they have any imperfect apples. Sometimes you can get a great deal on a box of slightly bruised apples.

INSTRUCTIONS

1. Peel* and core the apples then chop them into 2-inch pieces.
2. Combine the apples with ¼ cup water, the lemon zest and juice if using, cinnamon, syrup (or honey), and salt.
3. Heat the cinnamon-lemon mixture over low heat while stirring the apples so they are evenly coated.
4. Cover and cook over low heat for about 15–20 minutes until apples have softened.
5. Remove lid and allow the apples to cool.
6. You can mash them if you like a chunkier applesauce, or use an immersion blender to blend. The apples can also be puréed in a food processor or high-speed blender.

Store covered in the fridge for 5 days or in the freezer for several months.

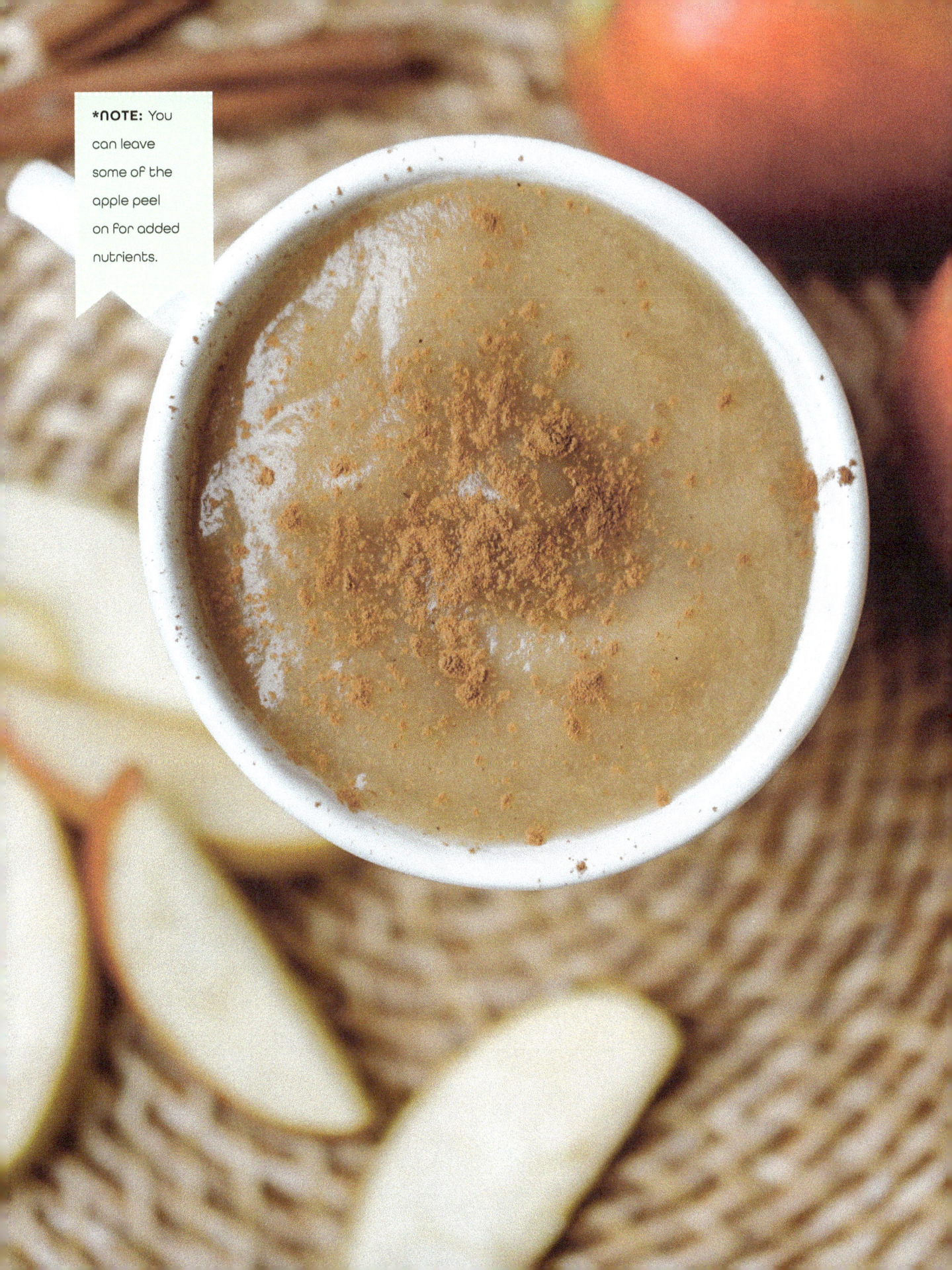

*NOTE: You can leave some of the apple peel on for added nutrients.

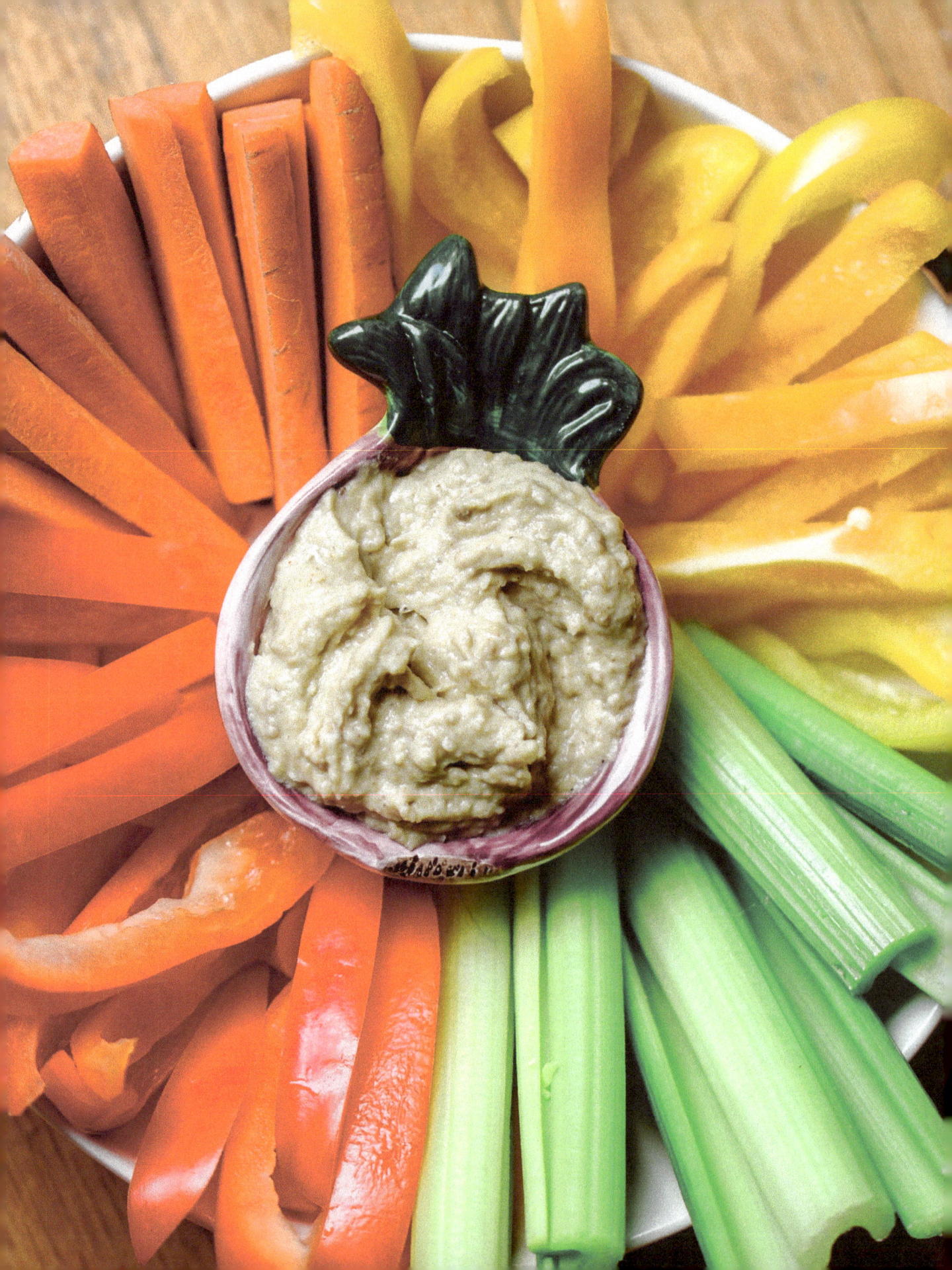

Baba Ghanoush

I love snacking on this dip with carrot slices, cucumbers, and pita chips. If you have leftovers, it can be used as a spread on a sandwich, and a spoonful can elevate many pasta sauces. (And bonus points to you if you reference the movie "Wedding Crashers" after hearing the words "baba ghanoush"!)

YIELD: ABOUT 2½ CUPS

INGREDIENTS

1 medium–large eggplant

Olive oil for drizzling

1 clove garlic, peeled

Juice of ½ lemon (optional)

2 tablespoons tahini

1 teaspoon ground cumin

½ teaspoon smoked paprika

2 tablespoons extra virgin olive oil

1 (15 oz) can chickpeas, drained and rinsed

Kosher salt and freshly ground pepper

INSTRUCTIONS

1. Preheat oven to 375°F.
2. Cut the eggplant in half lengthwise. Drizzle with olive oil and sprinkle with salt. Place flesh side down on a parchment- or Silpat mat-lined baking sheet.
3. Bake for about 30 minutes, until soft and it can easily be pierced with a fork. Remove from oven and allow it to rest until it's cool enough to handle.
4. Scoop out the flesh and place in a high-speed blender along with the rest of the ingredients. You should get approximately 1¼ cups of eggplant once scooped out.
5. Blend until almost smooth or desired smoothness. If you are having trouble blending or would like a thinner consistency, you can add up to 2 tablespoons water.
6. Adjust seasoning if needed and enjoy.

Blueberry Bites

Freeze-dried fruit is light and crisp, unlike dehydrated fruit, which can be chewy. You can find it in most grocery stores.

YIELD: 16–18 BALLS

INGREDIENTS

2 cups rolled oats

¼ cup pumpkin seeds, raw

⅛ teaspoon or less kosher salt, depending on if the sunflower seed butter includes salt

2 tablespoons hemp hearts

1 (1.2 oz) bag freeze-dried blueberries

⅓ cup sunflower seed butter

¼ cup honey

1 tablespoon coconut oil, melted

INSTRUCTIONS

1. Place the oats, pumpkin seeds, salt, and hemp hearts in a food processor and pulse a few times until you see only a few whole oats remaining, but it is not as fine as oat flour. Then add the freeze-dried blueberries and pulse once more for about 3 seconds.

2. Add the sunflower seed butter, honey, and coconut oil and pulse until combined.

3. Scrape the mixture into a bowl.

4. Roll into about 18 balls.* If the mixture doesn't easily pack into small balls, you can add 1 teaspoon of water to the mixture. It also helps to wet your hands when rolling.

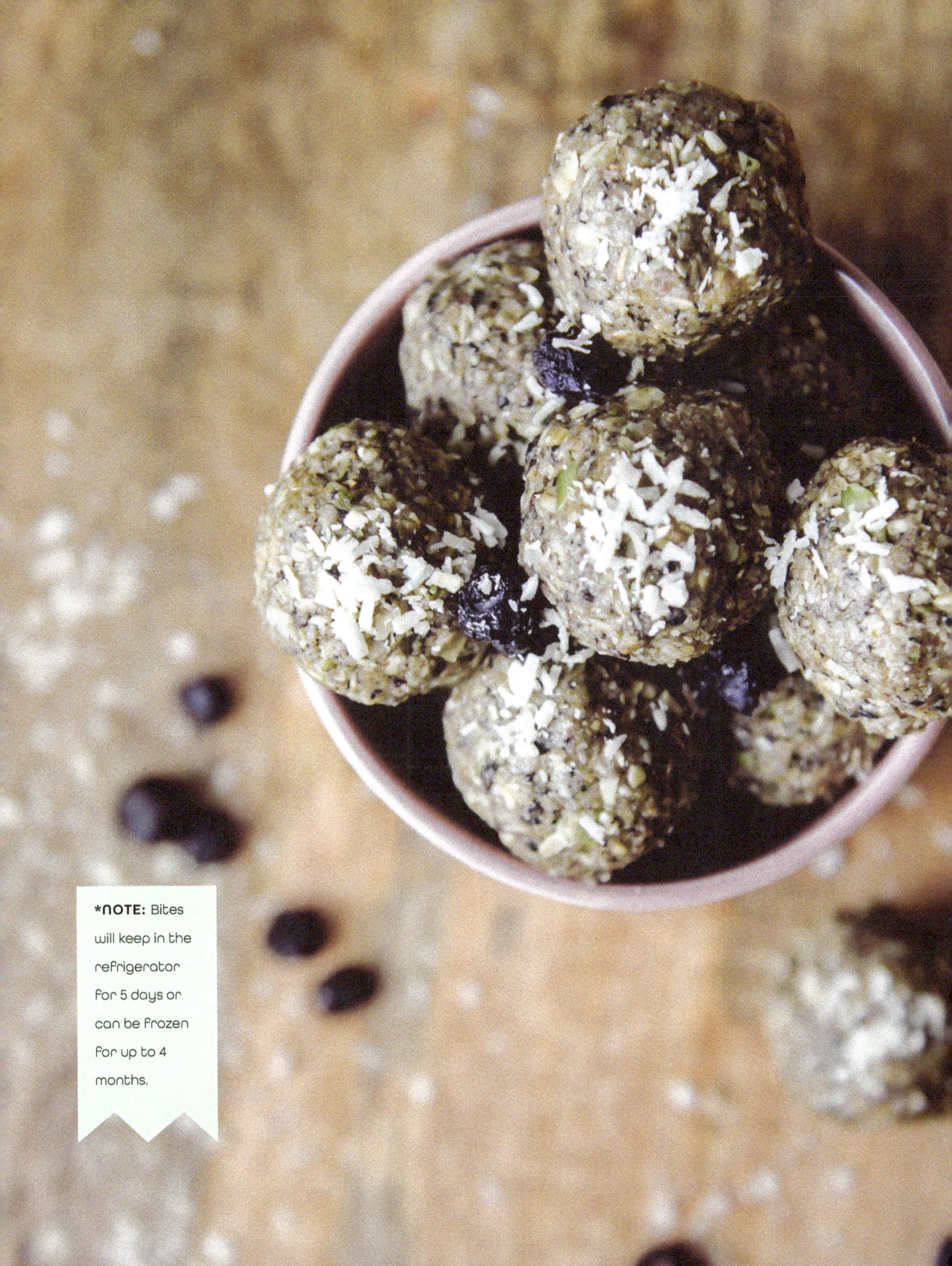

*NOTE: Bites will keep in the refrigerator for 5 days or can be frozen for up to 4 months.

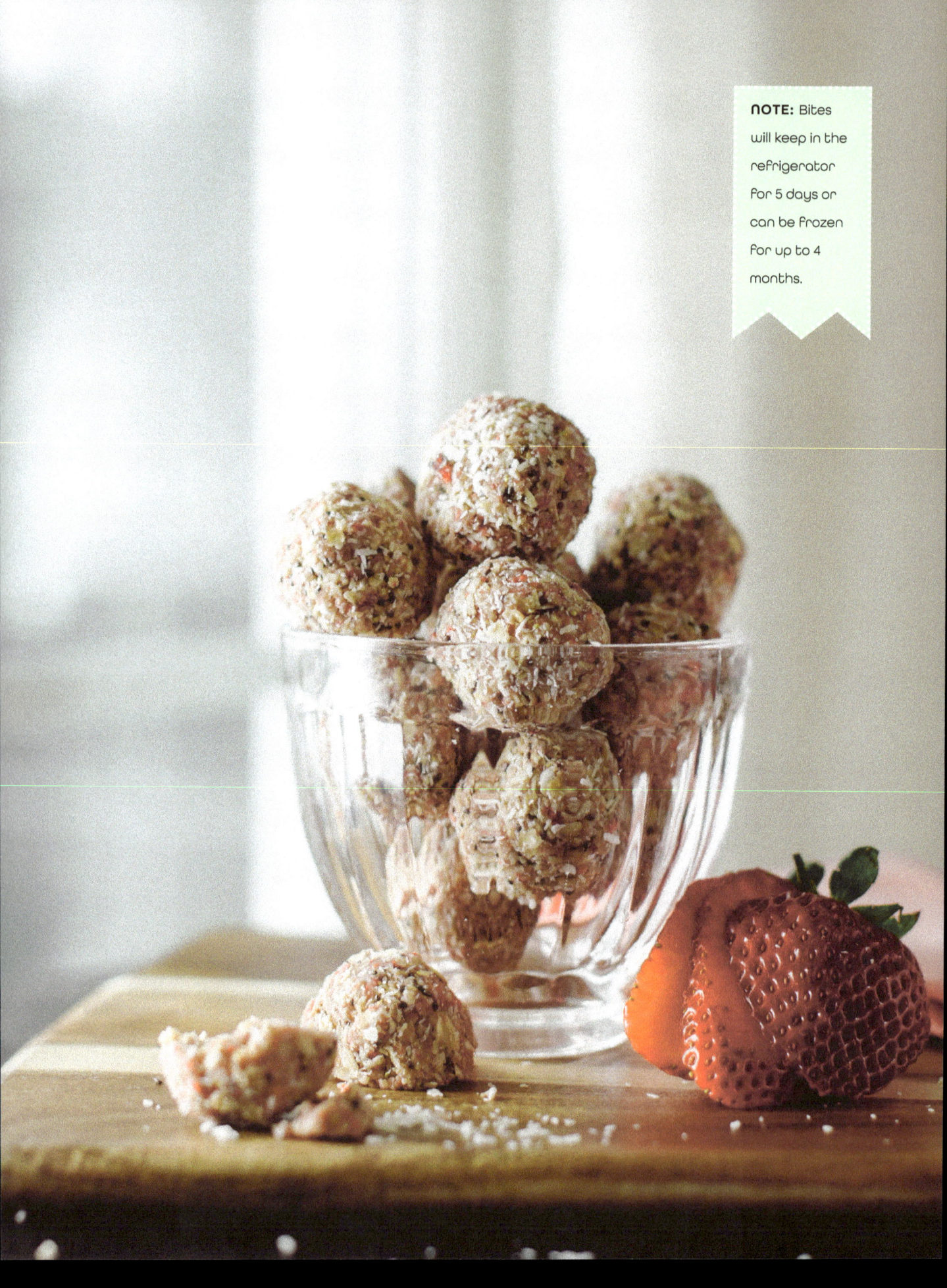

Strawberry Coconut Bites

YIELD: 16 BALLS

INGREDIENTS

1 tablespoon coconut oil

⅓ cup maple syrup

3 tablespoons sunflower seed butter

1 tablespoon chia seeds

1½ cups rolled oats

½ cup finely shredded coconut, plus about 2 tablespoons for rolling

⅛ teaspoon kosher salt

1 (1.2 oz) bag freeze-dried strawberries

INSTRUCTIONS

1. Place the coconut oil, syrup, sunflower seed butter, and chia seeds in a small pot and bring to a boil. Stir the mixture. Turn off heat and allow it to sit for 10 minutes.

2. Meanwhile, add the oats, ½ cup shredded coconut, and salt in a food processor and pulse for about 5–8 seconds until almost all the oats are broken up.

3. Add the strawberries and pulse another 2 times. Then add the wet ingredients in the food processor and pulse until combined.

4. Scrape the mixture into a bowl.

5. Roll into about 16 balls. If the mixture doesn't easily pack into small balls, you can add 1 teaspoon of water to the mixture. It also helps to wet your hands when rolling. Then lightly roll each ball in the extra shredded coconut.

Pumpkin Seeds Two Ways

High in zinc, magnesium, and a good source of healthy fats, pumpkin seeds are a delicious staple to keep in your kitchen. I love to top a big bowl of warm soup with these pumpkin seeds or enjoy with some fruit for a satisfying snack.

YIELD: 1 CUP

INGREDIENTS

Maple Chili

1 cup pumpkin seeds, raw

1 tablespoon maple syrup

½ teaspoon chili powder

¾ teaspoon kosher salt

Maple Curry

1 cup pumpkin seeds, raw

2 teaspoons maple syrup

1 teaspoon olive oil

2 teaspoons curry power

¾ teaspoon kosher salt

INSTRUCTIONS

1. Preheat oven to 275°F and line a sheet tray with parchment paper or a Silpat mat.

2. Add the ingredients to a bowl and stir.

3. Spread out in a single layer on the tray. Roast for 25–30 minutes. Allow it to cool completely before breaking apart and storing.

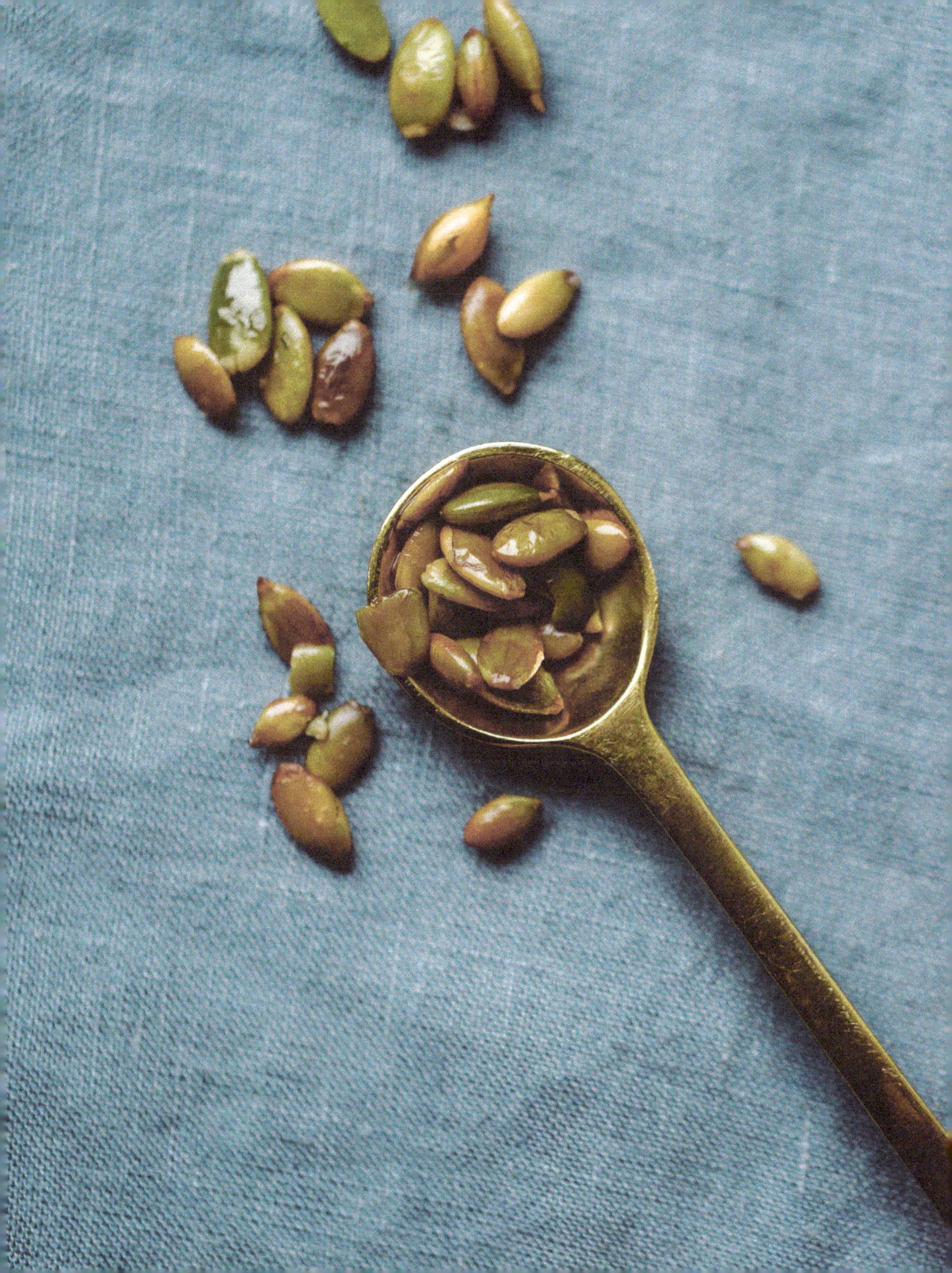

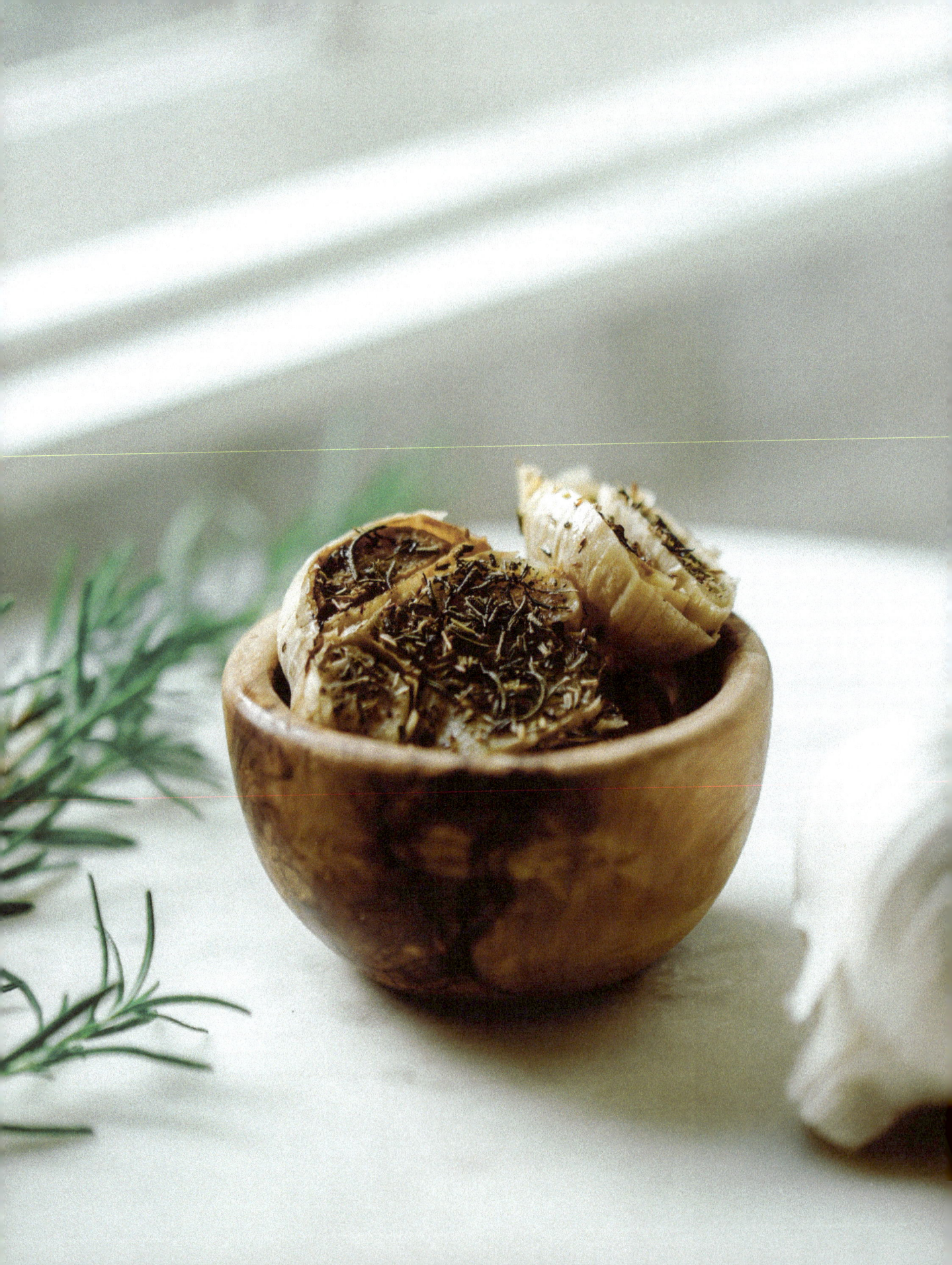

Herb-Roasted Garlic

When I roast garlic, I usually make a triple batch and keep some in the freezer to save time on future recipes. It makes the entire house smell delicious, assuming you like the smell of roasted garlic. Extra can be added to pasta sauces or pesto.

YIELD: 1 HEAD GARLIC

INGREDIENTS

1 head garlic, unpeeled

1 teaspoon fresh rosemary, chopped

½ teaspoon fresh or dried thyme, chopped

Olive oil

INSTRUCTIONS

1. Preheat oven to 400°F.
2. Cut the garlic in half so you slice through all the cloves.
3. Place the garlic halves root side down side by side on a piece of foil.
4. Top with the herbs and a drizzle of olive oil. Fold the foil into a packet over the garlic, crimping it shut at the top and on the sides.
5. Place in the oven and roast for 35–40 minutes.
6. Carefully open foil packet and allow to cool slightly.
7. Squeeze the garlic out of its peel.

Roasted garlic can be used in the Roasted Garlic White Bean Dip (page 74), mixed with room temperature butter for a compound butter, or kept on hand to mix into soups or other dishes.

Roasted Garlic White Bean Dip

YIELD: 3 CUPS

INGREDIENTS

1 recipe Herb-Roasted Garlic (page 73)

¼ cup extra virgin olive oil

Juice of ½ (about 1 tablespoon) lemon (optional)

⅛ teaspoon cayenne or to taste (optional)

2 (15 oz) cans cannellini beans, drained and rinsed

2 tablespoons water

2 tablespoons parsley, chopped (some stems OK)

A few chives or 1 scallion, sliced

Kosher salt and freshly ground black pepper

INSTRUCTIONS

1. Place the first 5 ingredients into a food processor or high-speed blender along with 2 tablespoons water and some salt (I use about 1 teaspoon) and pepper.
2. Blend until almost smooth. Add the parsley and chives (or scallion). Blend just a bit longer to incorporate the herbs. Adjust seasoning if needed.

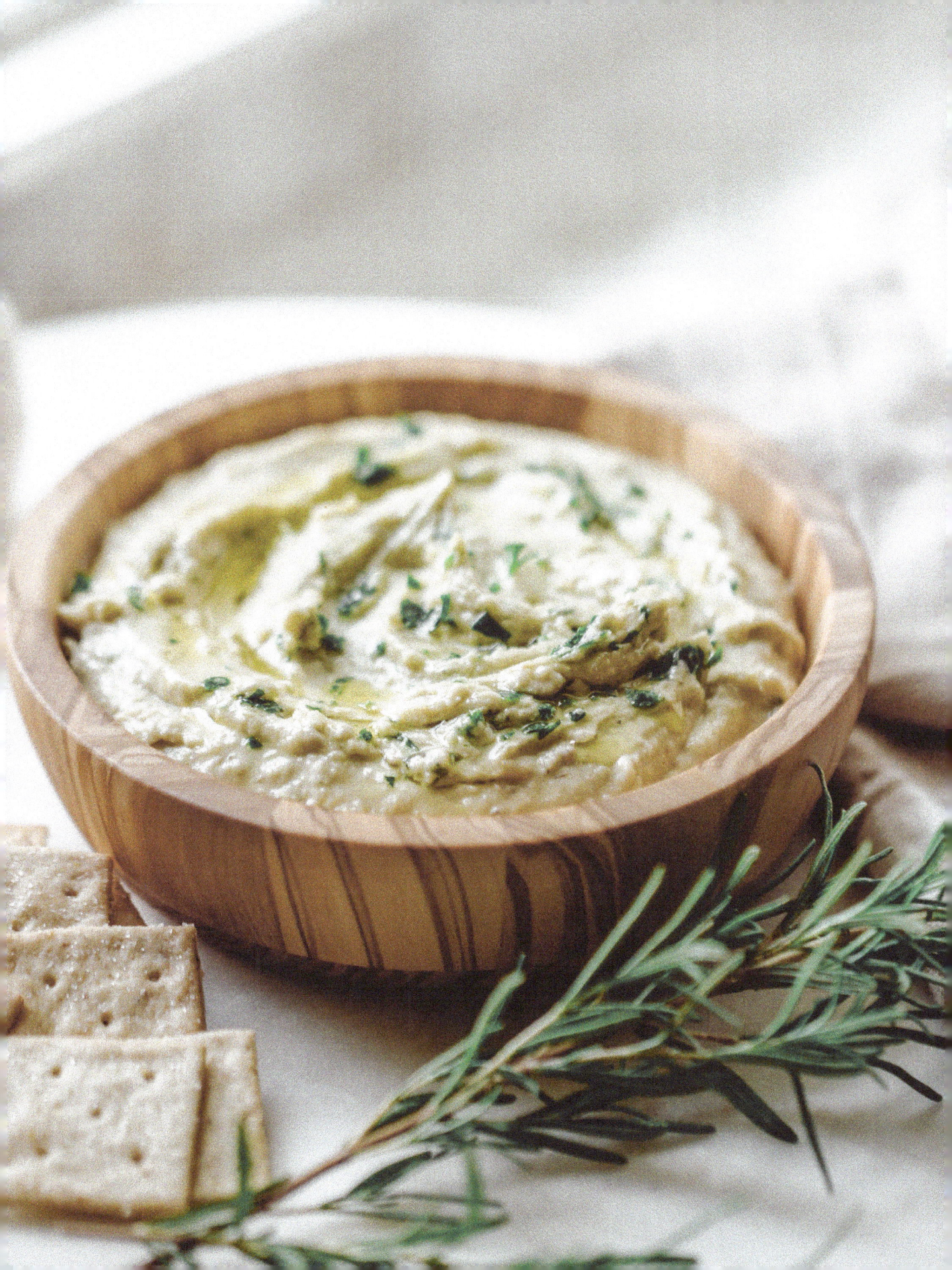

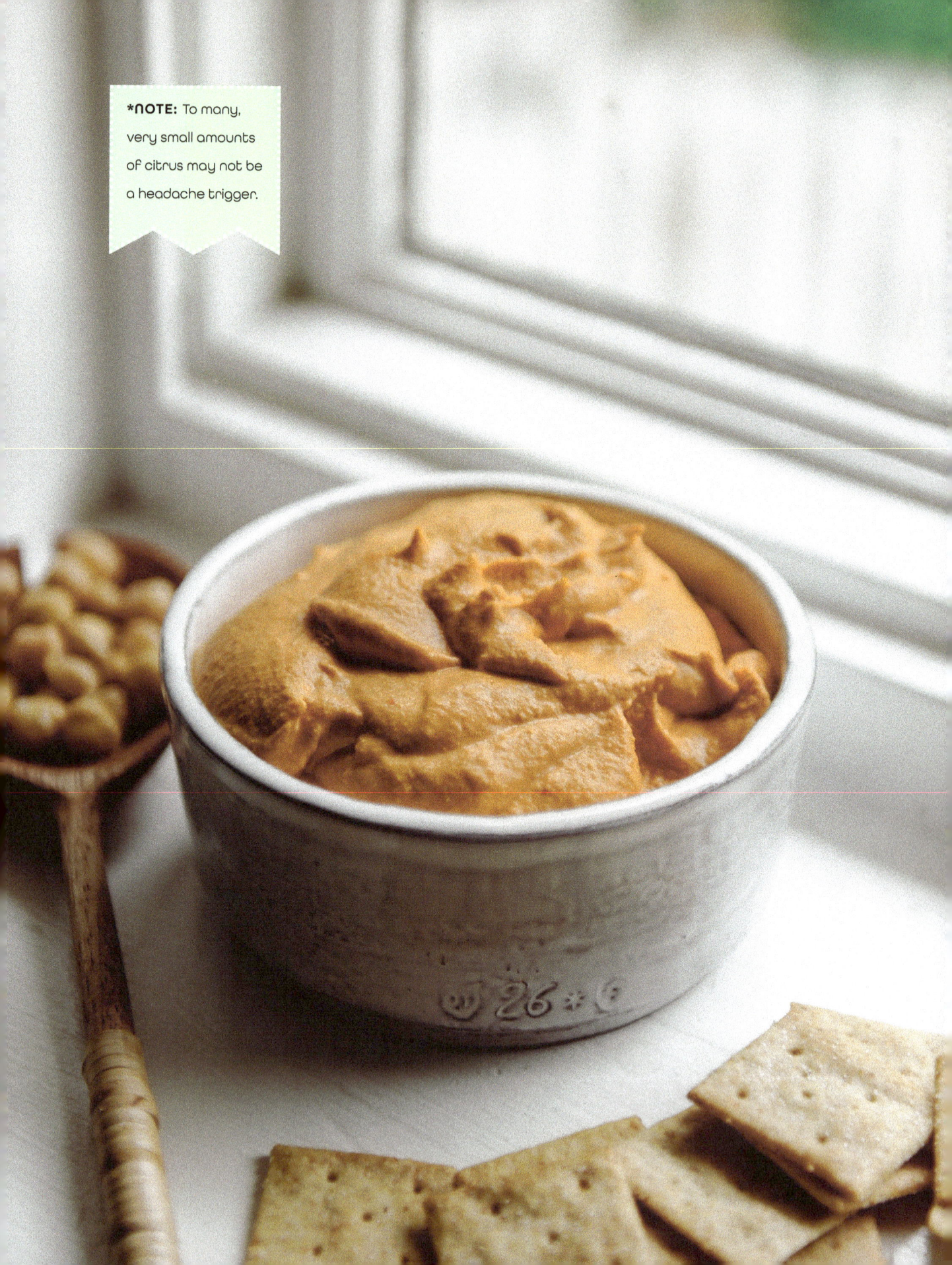

*NOTE: To many,
very small amounts
of citrus may not be
a headache trigger.

Roasted Red Pepper Hummus

This dip is creamy, slightly sweet, and a little smoky. To save time, you can use jarred roasted red peppers.

YIELD: ABOUT 2 CUPS

INGREDIENTS

1 (15.5 oz) can chickpeas, drained and rinsed

½ cup roasted red peppers from jar or one whole roasted red pepper, seeded and cleaned

1 garlic clove, peeled

2 tablespoons extra virgin olive oil

Juice of ½ (about 1 tablespoon) lemon* (optional)

1 teaspoon coconut aminos

2 tablespoons tahini

½ teaspoon kosher salt

½ teaspoon ground cumin

½ teaspoon paprika or smoked paprika

⅛ teaspoon cayenne, or more to taste (optional)

Freshly ground black pepper

INSTRUCTIONS

1. Place all the ingredients into a high-speed blender along with some pepper and 1 tablespoon water.

2. Blend until smooth and creamy.

3. Taste and adjust seasoning if needed.

Sweet Pea and Basil Hummus

This recipe came together one day when I needed some baby purée—fast! Parker, my daughter, was getting "hangry," and I didn't have any purée made. I tossed some peas in a blender and grabbed a big handful of basil from outside. She devoured it, and this simple mixture quickly became a staple in our kitchen.

YIELD: ABOUT 1½ CUPS

INGREDIENTS

2 cups thawed frozen sweet peas or fresh peas that have been lightly cooked and cooled

1½ cups fresh basil leaves

2 tablespoons extra virgin olive oil

1 small clove garlic, peeled

2 tablespoons tahini

½ teaspoon kosher salt

Freshly ground pepper

INSTRUCTIONS

Add the ingredients into a high-speed blender in the order listed and blend until smooth.

You can add up to 2 tablespoons water if the mixture is having trouble blending.

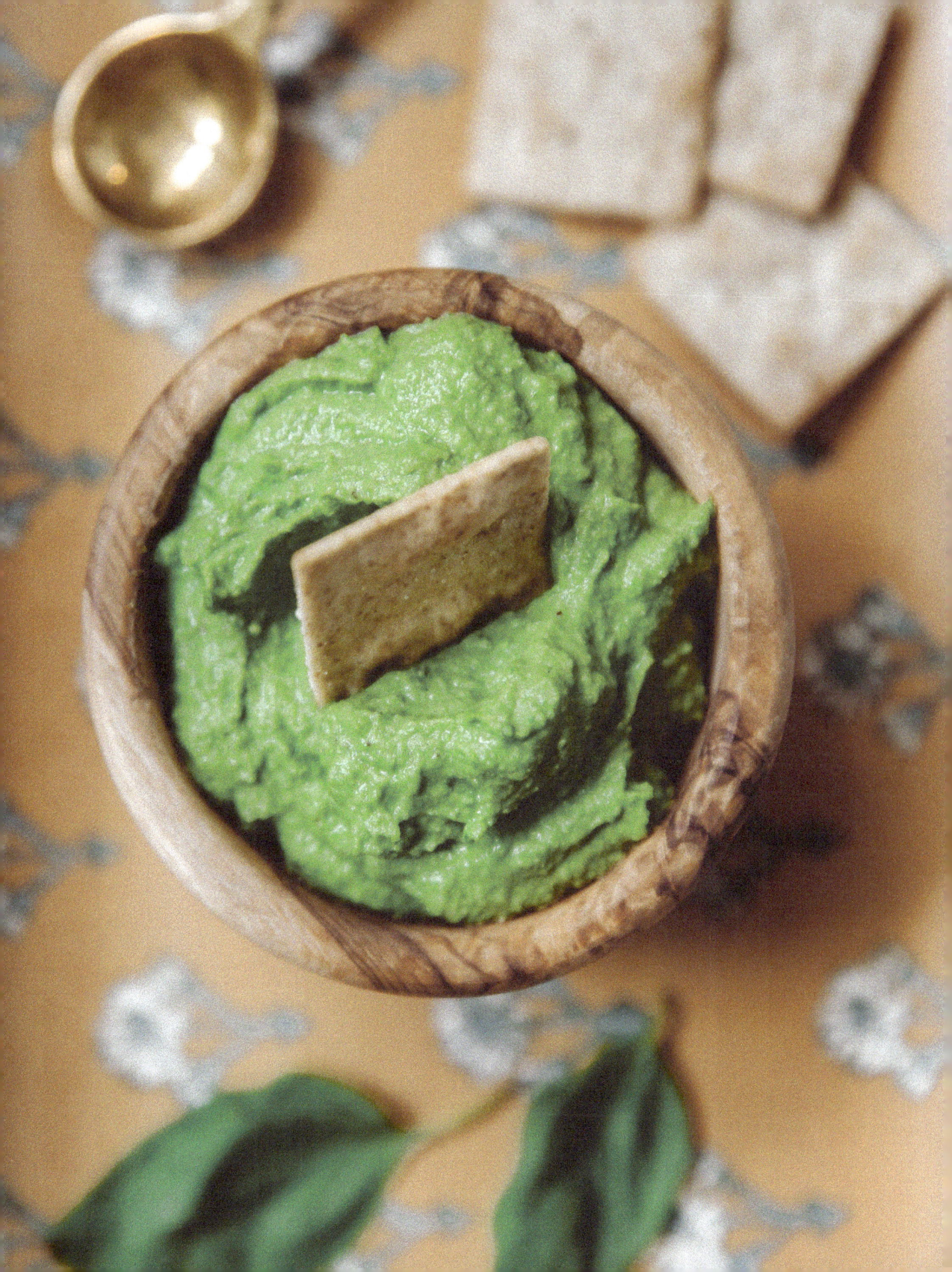

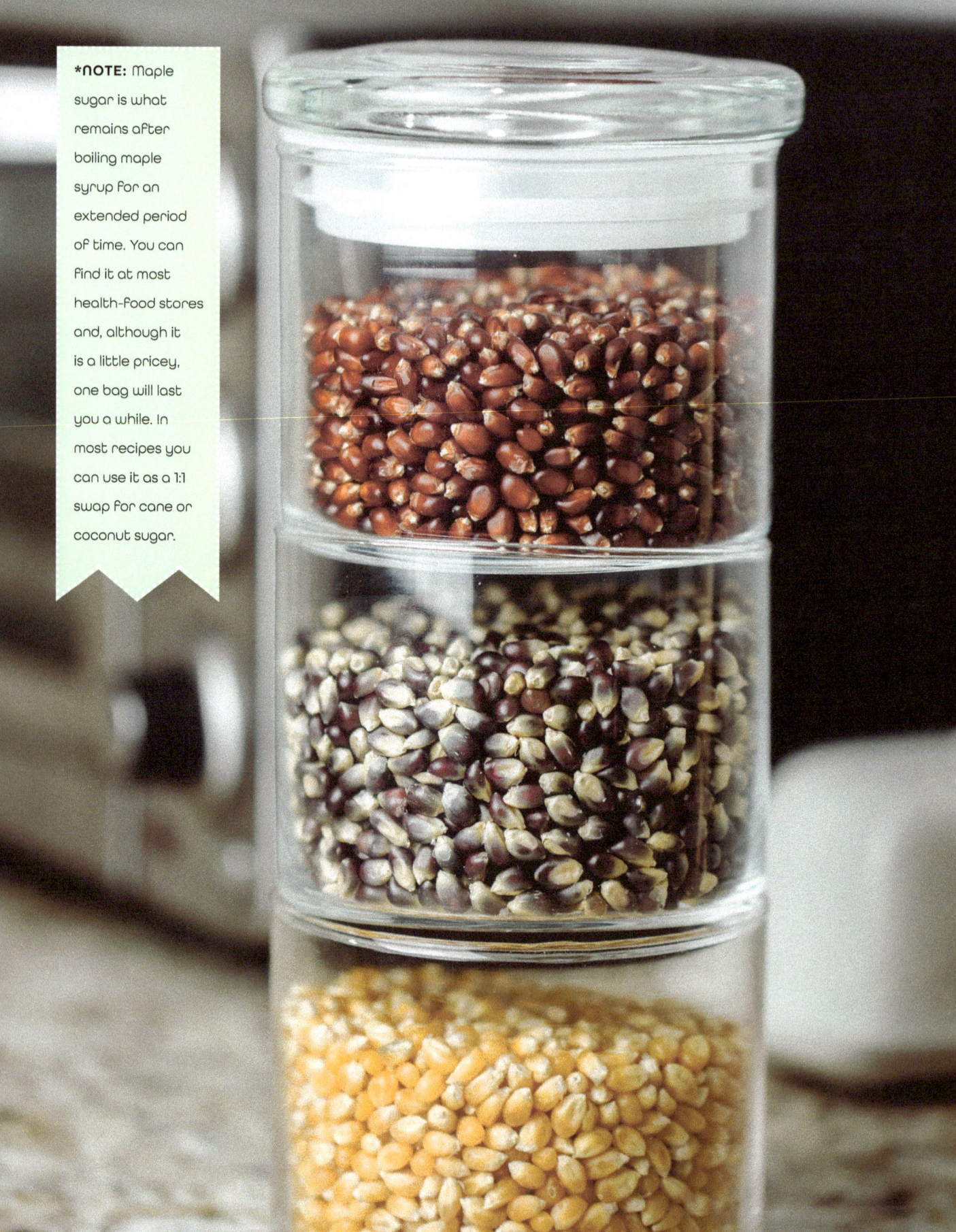

*NOTE: Maple sugar is what remains after boiling maple syrup for an extended period of time. You can find it at most health-food stores and, although it is a little pricey, one bag will last you a while. In most recipes you can use it as a 1:1 swap for cane or coconut sugar.

Sweet and Savory Popcorn Toppings

These popcorn toppings are two fun and different twists on the classic buttery snack. The savory idea comes from my good friend and culinary school classmate Christina. She loves popcorn as much as I do. The cinnamon maple one is great for a sweet and salty craving. You can substitute coconut sugar for the maple sugar, but I highly recommend the maple sugar.

YIELD: 7 CUPS

INGREDIENTS

Sweet: Cinnamon Maple

½ teaspoon ground cinnamon

2 teaspoons maple sugar*

¼–½ teaspoon kosher salt

¼ cup popcorn kernels, popped (approximately 7 cups popped popcorn)

Olive oil, coconut oil, or butter

INGREDIENTS

Savory: Rosemary Garlic

2 tablespoons olive oil

2 cloves garlic, peeled and smashed

1 sprig rosemary, stem removed and leaves chopped (about ½ tablespoon)

¼–½ teaspoon kosher salt

Freshly ground black pepper

¼ cup popcorn kernels, popped (approximately 7 cups popped popcorn)

INSTRUCTIONS

Sweet: Cinnamon Maple

1. Combine the cinnamon, maple sugar, and salt in a small bowl and stir.
2. Place the popcorn in a large bowl and lightly coat it with some oil. I like to keep some oil in a small spray bottle and spritz the cooked popcorn.
3. Toss the popcorn with the maple sugar mixture. Adjust seasoning if needed.

INSTRUCTIONS

Savory: Rosemary Garlic

1. In a small sauce pot heat the olive oil and garlic over medium-low heat.
2. Heat a few minutes until the garlic has infused the olive oil. It will begin to sizzle. Turn off heat and allow the garlic to sit in the oil for a few more minutes.
3. Remove the garlic from the oil with a slotted spoon.
4. Add the rosemary, salt, and pepper.
5. Place the cooked popcorn in a large bowl and drizzle with rosemary mixture.
6. Toss to coat. Adjust salt and pepper if needed.

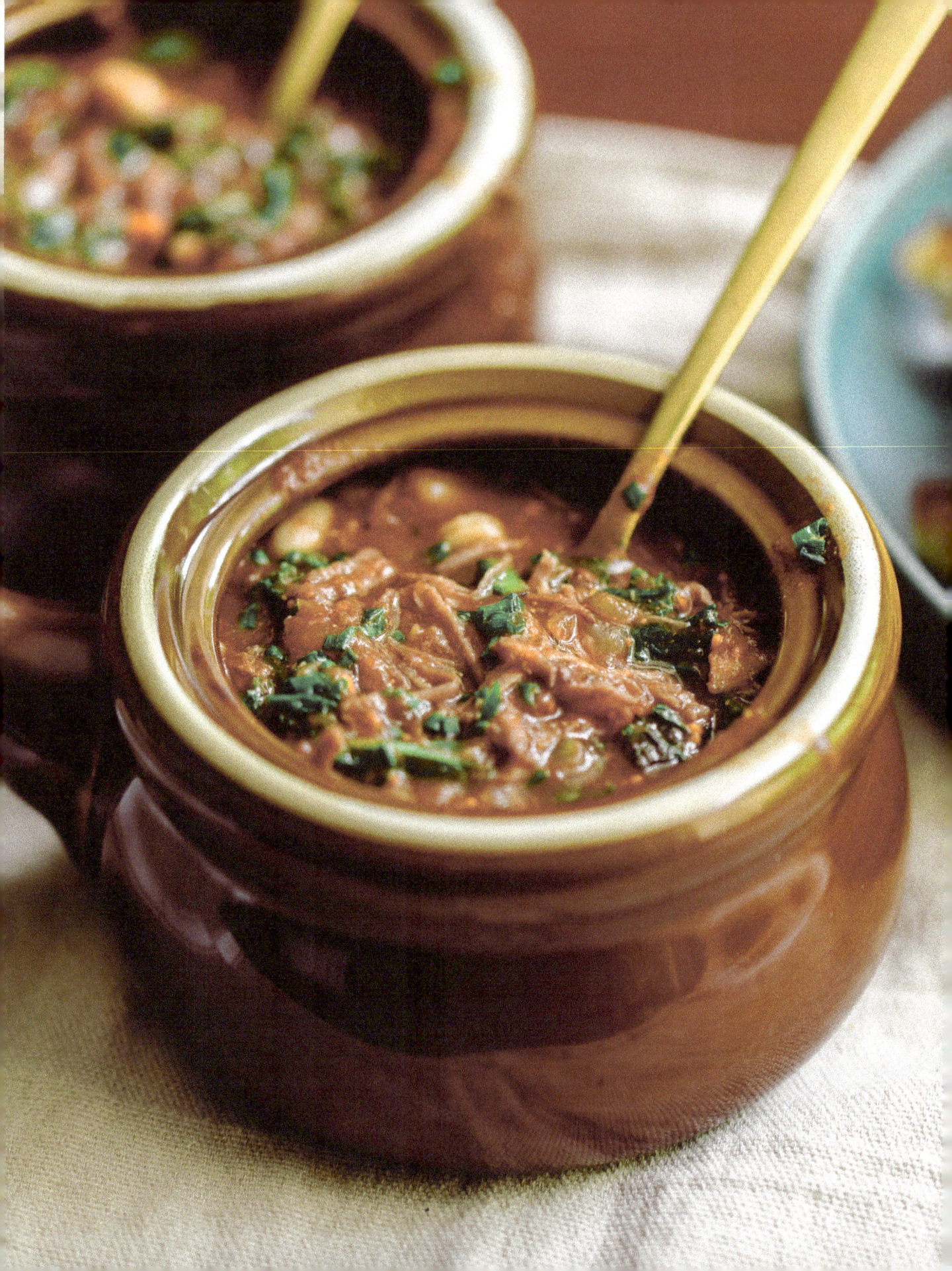

Stocks, Soups, Stews, and Salads

Vegetable Stock 84

Chicken Stock.. 86

Autumn Squash and Apple Cider Soup 87

Root Vegetable Soup.. 91

Chicken Orzo Soup with Ginger 92

Duck Gumbo 95

Beans and Greens Turkey Stew 96

Short Rib and White Bean Stew.. 99

Roasted Grape and Radicchio Salad 100

Roasted Chickpea and Cauliflower Salad 103

Seasonal Quinoa and Mixed Greens Salad........................104

Spring Strawberry and Arugula Salad 107

Chicken Salad with Grapes 108

Vegetable Stock

Homemade stocks are a delicious staple to have on hand. They are far superior in flavor and nutrition than most of the boxed options out there and cost a lot less. If you are new to making stock or are short on time, a vegetable stock is a great place to start.

YIELD: 1 GALLON

INGREDIENTS

5 pounds of non-starchy vegetables*

5 garlic cloves, smashed

8 black or white peppercorns

Herbs such as bay leaf, thyme, and parsley stems

5 quarts water

*NOTE: I keep stock-friendly vegetable scraps in the freezer until I have enough to make a big batch of stock.
Some stock-friendly vegetables include onions, carrots, celery, leeks, mushrooms, fennel, and turnips.
Vegetables to avoid include potatoes (due to their high starch content), beets and peppers (since they overpower the stock), and green beans, broccoli, and zucchini (since they turn bitter).

INSTRUCTIONS

1. Place all the ingredients into a large stock pot.
2. Bring to a light boil then turn down to a simmer. Cook for about 45 minutes then turn off the heat.
3. Pour the stock through a fine mesh strainer and cool.

Store covered in the fridge and use within 5 days or package in containers to freeze for several months.

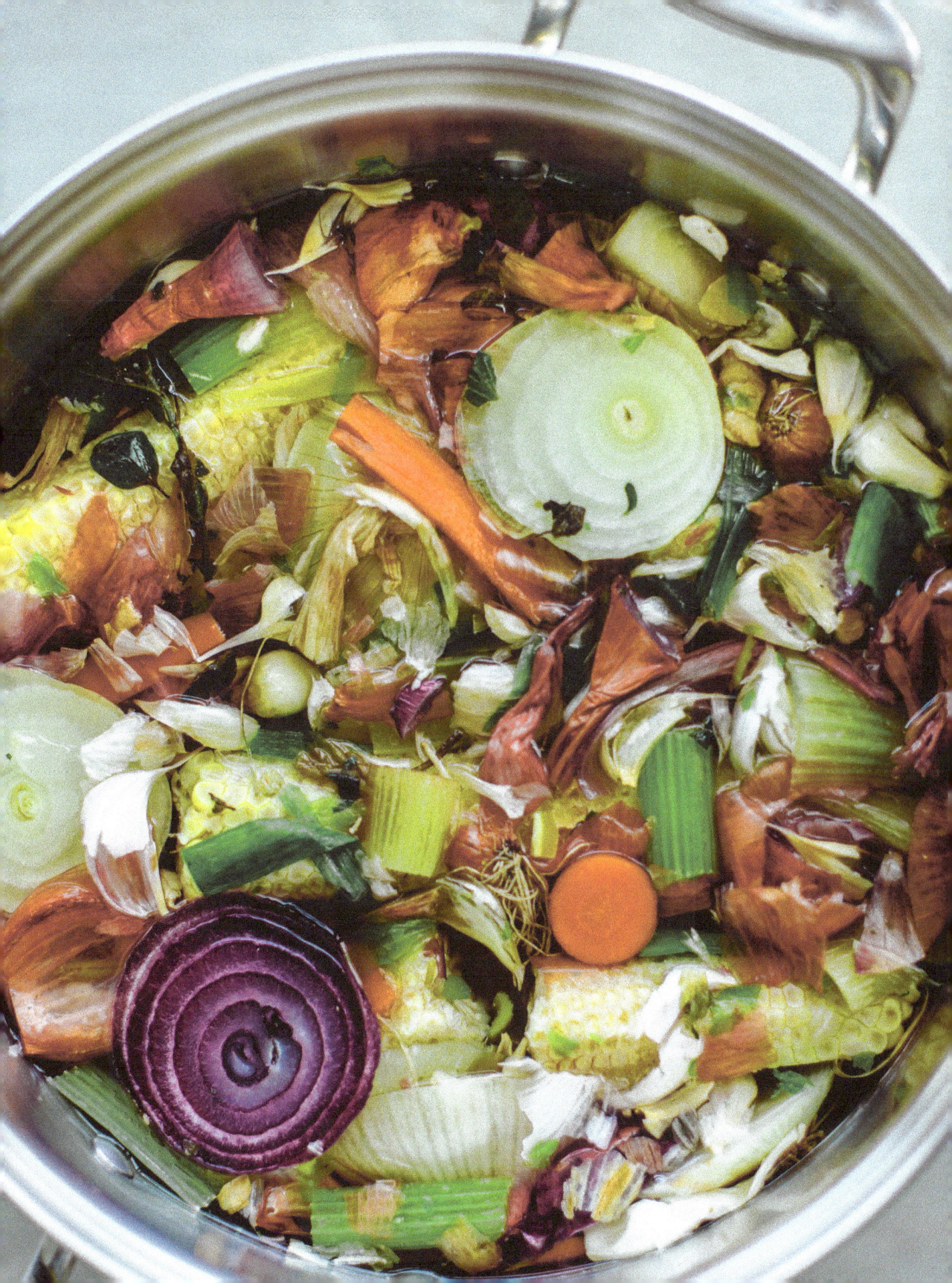

Chicken Stock

Some chicken stock recipes call for adding the vegetables at the beginning, while others say to add them in the last hour of cooking. I have done both but find that adding them at the beginning results in a more concentrated flavor.

YIELD: 1 GALLON

INGREDIENTS

About 4 pounds of chicken bones/parts such as a carcass, neck, backs and wings, preferably local

About 1 pound of non-starchy vegetables, such as 1 onion, 1 carrot, 1 celery rib, and a few cloves smashed garlic, chopped

8 black or white peppercorns

Herbs such as bay leaf, thyme, and parsley stems

About 5 quarts water

INSTRUCTIONS

1. Place all the ingredients into a large stock pot and cover with the water.
2. Bring to a boil then turn down to a simmer and keep partially covered for about 4 hours. After the first hour you can skim off the top then continue to cook.
3. Turn off heat, strain, and cool.

Store covered in the fridge and use within 5 days or package in containers to freeze for up to 6 months.

> **TIP:** I keep stock-friendly vegetable scraps in the freezer until I have enough to make a big batch of stock.
> Some stock-friendly vegetables include onions, carrots, celery, leeks, mushrooms, fennel, and turnips.
> Vegetables to avoid include potatoes (due to their high starch content), beets and peppers (since they overpower the stock), and green beans, broccoli, and zucchini (since they turn bitter).
> For a brown chicken stock, you can rub the bones/carcass with a little oil and roast in the oven at 425°F for about 45 minutes before making the stock.

Autumn Squash and Apple Cider Soup

The idea for this soup came from Chef Larry Forgione, who I worked for at The Culinary Institute of America in St. Helena, California. We made a similar soup for hundreds of people at one of their annual conferences, Worlds of Flavor. He topped his with crème fraiche, but you can also top it with either of the two pumpkin seed recipes on page 70.

YIELD: 4–6 SERVINGS

INGREDIENTS

Squash

1 medium butternut (or similar) squash, peeled, deseeded, and cubed in 2-inch pieces (approx. 7 cups cubed squash)

2 tablespoons unsalted butter, can substitute coconut oil or olive oil

2 teaspoons coconut sugar or light brown sugar

1¼ teaspoons ground cinnamon

1½ teaspoons ground cumin

¼ teaspoon ground nutmeg

Kosher salt and freshly ground pepper

Soup

1 tablespoon olive oil

3 large shallots, peeled and chopped

1 cup carrots, chopped (approx. 1–2 carrots)

3 cloves garlic, peeled and chopped

1½ teaspoons curry powder

4 cups vegetable stock, preferably homemade (page 84) or other non-MSG stock

1½ cups apple cider (not apple cider vinegar)

½ cup canned coconut milk, full fat

Kosher salt and freshly ground pepper

CONTINUES NEXT PAGE

INSTRUCTIONS

1. Preheat oven to 400°F. Line a baking sheet with parchment paper or a Silpat mat.

2. For the squash, melt the butter and combine in a small bowl with the coconut sugar and spices along with some salt and pepper. Rub the cubed squash with the butter/spice mixture to evenly coat, then spread out evenly on the baking sheet.

3. Roast 30–40 minutes or until the squash is almost fork-tender. Remove and set aside.

4. While the squash is roasting, heat the olive oil in a large Dutch oven or pot and once hot add the shallots. Cook a few minutes, stirring occasionally then add the carrots and garlic.

5. Cook for a few minutes and add the curry powder along with a large pinch of salt.

6. Next add the stock and cider. Bring to a boil, then turn the heat down and simmer for 15–20 minutes or until the vegetables are almost fork-tender.

7. Add the roasted squash and simmer for an additional 5–10 minutes.

8. Turn off heat and add the coconut milk.

9. Purée with an immersion blender or allow to cool slightly and blend in a high-speed blender. Adjust seasoning if needed.

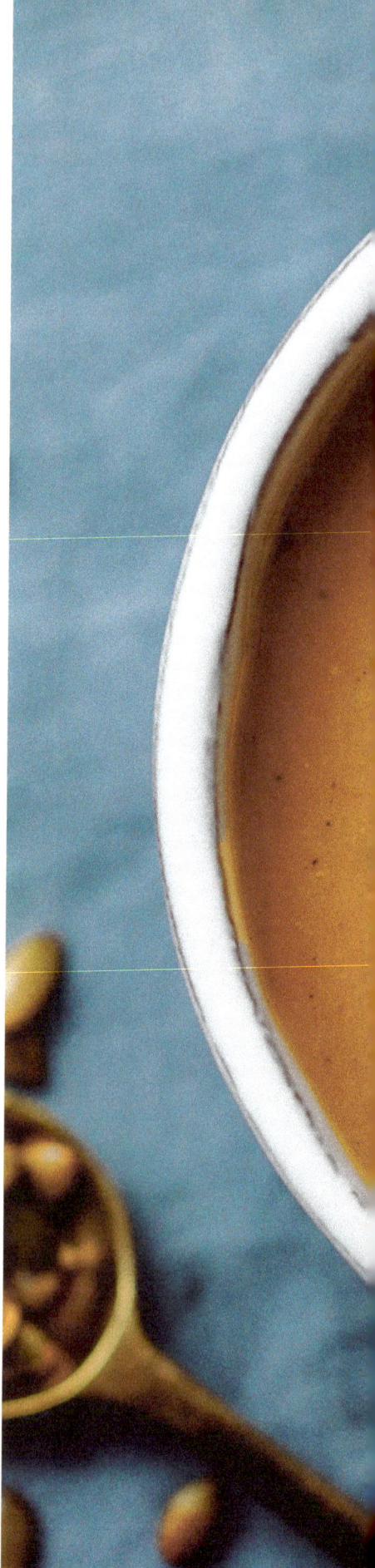

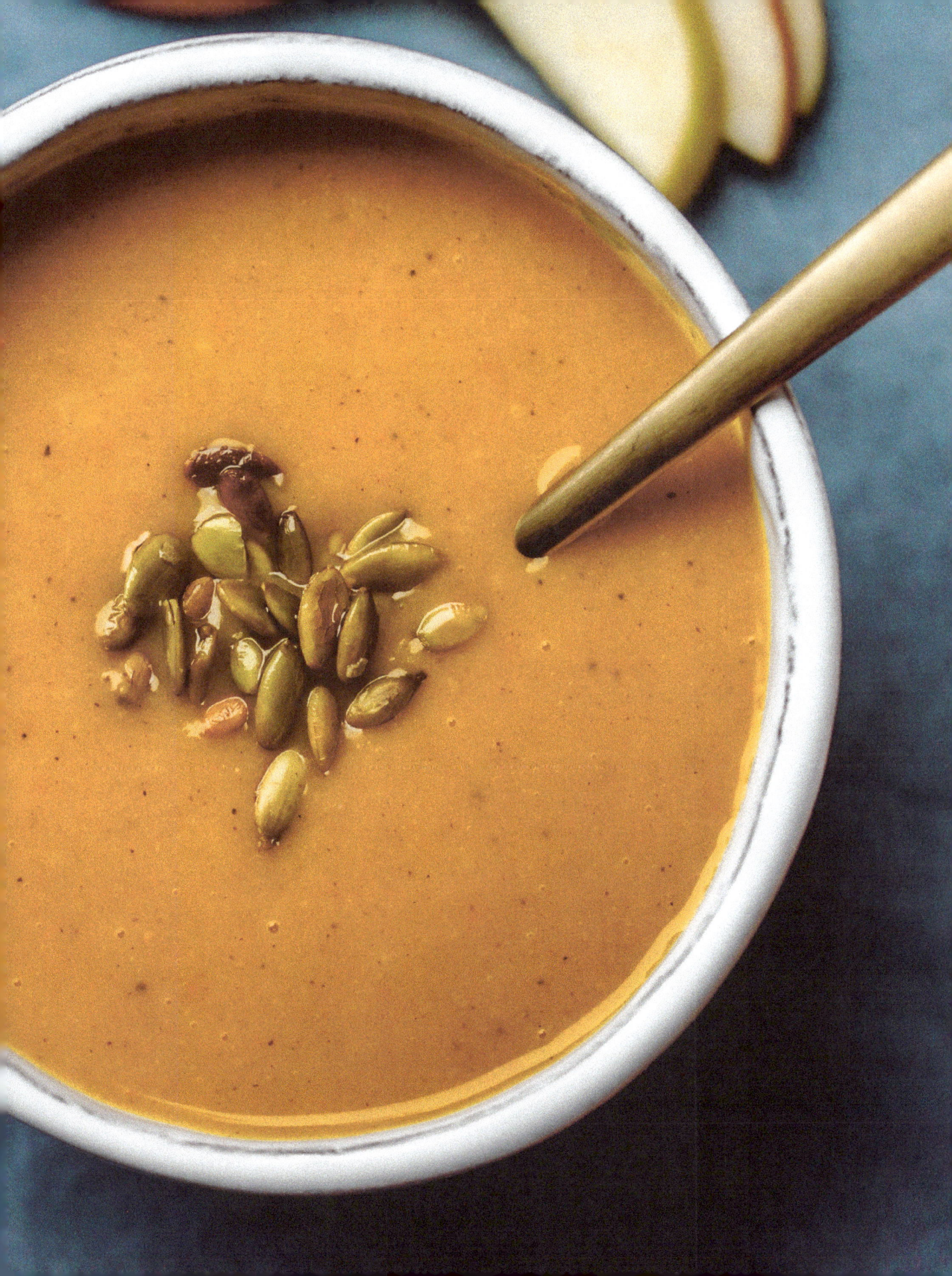

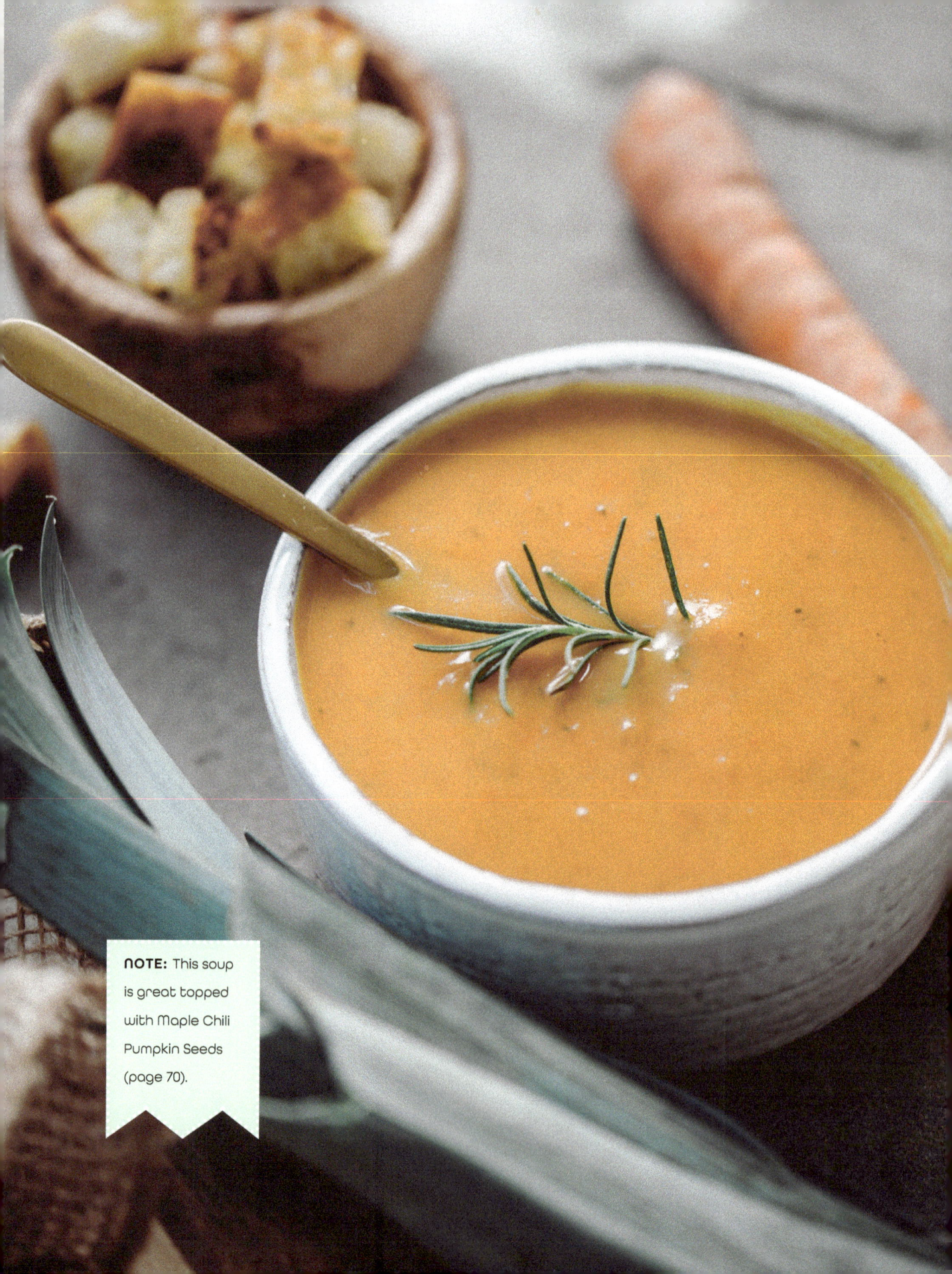

NOTE: This soup is great topped with Maple Chili Pumpkin Seeds (page 70).

Root Vegetable Soup

This soup was created one night when I was playing "clean out the fridge" for dinner. Everyone enjoyed it so much that it became a winter staple at our house. Feel free to play around with different root vegetables based on what you have or what you find at the local farmers market.

YIELD: 4–6 SERVINGS (ABOUT 9 CUPS)

INGREDIENTS

2 tablespoons unsalted butter or olive oil

2 leeks, chopped and rinsed, white parts only

2 large carrots, chopped

1 small rutabaga, peeled and chopped, can substitute 1 medium turnip

1 medium russet potato, peeled and chopped

1 medium sweet potato, peeled and chopped

3 cloves garlic, peeled and chopped

1 sprig rosemary, destemmed and leaves chopped

1½ teaspoons fresh thyme

½ teaspoon dried parsley

¼ teaspoon dried dill

1 bay leaf

1 quart vegetable or chicken stock, preferably homemade (pages 84, 86), or other non-MSG stock

1 cup water or additional stock

⅓ cup canned coconut milk (optional)

Kosher salt and freshly ground pepper

INSTRUCTIONS

1. In a large Dutch oven heat the olive oil over medium heat. Once hot add the leeks. Give them a stir and allow them to cook a minute until they begin to soften.

2. Add the carrots, rutabaga, potatoes, and garlic along with 2 large pinches of salt and pepper. Stir and cook for 5–10 minutes. Then add the herbs and bay leaf.

3. Add the stock along with 1 cup water and bring to a boil. Once at a boil, reduce to low and cover for 15–20 minutes or until the vegetables are fork-tender. Turn off heat and remove the bay leaf. Add coconut milk, if using.

4. Purée using an immersion blender or allow to cool slightly and blend the soup in a high-speed blender. Adjust seasoning if needed.

Chicken Orzo Soup with Ginger

My take on the classic chicken noodle soup, this version is full of nutritious and filling ingredients like cannellini beans, vegetables, and ginger. Homemade stock takes this soup to the next level, so I always make sure to have some on hand.

YIELD: 4–6 SERVINGS

INGREDIENTS

1 tablespoon olive oil or butter

3 shallots, peeled and diced

2 carrots, diced

2 stalks celery, diced

1 (2-inch) piece fresh ginger, peeled and finely grated

3 garlic cloves, peeled and minced or grated

½ teaspoon dried basil

½ teaspoon dried oregano

1 bay leaf

6 cups stock, preferably homemade, such as vegetable or chicken (pages 84, 86), or non-MSG stock

1 (15 oz) can cannellini beans, drained and rinsed

½ cup orzo

1 pound cooked and shredded chicken

½ cup fresh parsley (some stems OK), chopped

INSTRUCTIONS

1. Heat the olive oil or butter in a Dutch oven over medium heat. Once hot add in the shallots with a couple pinches of salt. Cook for a few minutes until they begin to soften and add in the carrot and celery. Cook a few more minutes, stirring occasionally.

2. Next add the ginger and garlic. Cook until fragrant, about 1 minute.

3. Add the herbs, stock, and beans. Bring to a boil and then reduce to a simmer. Cover and cook for 20 minutes.

4. Remove the lid, then remove and discard the bay leaf.

5. Using an immersion blender, pulse the soup a few times to blend about ⅓ of it. (Alternatively, you can place about 1½ cups of soup, once cooled slightly, in a blender and blend. Then add it back to the pot.)

6. Stir in the orzo and chicken. Simmer for another 6 minutes or until the orzo is almost done.

7. Turn off heat and add the parsley. Adjust seasonings if needed.

Enjoy right away or store it in the fridge for up to 5 days or in the freezer for several months. The orzo will thicken as it sits so you might need to thin the soup with a little water or stock when heating it up.

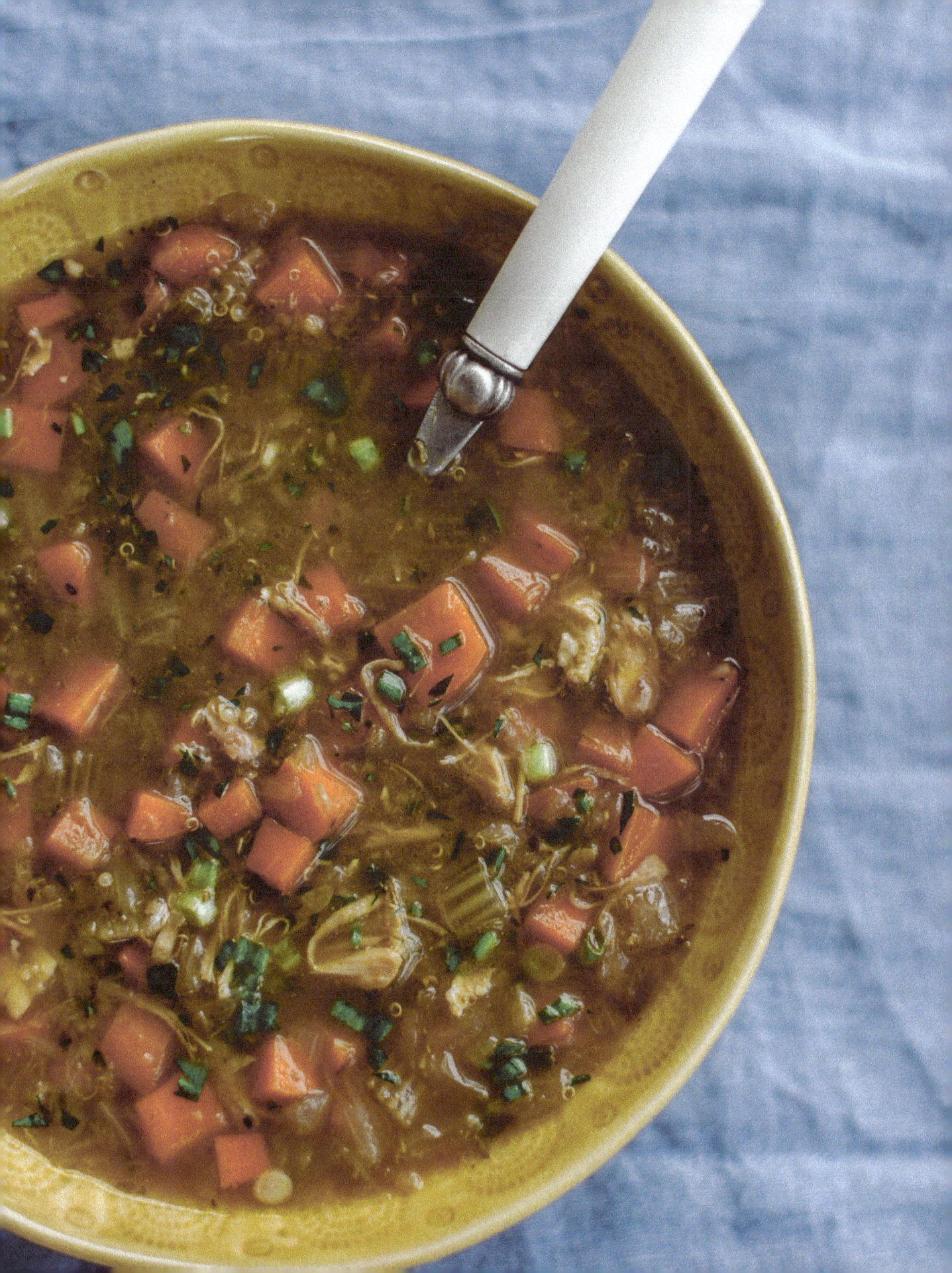

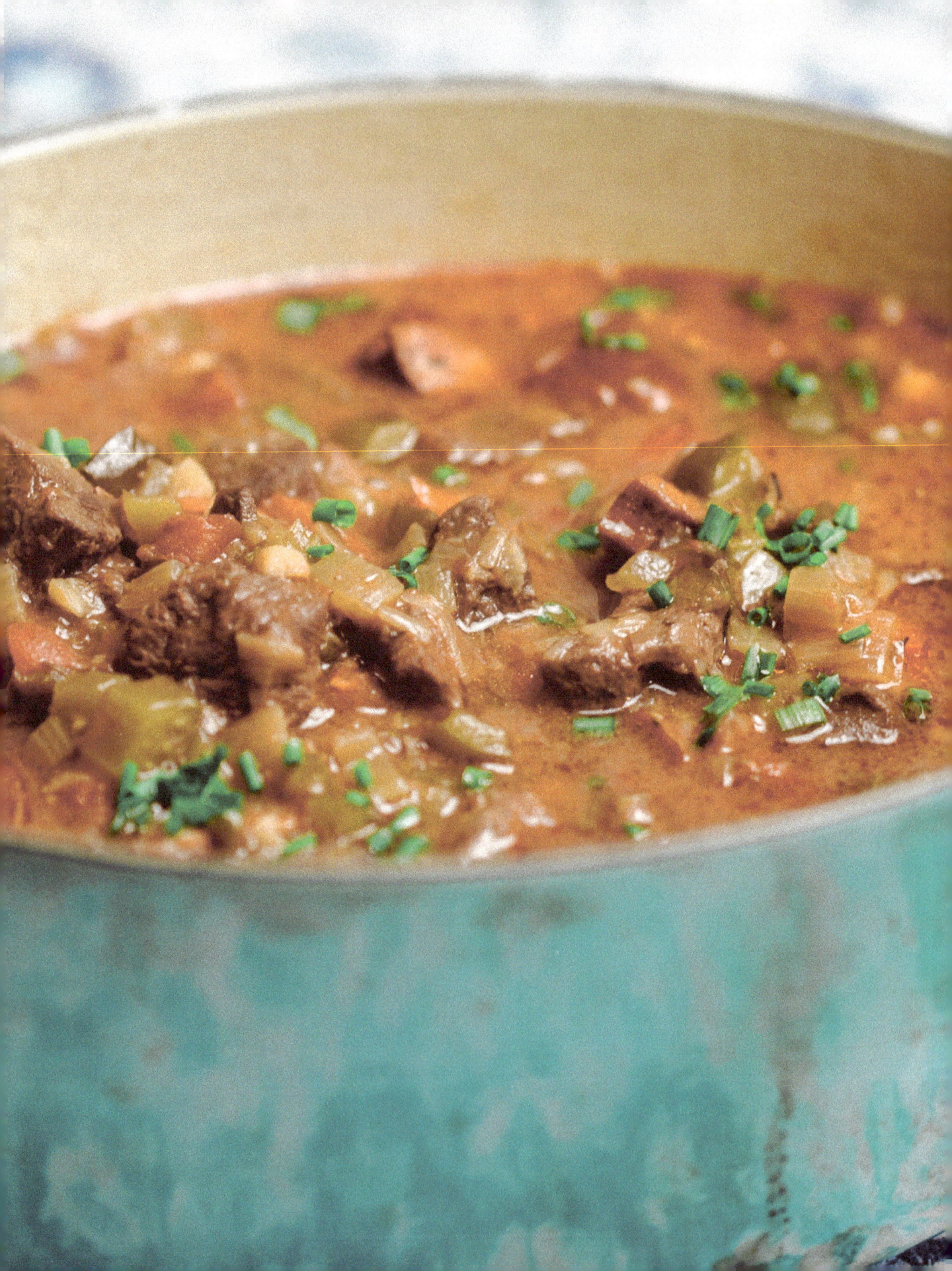

Duck Gumbo

INGREDIENTS

1 pound wild duck meat, cut
into about 1½ inch cubes, can
substitute chicken thighs

½ cup crushed tomatoes or
tomato sauce

1 tablespoon olive oil

3 large shallots, diced

1 stalk celery, diced

1 bell pepper, green or red,
diced

1 jalapeño, deseeded,
destemmed, and minced

3 gloves garlic, peeled and
minced

¼ cup unsalted butter

¼ cup all-purpose flour or
gluten-free flour blend such
as Bob's Red Mill

3 cups chicken stock,
preferably homemade (page
86), or non-MSG stock

2 teaspoons Cajun seasoning

1 teaspoon fresh thyme leaves,
chopped

1 bay leaf

2 links andouille sausage,
diced, or cooked and
crumbled migraine friendly
sausage (approx. 6 oz)
(page 53)

2 green onions, trimmed and
sliced thin

¼ cup fresh parsley, chopped
fine

Kosher salt and freshly ground
pepper

INSTRUCTIONS

1. Place the duck, crushed tomatoes, 1 teaspoon salt, and some pepper in a pressure cooker or slow cooker.

2. In a skillet heat the olive oil over medium heat. Add the shallots and a pinch of salt. Sauté for a few minutes.

3. Next, add the celery, bell pepper, and jalapeño. Cook for 5–8 minutes, stirring occasionally. Add the garlic and cook for about a minute.

4. Transfer the mixture to the pressure cooker or slow cooker and place the pan back on the stove.

5. Add the butter and once melted, whisk in the flour to make a roux.

6. Continue to cook over medium heat, whisking constantly, until the roux has turned a medium brown. This will take 10–15 minutes.

7. Slowly whisk in the stock.

8. Once combined pour the mixture into the pressure cooker or slow cooker along with the Cajun seasoning, thyme, bay leaf, and sausage.

9. Set the pressure cooker on manual for 45 minutes (for an Instant Pot you can set it to the stew setting) and allow to vent naturally. If you're using a slow cooker, cook on high for 4 hours or low for 7–8 hours.

10. Remove the lid, remove and discard bay leaf, and stir in the green onions and parsley, leaving a little to garnish. Adjust seasoning if needed.

11. Divide into bowls and garnish with remaining green onions and parsley.

Beans and Greens Turkey Stew

I knew this recipe was a hit after my dad tried it and said he could eat this every single day. It's even better the next day, so make a large batch to enjoy all week long.

YIELD: 4 SERVINGS

INGREDIENTS

2 tablespoons olive oil

1 pound ground turkey or chicken, preferably local

2 shallots, peeled and diced

3 garlic cloves, peeled and minced or grated

1 tablespoon ground cumin

1 tablespoon fennel seeds

1 tablespoon Italian seasoning

⅛ teaspoon cayenne (optional)

3 tablespoons all-purpose or gluten-free flour

1 (8 oz) can mild green chilies

1 (15 oz) can cannellini beans, drained and rinsed

4 cups vegetable or chicken stock, preferably homemade (pages 84, 86), or non-MSG stock

1 bunch Swiss chard, chopped and washed, about 3 cups*

Kosher salt and freshly ground pepper

INSTRUCTIONS

1. Heat the oil in a large Dutch oven over medium-high heat. Once hot add the turkey or chicken with some salt, breaking it apart as it cooks. When it is cooked add the shallots and garlic. Continue cooking until the shallots begin to soften.

2. Then add the cumin, fennel seeds, Italian seasoning, and cayenne.

3. Once all the spices are mixed in, add the flour, stirring to incorporate so you do not see any white bits. Turn heat down to medium and cook a few minutes. This helps to remove the "floury" taste. If the bottom starts to turn dark brown at any point, you can add a tablespoon or 2 of water.

4. Then add the green chilies, beans, stock, and Swiss chard. Season with salt and pepper and bring to a boil. Turn the heat to low and simmer, covered, for about 2 hours.

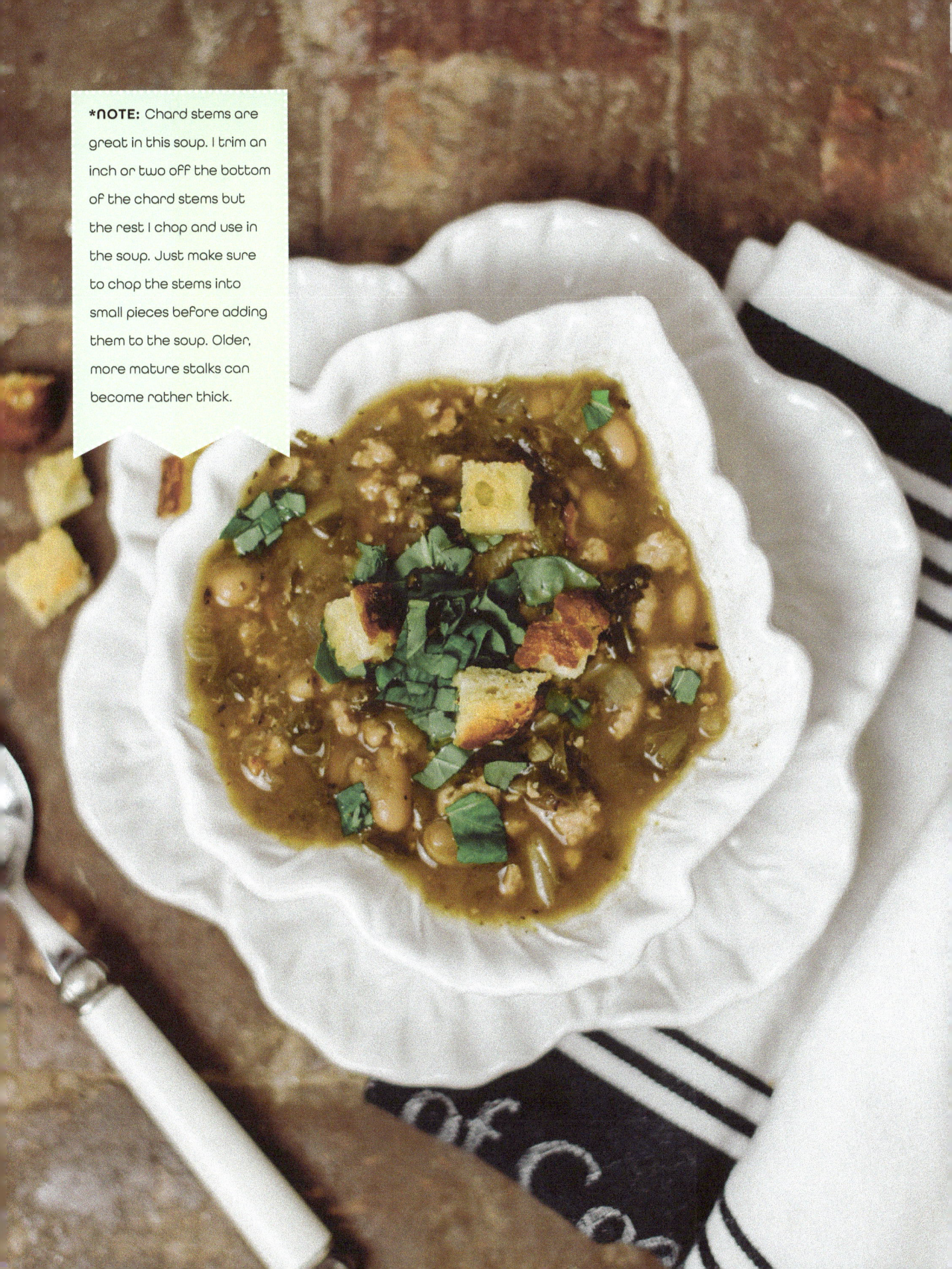

*NOTE: Chard stems are great in this soup. I trim an inch or two off the bottom of the chard stems but the rest I chop and use in the soup. Just make sure to chop the stems into small pieces before adding them to the soup. Older, more mature stalks can become rather thick.

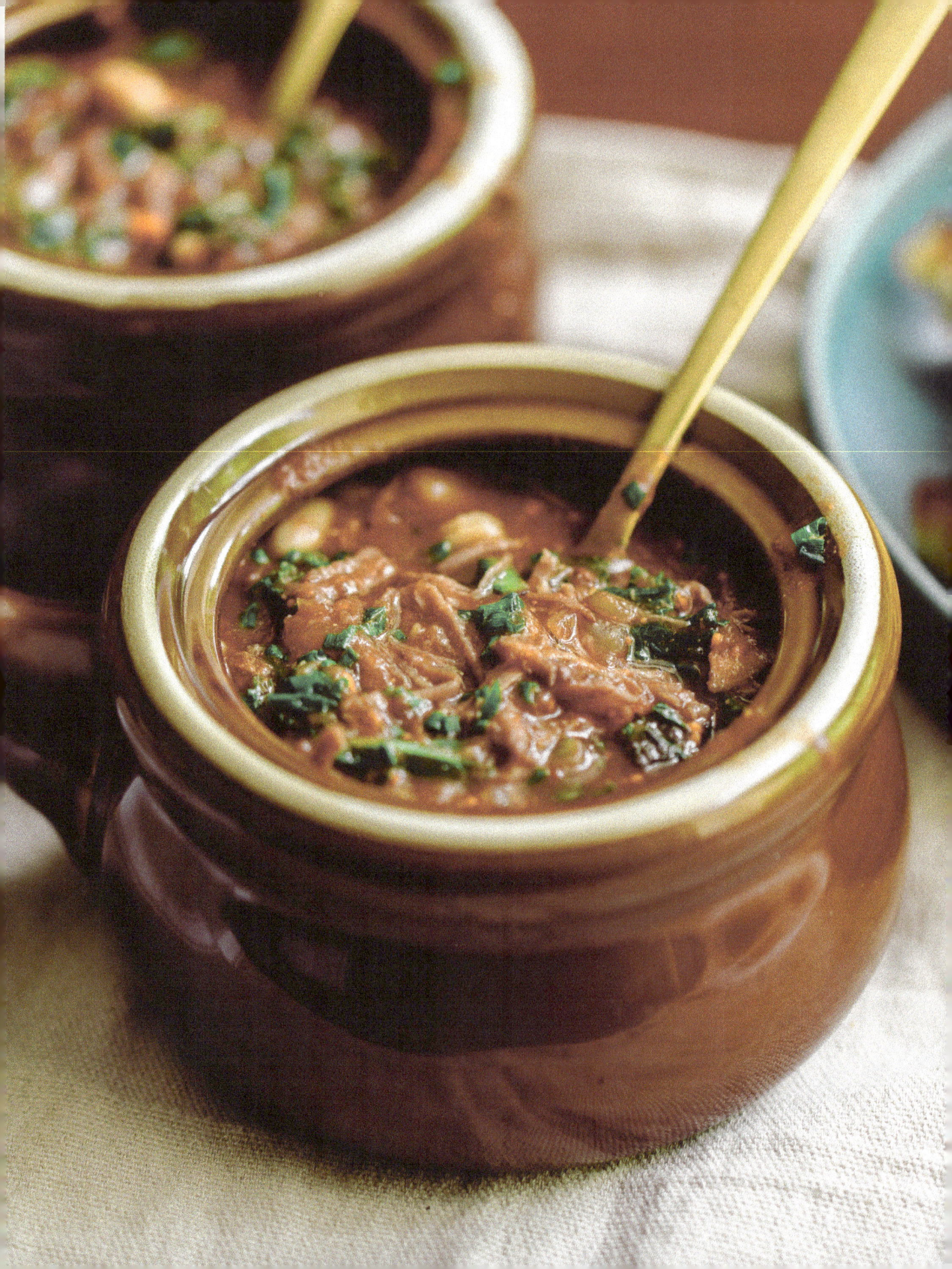

Short Rib and White Bean Stew

YIELD: 4—6 SERVINGS

INGREDIENTS

2 pounds bone-in beef short ribs, preferably local

1 tablespoon ghee or high-heat oil for searing (such as avocado oil)

2 large shallots, peeled and diced

2 stalks celery, diced

3 cloves garlic, peeled and minced

2 tablespoons tomato paste

1 (14.5 oz) can crushed tomatoes

½ tablespoon fresh thyme, chopped

2 teaspoons fresh sage, chopped

1 bay leaf

3 cups stock such as beef or chicken, preferably homemade (page 86), or non-MSG stock

1 (15.5 oz) can cannellini beans, drained and rinsed

3 cups chopped kale, or one small bunch, such as lacinato, stemmed and chopped

Kosher salt and freshly ground pepper

INSTRUCTIONS

1. Pat the short ribs dry with a paper towel and season with salt and pepper.

2. Heat a little oil in a large skillet or Dutch oven. Once the oil is very hot, add the short ribs, making sure they are spread out and not touching. Sear the short ribs on all sides. This might have to be done in batches.

3. Place the short ribs in an Instant Pot or other pressure cooker.

4. In the same skillet or Dutch oven add a small amount of oil, if needed, and sauté the shallots. Stir and cook until they begin to soften then add celery and garlic along with some salt and pepper.

5. Cook another couple of minutes and add the tomato paste. Stir to coat the vegetables. Continue to cook a few minutes, stirring so the tomato paste doesn't burn on the bottom of the pan.

6. Add the tomatoes, scraping any bits off the bottom of the pan. Turn off heat.

7. Add the tomato mixture along with the herbs, bay leaf, stock, beans, and kale to the Instant Pot.

8. Stir and add some salt and pepper. Set the Instant Pot for 55 minutes. Alternatively, the stew can cook in a slow cooker for 7—8 hours on low.

9. Once done, steam naturally and remove the lid. Skim any fat off the top if necessary and remove and discard the bay leaf. Allow to cool for a few minutes and remove the short ribs. When they are cool enough to handle, take the meat off the bones and shred, discarding any fat. The bones can be saved for future stock.

10. Add the meat back to the pot and adjust seasoning if needed.

Roasted Grape and Radicchio Salad

YIELD: 4–6 SERVINGS

INGREDIENTS

1 cup farro, uncooked

2 cups seedless red grapes or similar

Olive oil

Salt

1 small head radicchio, thinly sliced

4–6 cups arugula, iceberg, or other mixed greens

¼ cup roasted sunflower seeds

¼ cup migraine-friendly cheese, such as Boursin

Lemon Dijon Vinaigrette (page 233)*

Pomegranate seeds

INSTRUCTIONS

1. Preheat oven to 425°F.

2. While oven is preheating, cook the farro according to the package.

3. Combine grapes with a drizzle of olive oil and a pinch of salt. Toss to coat and place on a Silpat mat- or parchment-lined sheet tray. Roast for about 10–15 minutes. Remove from oven and set aside to cool.

4. Add the cooked farro, grapes, radicchio, greens, sunflower seeds, and cheese to a large bowl.

5. Season with a pinch of salt and drizzle with some vinaigrette. Toss and adjust seasoning if needed. Top with pomegranate seeds.

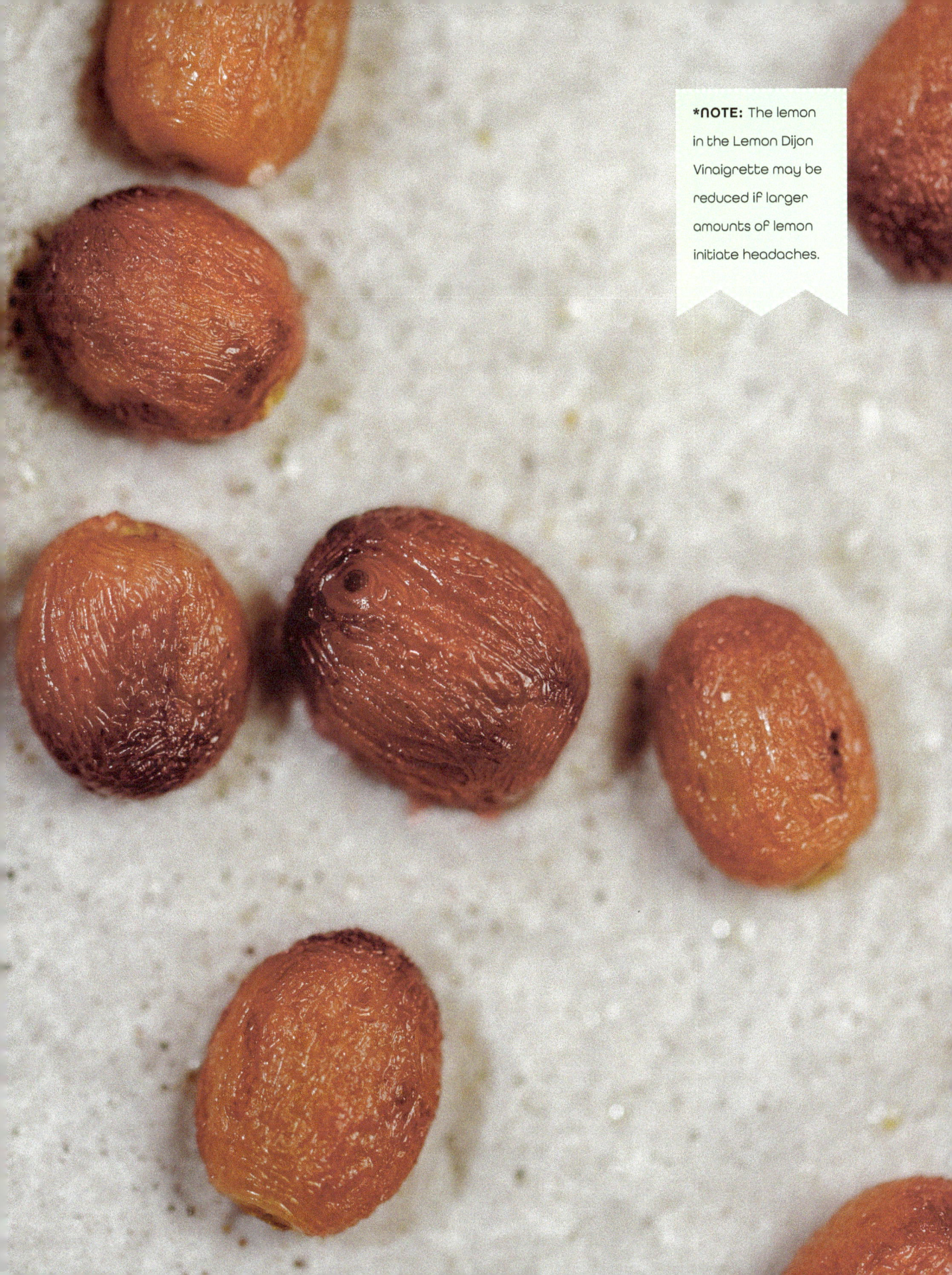

*NOTE: The lemon in the Lemon Dijon Vinaigrette may be reduced if larger amounts of lemon initiate headaches.

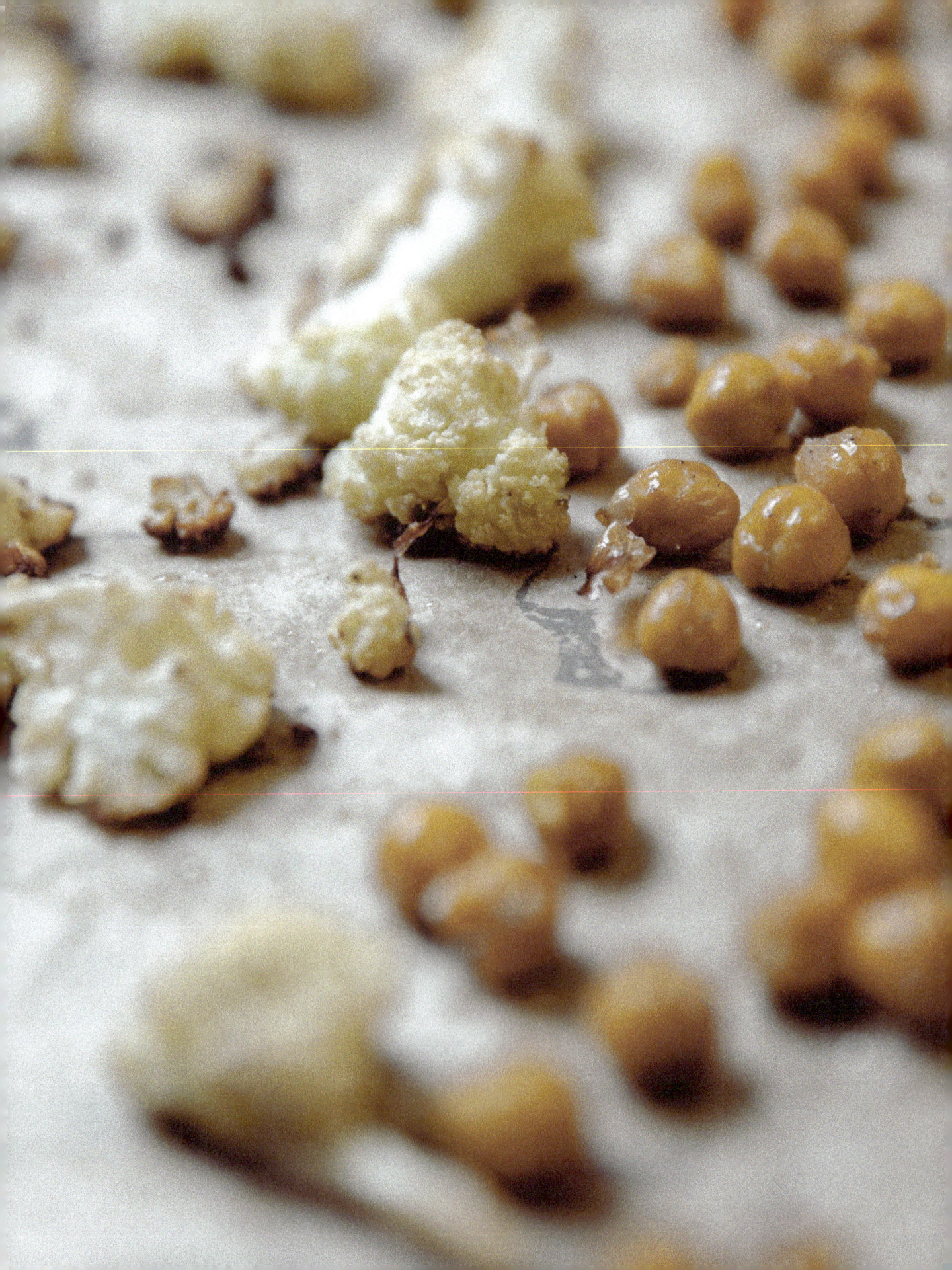

Roasted Chickpea and Cauliflower Salad

INGREDIENTS

1 small head of cauliflower, cut into small florets

1 (15 oz) can chickpeas, drained and rinsed

1 tablespoon olive oil

2–3 teaspoons of seasoning of your choice. I like to use a combination of cumin, onion granules, red pepper flakes, dry parsley, and dry chives

Salt and freshly ground pepper

6–8 ounces of mixed greens, such as spinach and arugula

½ cucumber, chopped

1 recipe Beet Tahini Dip (page 229)

Croutons (optional)

INSTRUCTIONS

1. Preheat oven to 425°F.

2. Place the cauliflower and chickpeas on separate small sheet trays and drizzle with olive oil and add seasoning (dividing evenly between each sheet) along with salt and pepper.

3. Toss to combine then spread the cauliflower and chickpeas out evenly on their own sheet trays so not many pieces are touching.

4. Bake for 20–24 minutes then check the cauliflower. It should be starting to brown in places. Remove the cauliflower and bake the chickpeas for another 5 minutes. They should be crispy when they come out. Allow them to cool slightly.

5. To assemble, add mixed greens, cucumber, roasted cauliflower, and chickpeas in a large bowl with a pinch of salt. Toss with Beet Tahini Dip and croutons.

Seasonal Quinoa and Mixed Greens Salad

This salad is a blank canvas for you to get creative and add your favorite vegetables, fruits, and dressing.

YIELD: 4–6 SERVINGS

INGREDIENTS

1 cup quinoa, uncooked

2 cups diced seasonal vegetables, such as butternut squash, beets, sweet potatoes, and/or fruit, such as apples

1 cucumber, diced

4–6 cups mixed greens, such as arugula, spinach, and baby kale

Olive oil

Kosher salt and freshly ground pepper

Dressing such as Beet Tahini (page 229) or Honey Mustard (page 234)

INSTRUCTIONS

1. Bring the quinoa to a boil with 2 cups of water and some salt in a pot. Then cover and turn down to simmer for about 15 minutes or until the quinoa is fluffy and all the water has been absorbed.

2. While the quinoa cooks, roast the vegetables (if using) with a little olive oil, salt, and pepper at 400°F until fork-tender.

3. Add the cucumber and vegetables (and/or fruit) to a large bowl.

4. Once the quinoa is done, allow it to cool then toss it with the cucumbers and vegetables/fruit.

5. Just before serving, add in the greens, some salt and pepper, and drizzle with some of the dressing.

6. Toss, check for seasoning once more and adjust if needed.

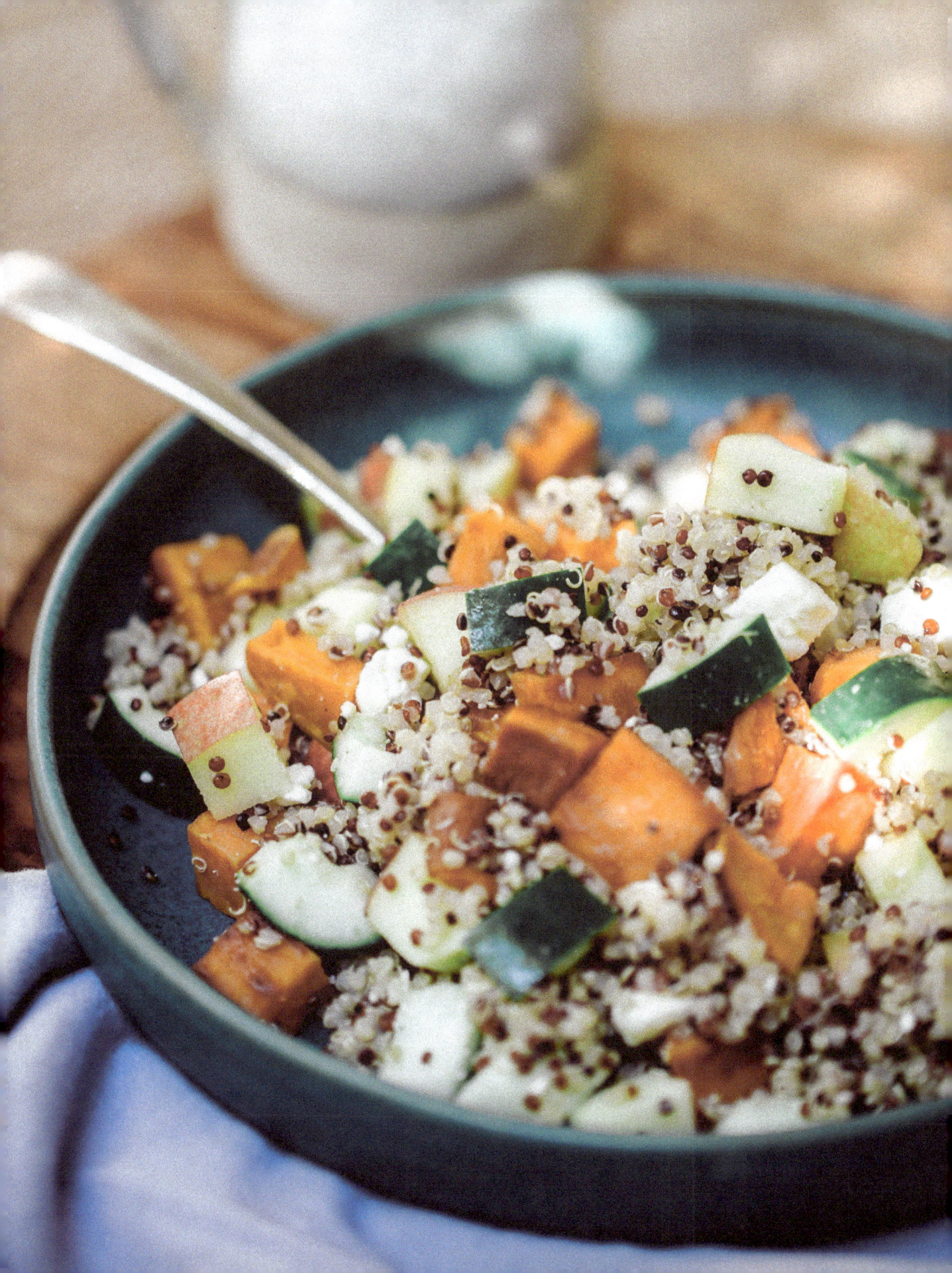

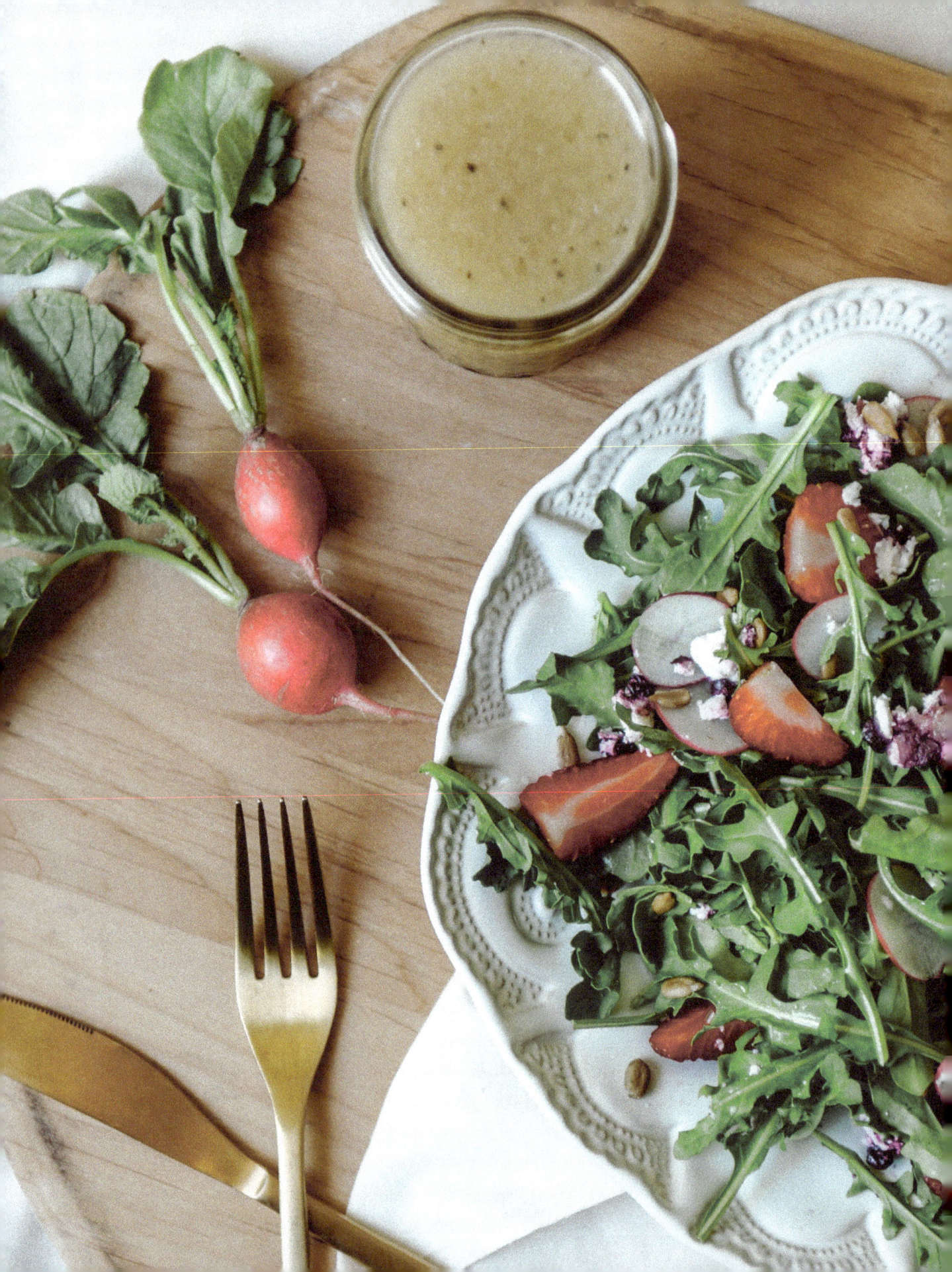

Spring Strawberry and Arugula Salad

Come springtime, we love to go strawberry picking, and every time we go, the kids run eagerly down the rows to find the largest strawberry.

YIELD: 4–6 SERVINGS

INGREDIENTS

4–6 cups arugula or mixed greens

1 cup strawberries, cored and chopped

½ cup thinly sliced radishes

Maple Chili Pumpkin Seeds (page 70)

2–3 oz goat cheese or feta (optional if they are not a trigger)

Kosher salt and freshly ground pepper

Extra virgin olive oil or dressing of choice

INSTRUCTIONS

1. Add the first 5 ingredients to a large bowl and sprinkle with a little salt and pepper.
2. Drizzle with some extra virgin olive oil or dressing of choice and toss. Best served immediately.

Chicken Salad with Grapes

There are endless recipes for chicken salad, but this simple version uses a creamy poppy seed dressing and lots of grapes. I like to serve this on a big pile of greens and drizzle with a little extra virgin olive oil.

YIELD: 4 SERVINGS

INGREDIENTS

2½ cups cooked shredded chicken (just over 1 pound of meat)

2 stalks celery, diced

1 cup red seedless grapes, cut in half or quartered if they are large

1 recipe Poppy Seed Dressing (page 235)

2 tablespoons mayonnaise

3 scallions, trimmed and sliced thin

⅓ cup parsley, chopped

¼ cup fresh dill, chopped

Kosher salt and freshly ground pepper

INSTRUCTIONS

Combine all ingredients in a large bowl. Mix well. Season to taste with salt and pepper.

> **TIP:** If walnuts are not a migraine trigger, ½ cup roasted and chopped walnuts are a great addition.

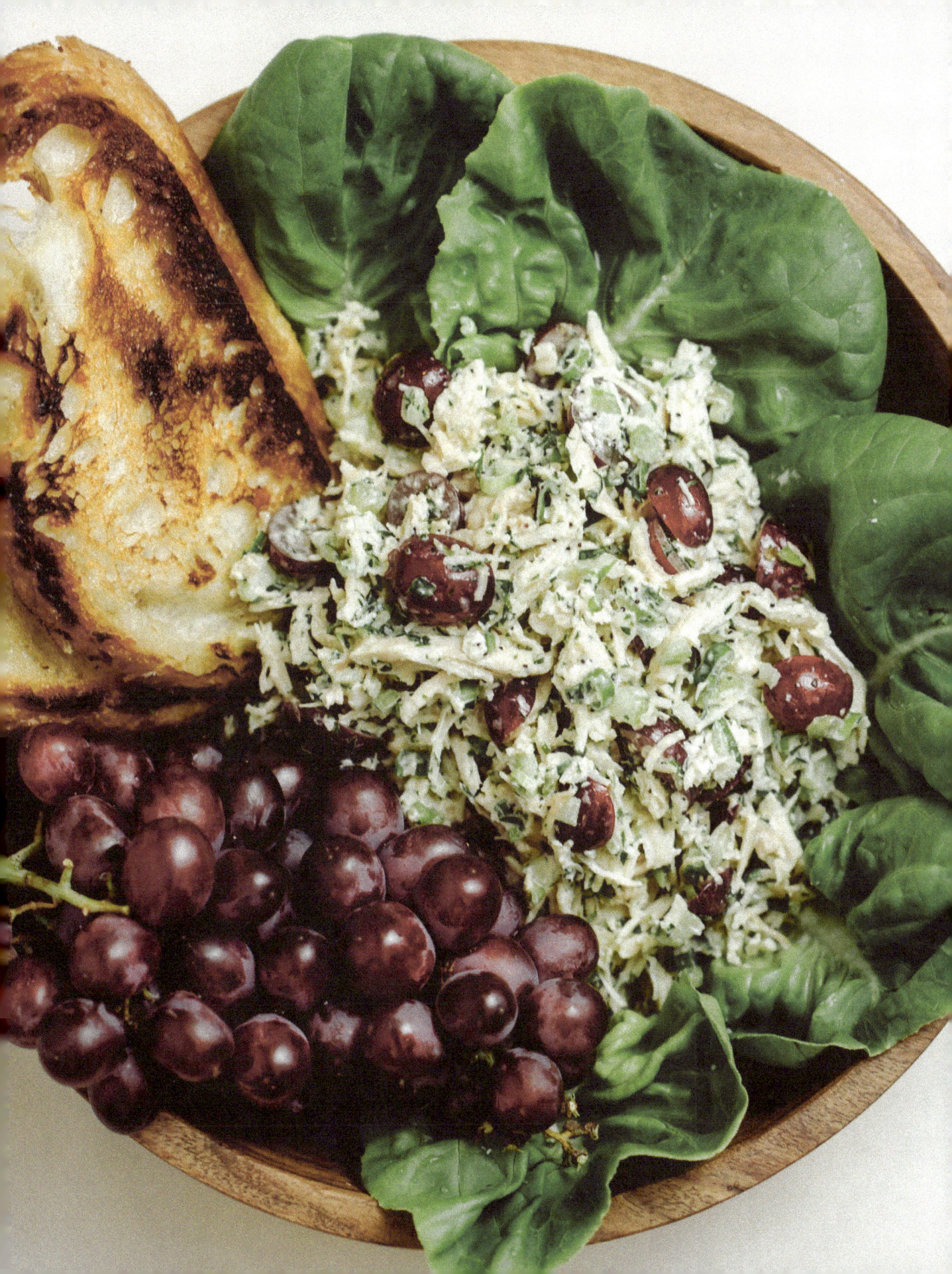

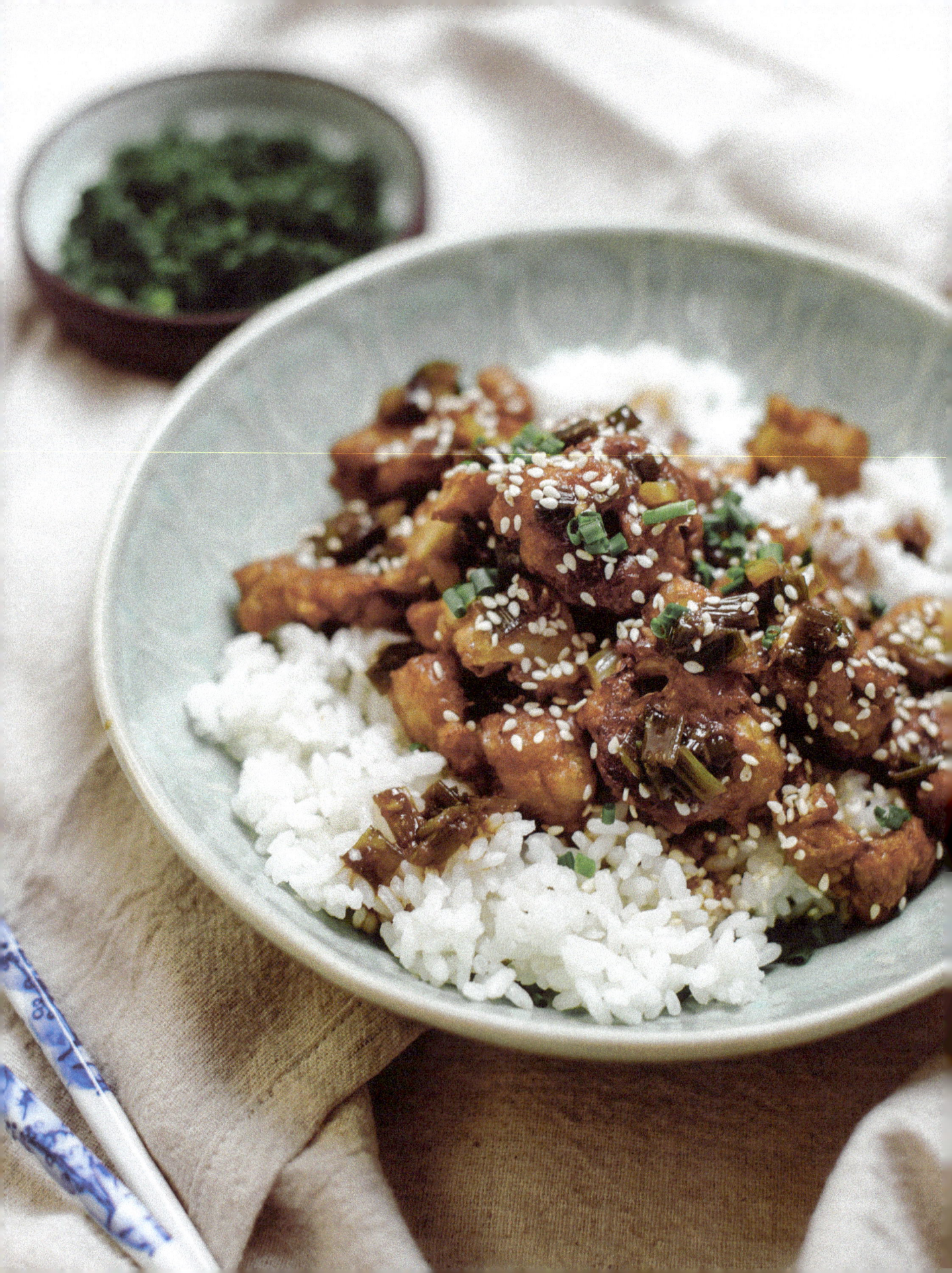

Vegetarian Mains

Banzo Balls..112

Black Bean Grain Bowl 115

General Tso's Cauliflower 116

Quinoa Taco Filling 119

Black Bean Burgers...120

Harvest Vegetable Pie 123

Cornmeal-Crusted Cauliflower Bites....................................124

Thai Vegetable Curry with Ramen..127

Banzo Balls

These are similar to falafel but with a slightly different flavor profile and baked instead of fried. I love to serve them with Instant Pot Marinara (page 224) and spaghetti squash or with Roasted Red Pepper Vodka Sauce (page 241) and pasta.

YIELD: 12–14 BALLS

INGREDIENTS

1–2 teaspoons olive oil

1 (15.5 oz) can chickpeas, drained and rinsed

2 shallots, peeled, diced small

2 garlic cloves, peeled and minced or grated

½ cup fresh basil leaves, chopped fine

2 tablespoons sun-dried tomatoes, minced

1 teaspoon dried oregano

⅓ cup breadcrumbs or oat flour (page 13)

1 egg

½ teaspoon kosher salt and freshly ground pepper

INSTRUCTIONS

1. Preheat oven to 400°F and line a baking sheet with parchment paper. Drizzle the olive oil on the parchment and smear a little with your fingers to cover most of the parchment.

2. Add the chickpeas to a large bowl and mash with a potato masher or fork until about halfway mashed.

3. Add the rest of the ingredients to the bowl and stir to combine.

4. Form the mixture into 12–14 balls and place on the baking sheet.

5. Bake for 22–28 minutes or until they are golden-brown.

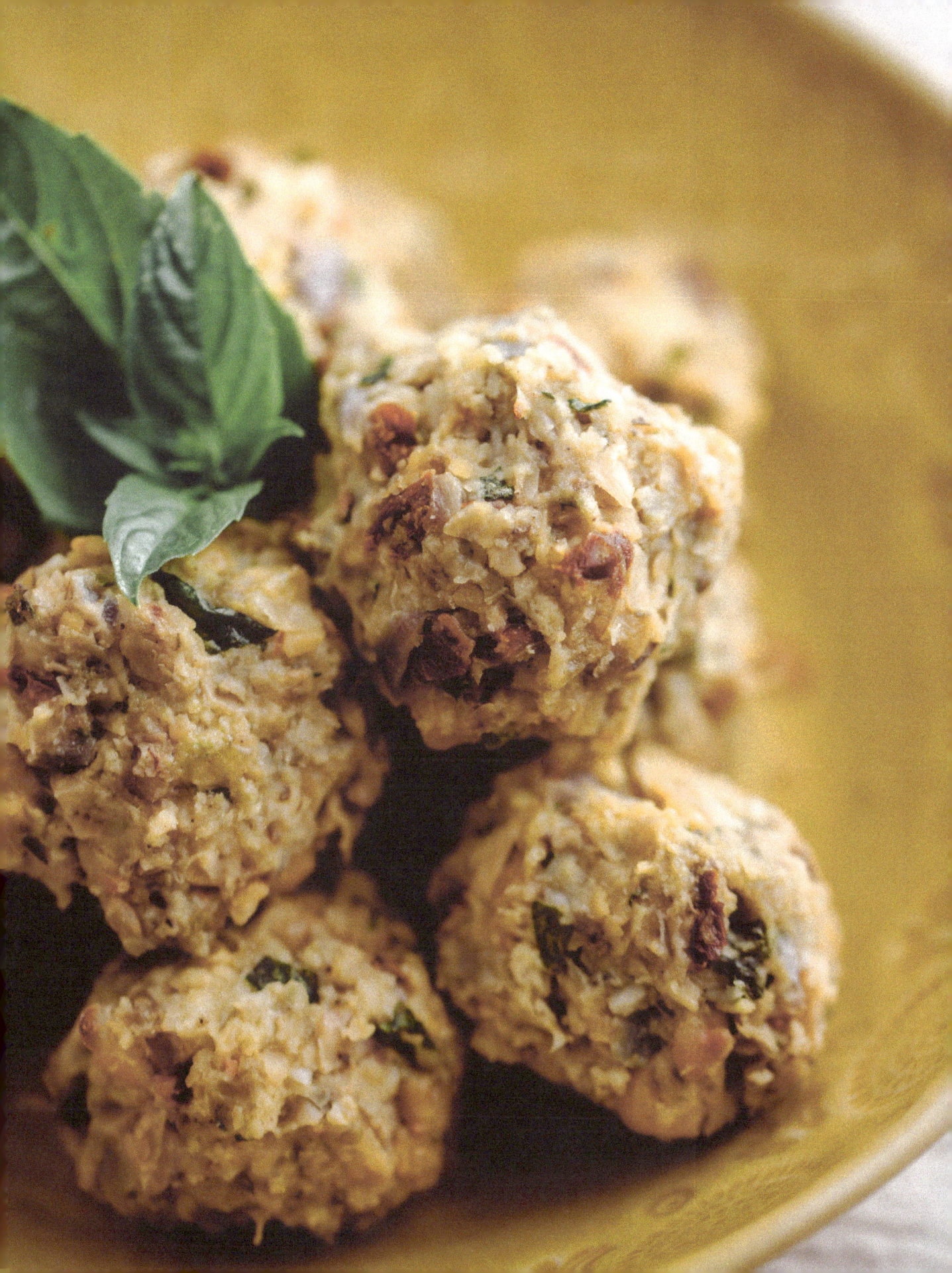

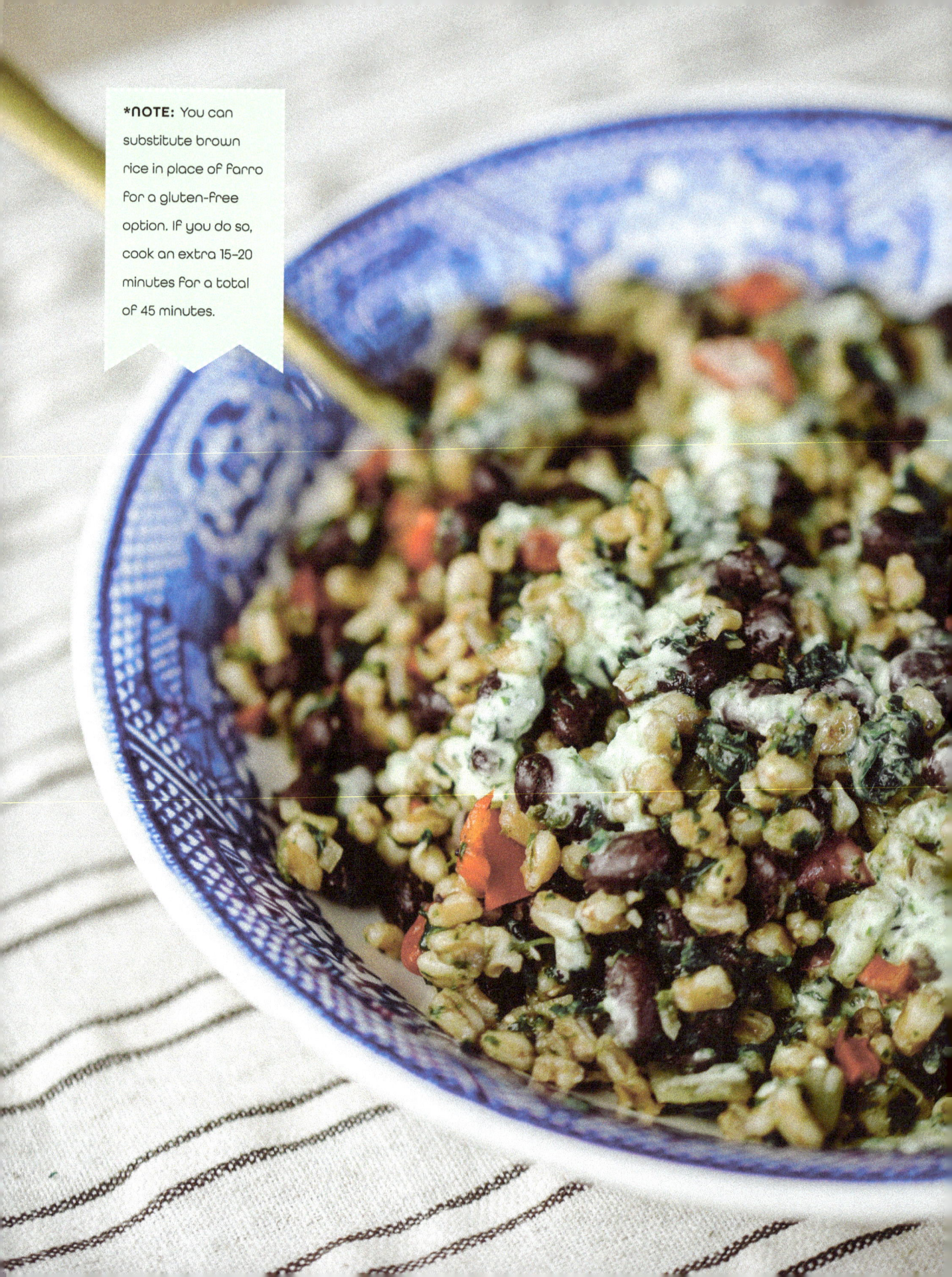

*NOTE: You can substitute brown rice in place of farro for a gluten-free option. If you do so, cook an extra 15–20 minutes for a total of 45 minutes.

Black Bean Grain Bowl

This bowl is a quick and easy meal for breakfast, lunch, or dinner. For even faster prep you can use prechopped kale from the freezer section.

YIELD: 4–6 SERVINGS

INGREDIENTS

1 cup farro (or brown rice*)

1 tablespoon olive oil

2 shallots, peeled and diced

1 bell pepper, seeded and diced

3 garlic cloves, peeled and minced or grated

2 cups finely chopped kale

2 (15 oz) cans black beans, drained and rinsed

2 tablespoons "everything bagel" seasoning

1 recipe Cilantro Lime Aioli (page 238)

Cherry tomatoes, halved, for topping (optional if they aren't a trigger)

Salt and freshly ground pepper

INSTRUCTIONS

1. Cook the farro by bringing 2¼ cups water to a boil. Add in the farro and simmer, covered, for 20–25 minutes. When done, the farro should be tender and chewy. Note that if you are using whole farro, you might need to increase the cooking time to 30 minutes. Drain off any excess liquid left in the pot after the farro has cooked.

2. Make the cilantro aioli and set aside.

3. Heat the olive oil over medium-high heat in a large skillet. Once the oil is hot, add the shallots and stir to coat.

4. Once the shallots start to soften slightly add in the bell pepper, garlic, and a large pinch of salt and some pepper. Continue cooking for another few minutes.

5. Add the kale and cook for a few more minutes until it has wilted.

6. Add the black beans and everything bagel seasoning.

7. Turn off heat. Fold in the farro (or rice) and adjust seasoning if needed.

8. Drizzle the cilantro lime aioli over and top with halved cherry tomatoes if not a trigger and serve.

General Tso's Cauliflower

We usually make this in place of take-out Chinese on a Friday night. While this recipe also works with chicken, we prefer to use cauliflower florets for a vegetarian option.

INGREDIENTS

Batter

½ cup all-purpose or gluten-free flour

⅓ cup arrowroot or cornstarch

¾ teaspoon baking powder

1½ teaspoons kosher salt

2 eggs

3 tablespoons coconut aminos

½ tablespoon distilled white vinegar

Cauliflower and Sauce

1 medium head cauliflower, cut into florets (about 1 pound)

High-heat oil for frying, such as avocado oil

1 bunch scallions, trimmed and thinly sliced

3 cloves garlic, peeled and minced or grated

1 recipe Ginger Glaze, mixed and uncooked (page 233)

½–1 teaspoon red pepper flakes (optional)

Rice to serve, such as sushi rice

Sesame seeds to garnish

INSTRUCTIONS

1. Line a sheet tray with a wire rack and set aside.
2. For the batter, combine the first 4 dry ingredients and whisk. Then add the eggs, coconut aminos, and vinegar. Stir with a spatula until the batter is smooth.
3. Add the cauliflower to the batter and toss to coat.
4. Heat the oil in a medium-sized sauté pan or wok until it reaches 350°F. You want the oil to cover the bottom and barely start to come up the sides of the pan.
5. Add the cauliflower in batches, making sure not to crowd the pan too much.
6. Flip the cauliflower over once brown on one side. Cook until the other side is brown and remove from pan.
7. Rest cauliflower on wire rack to cool. Repeat with remaining cauliflower.
8. After all cauliflower is cooked, discard almost all the oil, leaving 1 tablespoon in the pan.
9. Heat over medium-high then add the scallions. Cook a minute or so then add the garlic and cook another minute until fragrant.
10. Add the Ginger Glaze to the pan. Over medium heat, allow the sauce to thicken for a few minutes.
11. Add in the red pepper flakes if using and turn off heat. Adjust seasoning if needed. You can add ¼–½ cup water or stock to thin out the sauce a bit if needed.
12. To serve, add the cauliflower to the sauce and coat. Serve over rice and top with sesame seeds.

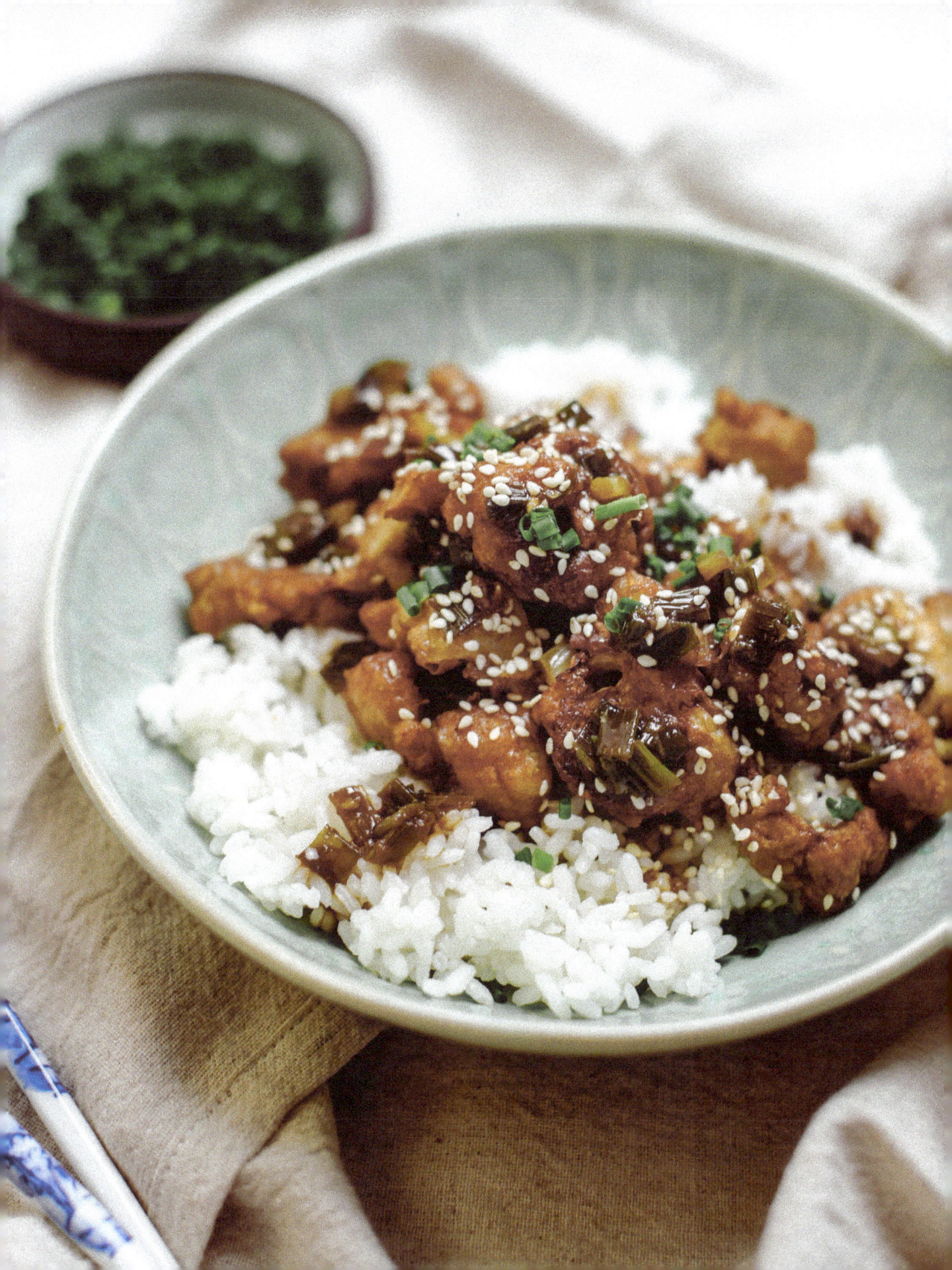

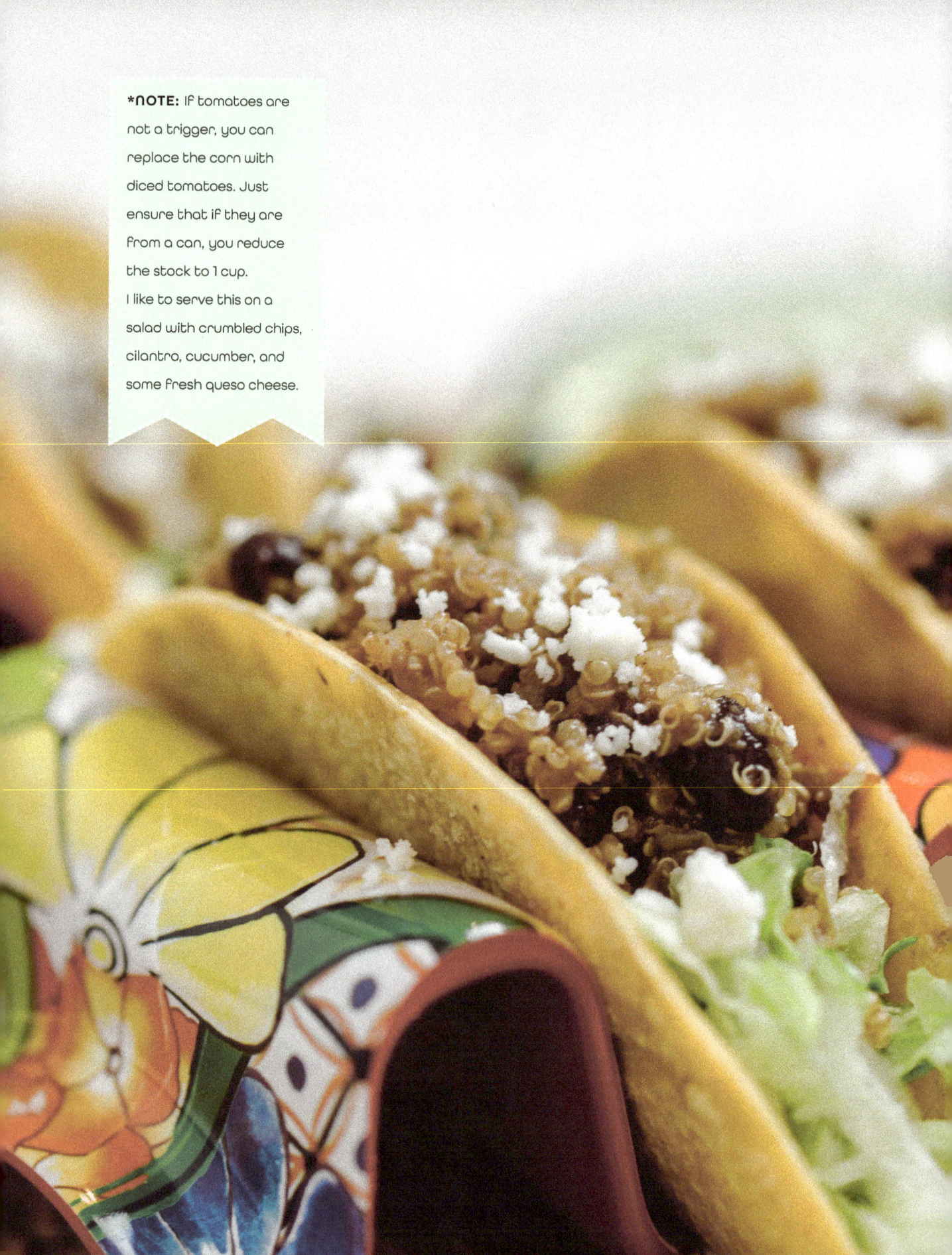

*NOTE: If tomatoes are not a trigger, you can replace the corn with diced tomatoes. Just ensure that if they are from a can, you reduce the stock to 1 cup.
I like to serve this on a salad with crumbled chips, cilantro, cucumber, and some fresh queso cheese.

Quinoa Taco Filling

On trips back home from culinary school, I usually cooked whatever I was learning in school for my friends and family. I will never forget my parents (who are excellent cooks) pulling out the bag of quinoa that I bought, looking at it and saying, "What is Qu-no?"

INGREDIENTS

2 teaspoons olive oil

1 large shallot, peeled and diced

½ bell pepper, seeded and diced

3 garlic cloves, peeled and minced or grated

¾ cup quinoa, uncooked

1¼ cups vegetable stock, preferably homemade (page 84), or other non-MSG stock or water

1 (4 oz) can diced green chilies

1 cup corn kernels*

1 (15.5 oz) can black beans or pinto beans, drained and rinsed

1 tablespoon plus 1 teaspoon Taco Seasoning (page 239)

1 teaspoon nutritional yeast (optional if not a trigger)

Kosher salt and freshly ground pepper

For serving: Bibb lettuce and taco shells or shredded lettuce for a taco salad

INSTRUCTIONS

1. Heat a medium-sized pot, fitted with a lid, over medium heat.

2. Drizzle a little olive oil in the pot and when the oil is hot add the shallot and stir. When the shallot begins to soften, add in the bell pepper. Cook for a few minutes then add in the garlic and stir until it becomes fragrant, about 1 minute.

3. Add the quinoa, stock or water, chilies, corn, beans, taco seasoning, nutritional yeast (if not a trigger), 2 large pinches of salt, and some pepper.

4. Stir to combine and bring to a boil. Once at a boil, cover with a lid and turn down to a simmer.

5. Cook for about 25–30 minutes or until the quinoa is cooked and there is no more liquid in the pot. If there is some liquid left in the pot, you can remove the lid for a few minutes at the end.

Black Bean Burgers

These are one of our go-to weeknight dinners that the entire family enjoys. You can serve them as a traditional burger or crumble them over a salad and drizzle with Herby Aioli (page 238).

YIELD: 4 BURGERS

INGREDIENTS

2 shallots, peeled

1 carrot

2 garlic cloves, peeled

Olive oil

1 (15.5 oz) can black beans, drained and rinsed

½ teaspoon ground cumin

½ teaspoon garlic granules

½ teaspoon paprika

½ teaspoon kosher salt

¼ cup breadcrumbs or oat flour (page 13)

1 egg

Freshly ground black pepper

Hamburger buns

Toppings of choice, such as lettuce, Herby Aioli (page 238), or high-quality cheese

INSTRUCTIONS

1. Preheat oven to 375°F.
2. Rough-chop the shallots and carrot. Add the shallots, carrot, and garlic to a food processor and pulse until minced. If you do not have a food processor, you can grate the carrot and mince the shallots and garlic.
3. Heat a little olive oil in a large, oven-safe skillet and once hot add the shallot mixture. Cook for a few minutes until softened, stirring occasionally.
4. Add the cumin, garlic granules, and paprika. Stir to combine and turn off heat.
5. Pulse the black beans in the same food processor until about half are mashed, or you can mash them in a large bowl by hand.
6. Combine the beans, shallot mixture, salt, breadcrumbs (or oat flour), egg, and some pepper in a large bowl and mix. Shape into 4 equal-sized patties.
7. In a clean pan over medium heat, add a little more olive oil. Once the oil is hot, sear the patties on one side for a few minutes until they start to brown. Flip and do the same on the other side.
8. Finish in the oven for about 10–15 minutes. Allow to cool slightly then serve on buns with toppings of choice.

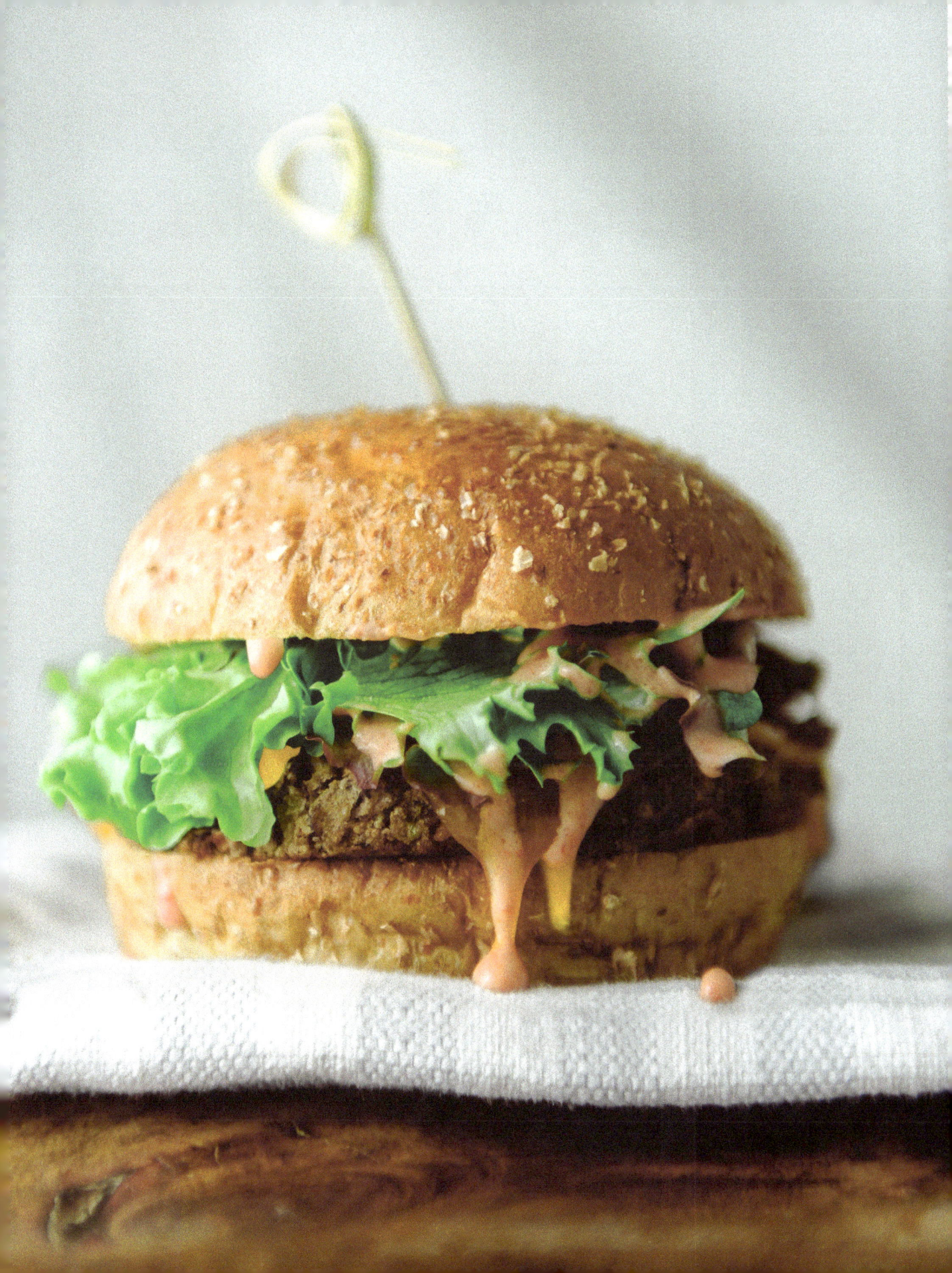

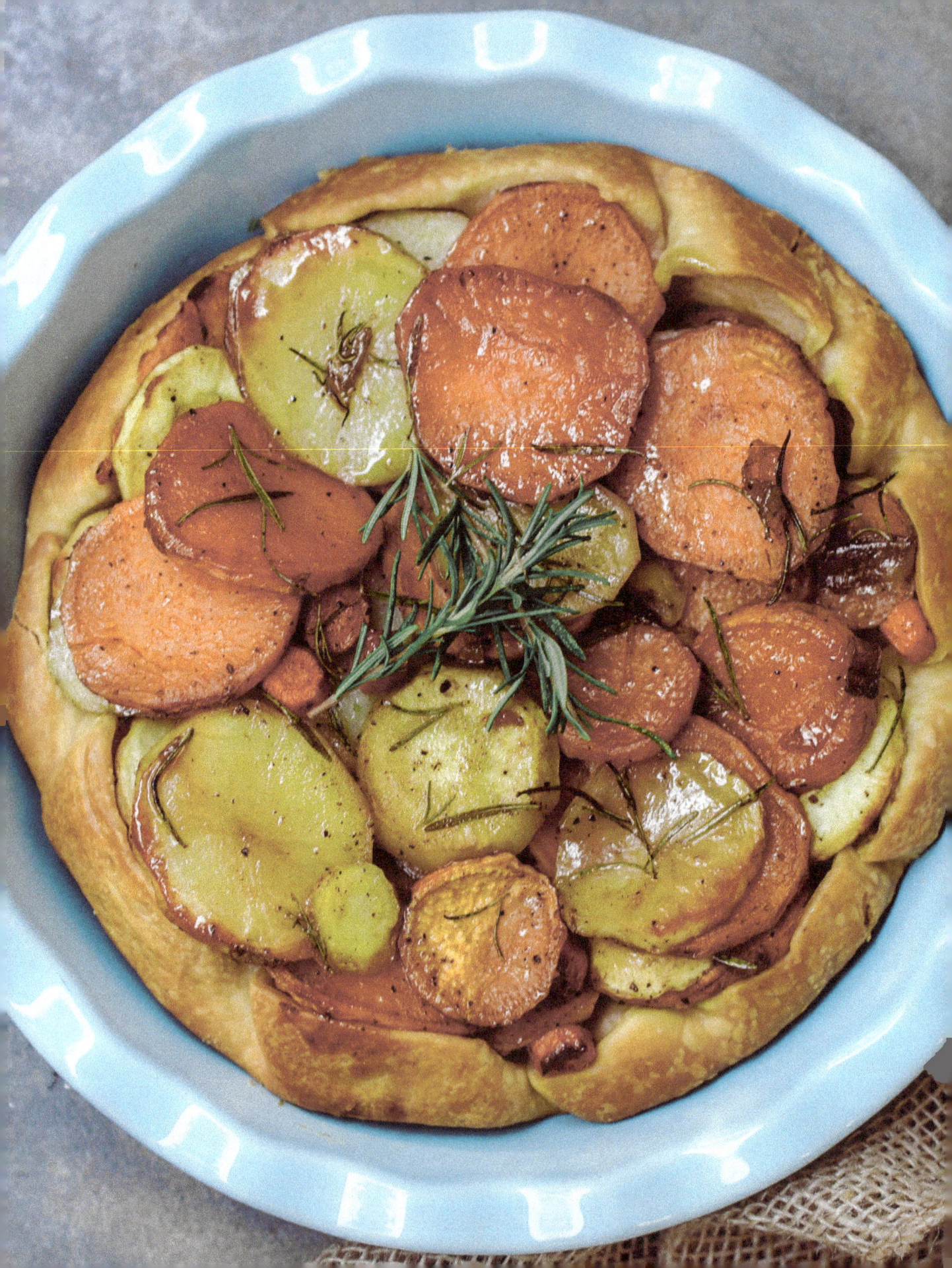

Harvest Vegetable Pie

This scrumptious inverted pie filled with caramelized root vegetables and flaky pie crust is my idea of vegetarian comfort food. Whether it's for a Thanksgiving feast or a chilly winter evening, you can't go wrong with this savory take on a classic.

YIELD: 8 SERVINGS

INGREDIENTS

1 Go-To Pie Crust recipe (page 260)

1 sweet potato

1 Yukon Gold potato

1 parsnip

2 carrots

1 shallot, peeled and sliced thin

2 tablespoons olive oil

Salt and freshly ground black pepper

2 tablespoons maple syrup

10 sage leaves

2 rosemary sprigs

3 oz Boursin cheese or goat cheese if not a trigger

INSTRUCTIONS

1. Preheat oven to 450°F.
2. Make the pie crust if you have not already, but don't roll out yet. Keep refrigerated until ready to use.
3. Peel the potatoes and parsnip and cut into ¼-inch slices along with the carrots.
4. Add the vegetables in a large bowl along with the shallot, olive oil, 1 teaspoon salt, and some pepper. Gently mix.
5. Add the vegetables to a parchment- or Silpat mat-lined sheet tray and spread into one layer. Bake for 20–25 minutes until almost fork-tender.
6. In a pie dish drizzle the syrup on the bottom and evenly distribute the sage and rosemary.
7. Once the vegetables are done, remove them from the oven.
8. Top the herbs with the cooked vegetables in a few layers then dollop the cheese if using on top.
9. Roll out the pie crust on a lightly floured surface and place it gently on top of the vegetables, being sure to tuck the edges into the inside of the dish.
10. Bake at 450°F for 15 minutes then lower the temperature to 375°F and continue baking until pie crust is golden brown, about 20–25 minutes. Remove and allow to cool for a few minutes before carefully inverting the pie into another pie dish so the crust is on the bottom.

Cornmeal-Crusted Cauliflower Bites

These are great served with Herby Aioli (page 238) for dipping or enjoyed in a vegetarian taco.

(page 238)

YIELD: 4–6 SERVINGS

INGREDIENTS

1 heaping tablespoon sunflower seed butter

½ tablespoon coconut aminos*

1 tablespoon honey

1 tablespoon olive oil or coconut oil, melted

1 head cauliflower, cut into small florets (about 12 oz total)

½ cup cornmeal

½ cup panko breadcrumbs

1 teaspoon ground cumin

½ teaspoon regular or smoked paprika

½ teaspoon chili powder

1 teaspoon garlic granules

1 teaspoon kosher salt

Freshly ground pepper

INSTRUCTIONS

1. Preheat oven to 400°F on convection. Line a baking tray with a Silpat mat or parchment paper.
2. In a large bowl combine the sunflower seed butter, coconut aminos, honey, and oil. Stir to combine.
3. Add the cauliflower and stir to coat evenly.
4. In a separate bowl combine the cornmeal, panko, spices, salt, and pepper. Stir to combine.
5. Add the cauliflower to the bowl with the dry ingredients and gently toss until there are hardly any crumbs at the bottom of the bowl.
6. Spread onto the baking tray. Bake for 20–25 minutes, flipping over halfway through, until the cauliflower is golden-brown. Remove from oven and allow to cool slightly.

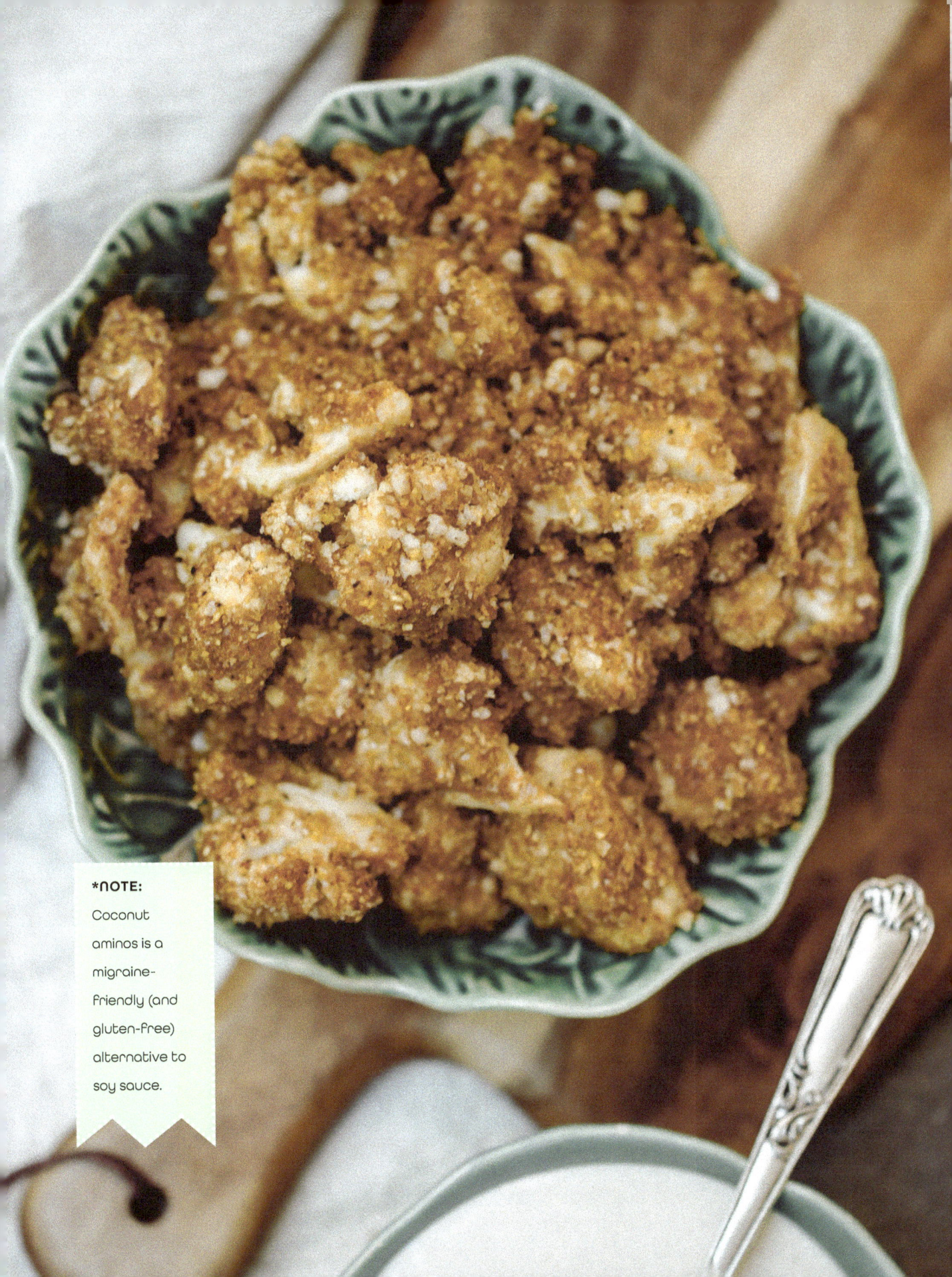

*NOTE:
Coconut aminos is a migraine-friendly (and gluten-free) alternative to soy sauce.

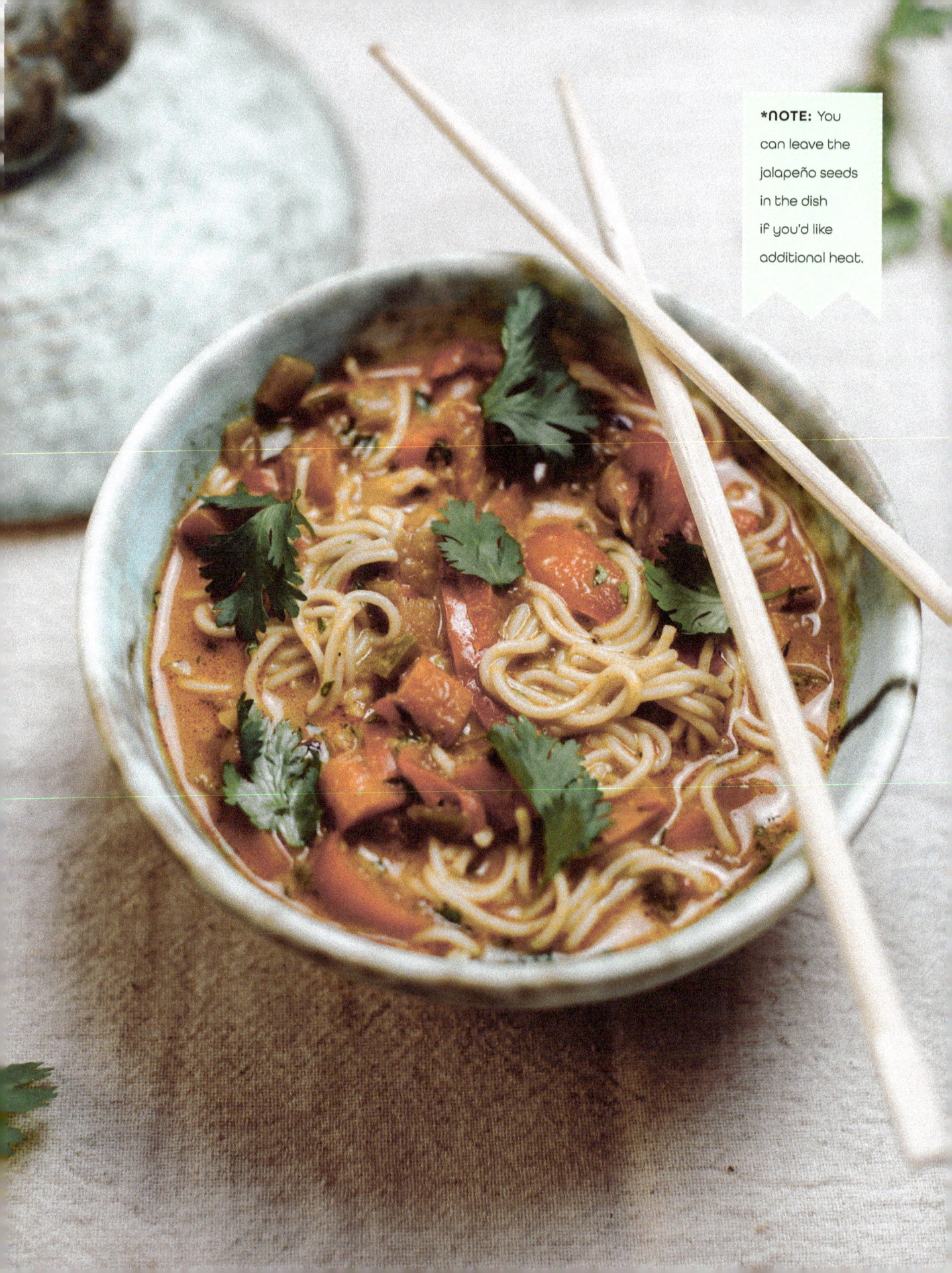

*NOTE: You can leave the jalapeño seeds in the dish if you'd like additional heat.

Thai Vegetable Curry with Ramen

"Globally beloved but difficult to define, curry is a testament to the creativity and resilience of the human spirit, drawing its spices and aromatics from a worldwide pantry." —Mari Uyehara, *Food & Wine*

YIELD: 4 SERVINGS

INGREDIENTS

1 tablespoon sesame oil or olive oil

2 shallots, peeled and diced

3 carrots, diced

1 bell pepper, stem and seeds removed, thinly sliced

1 jalapeño, stem and seeds removed, minced*

Salt

3 cloves garlic, peeled and grated or minced

2 tablespoons Thai red curry paste

1 (15 oz) can coconut milk, full fat

2 cups vegetable stock, preferably homemade (page 84), or non-MSG stock

2 teaspoons coconut sugar

1 tablespoon coconut aminos

2 teaspoons curry powder

1 (8 oz) package ramen noodles cooked according to package and rinsed with cold water

½ cup cilantro, chopped

Juice of ½ lime

INSTRUCTIONS

1. In a wok or large skillet heat a little oil over medium-high heat. Once hot, add shallots and cook for a couple of minutes.
2. Add the carrots, bell pepper, and jalapeño. Cook for a few minutes, stirring occasionally.
3. Add the garlic and a large pinch of salt. Cook another minute until the garlic is fragrant then add the curry paste. Mix to coat all the vegetables.
4. Add the coconut milk, stock, coconut sugar, coconut aminos, and curry powder. Bring to a boil, then turn down to a simmer for 20–25 minutes uncovered or until the vegetables are tender.
5. Turn off heat and add the cilantro and lime juice. Adjust seasoning if needed.
6. To serve, divide the cooked ramen among bowls and ladle the curry over top.

TIP: You can swap ramen noodles for rice noodles or rice to make this dish gluten-free.

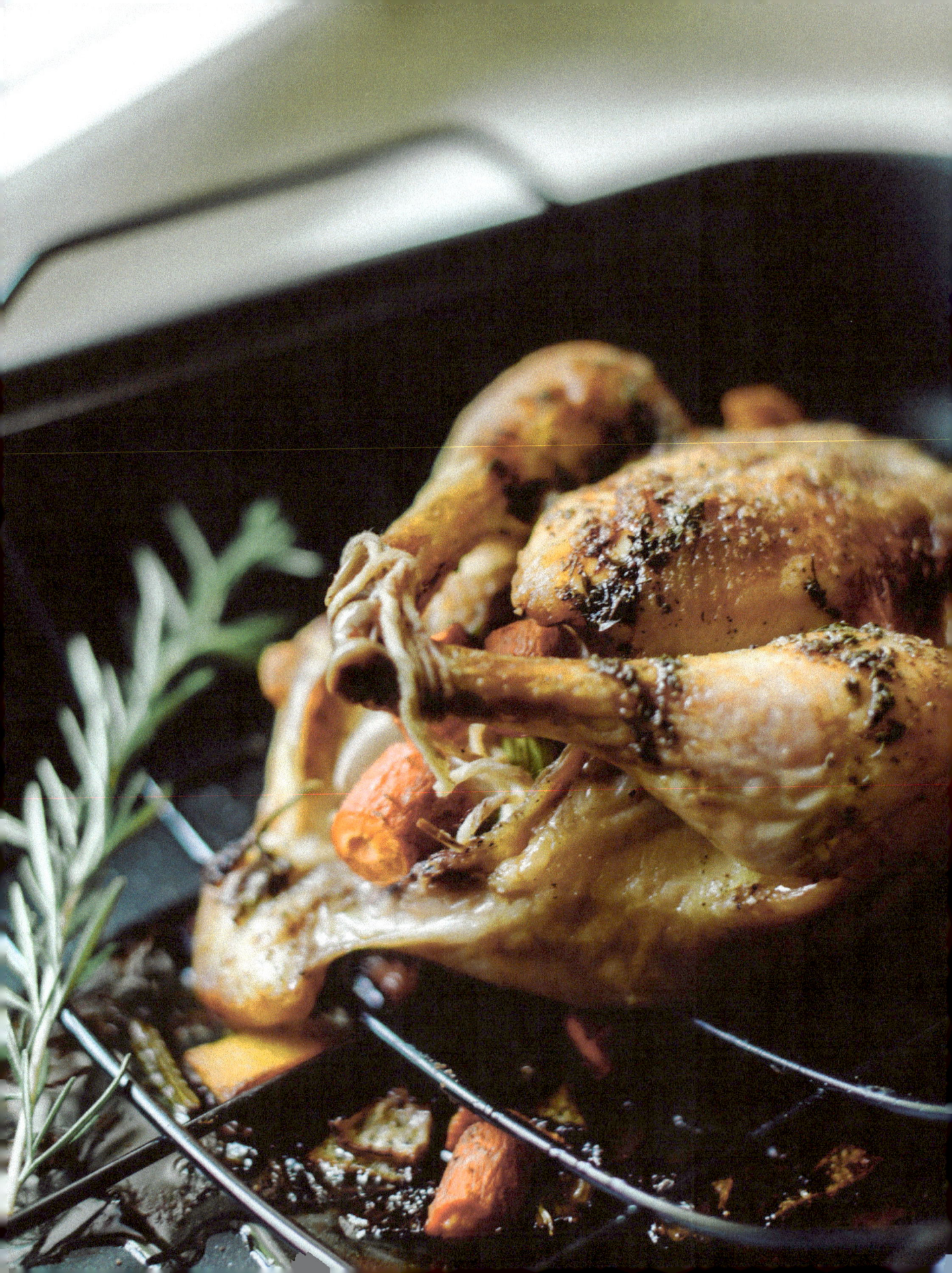

Meaty Mains

Stir-Fried Udon 130

Grown-Up Creamy Pasta Skillet 133

Chicken Lettuce Wraps 134

Mama's Chicken and Wild Rice Casserole 136

Chicken Empanadas with Zucchini and Corn 138

Classic Italian Beef Meatballs 141

Herby Turkey Meatballs 142

Chicken Sweet Potato Meatballs 145

Ginger Chicken with Lemongrass 146

Mediterranean Turkey Burgers 149

Delicious Roasted Chicken with Herb Butter 150

Quick Moo Shu Bowl 153

Sausage and Apple Stuffed Acorn Squash 154

Southwestern Stuffed Bell Peppers 157

Fully Loaded Sweet Potatoes 158

Shredded Taco Chicken 161

Pork Dumplings 162

Stir-Fried Udon

I have always been a big fan of all types of noodles, and udon noodles are no exception. They are a Japanese noodle made from wheat flour, which can be added to a stir fry or soup. There are brown rice udon noodles out there for those who can't eat gluten.

YIELD: 4 SERVINGS

INGREDIENTS

12 ounces udon noodles

1 recipe Thai "Peanut" Sauce (page 243)

1 teaspoon toasted sesame oil

1 pound grass-fed ground beef, can substitute ground turkey or pork, preferably local

Salt

1 (10–12 oz) bag of preshredded cabbage

1 bunch scallions, trimmed and sliced

½ teaspoon crushed red pepper flakes, more or less to taste

1 cup shredded carrots

2 tablespoons coconut aminos

Sesame seeds to top

INSTRUCTIONS

1. Cook noodles according to package. Rinse with cold water after draining.
2. Make the sauce if you haven't already. Toss the cooked noodles with the toasted sesame oil and set aside.
3. In a large skillet or wok add the ground meat over high heat with a large pinch of salt, breaking it apart as it cooks. Continue cooking until it's browned and crumbled.
4. Add the cabbage and cook until it begins to soften, about 5 minutes.
5. Add the sliced scallions and red pepper flakes. Cook for another minute. Then add the carrots, coconut aminos, and Thai "Peanut" Sauce.
6. Finish by adding the cooked udon noodles and turn off heat.
7. Stir and adjust seasoning if needed. Top with sesame seeds.

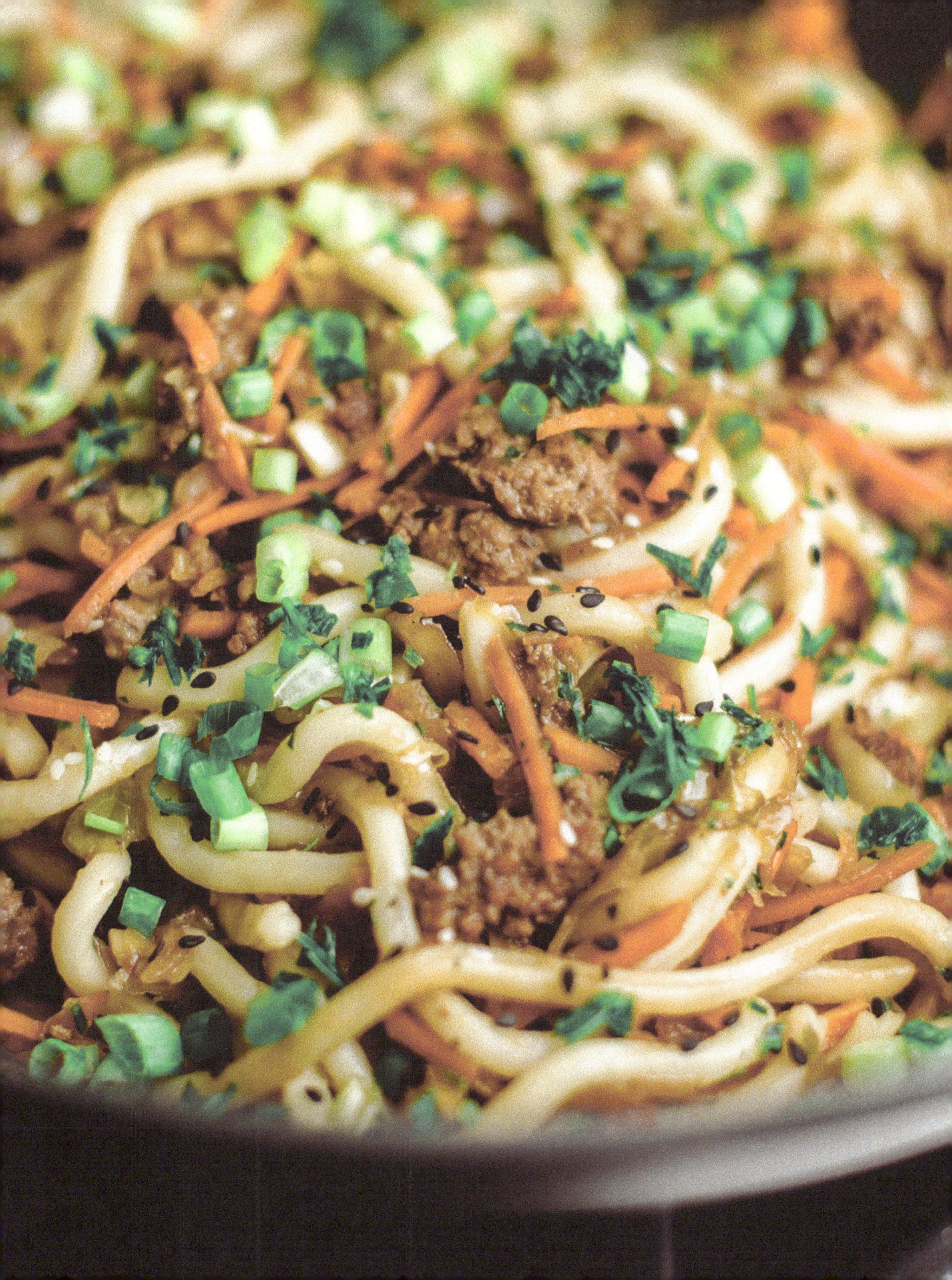

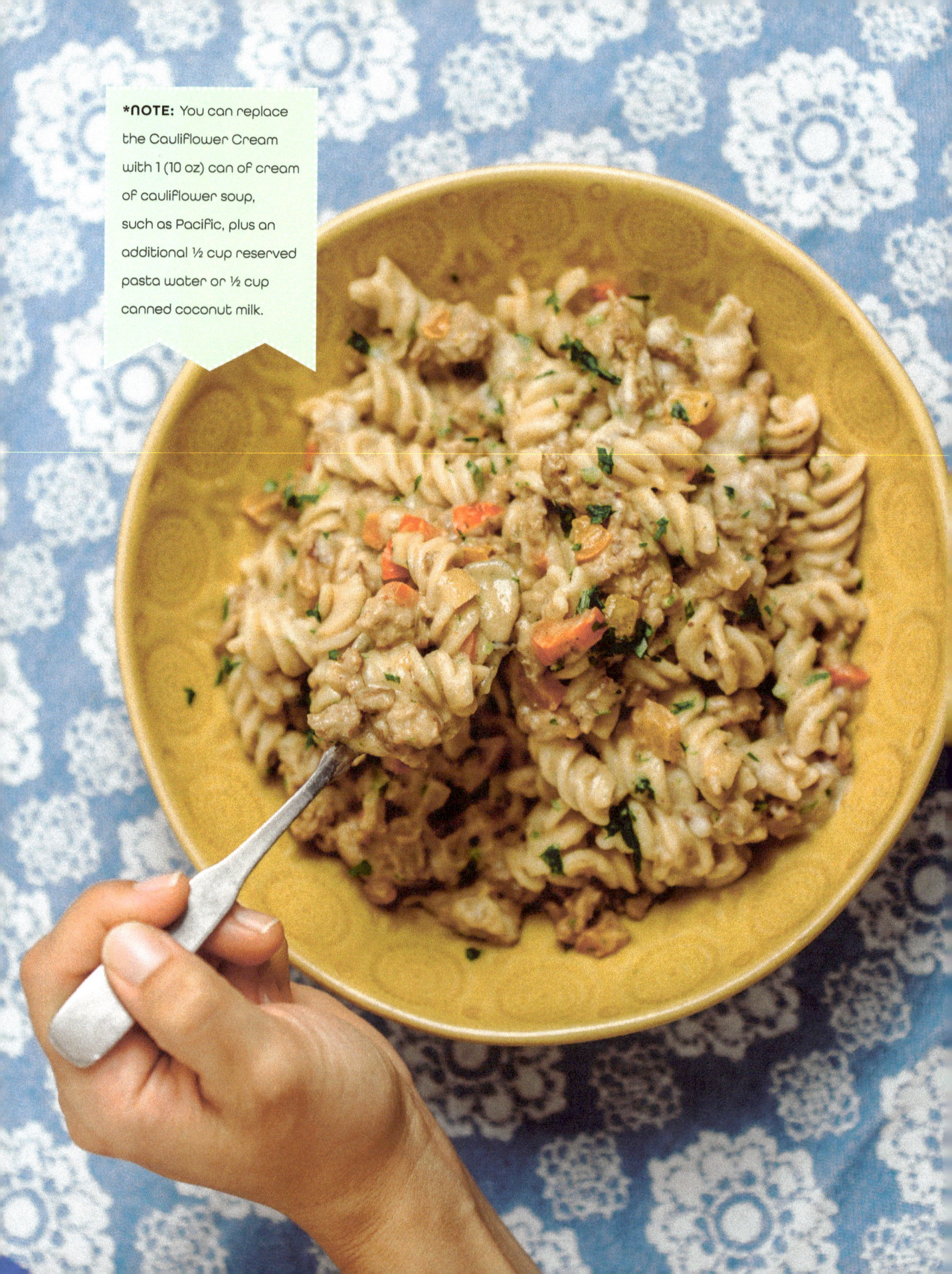

*NOTE: You can replace the Cauliflower Cream with 1 (10 oz) can of cream of cauliflower soup, such as Pacific, plus an additional ½ cup reserved pasta water or ½ cup canned coconut milk.

Grown-Up Creamy Pasta Skillet

I have loved pasta for as long as I can remember. Unfortunately for me (and my parents) I was a picky eater. When I was little and when we went out to eat, I would often order the most boring dish, noodles and butter, usually found only on the kids' menu. Thankfully, I grew out of my picky eating stage and will now try anything. And while a simple pasta dish will always remind me of my childhood, this updated version always hits the spot when I'm craving a big bowl of pasta.

YIELD: 4 SERVINGS

INGREDIENTS

12 oz dry pasta, such as fusilli (I prefer Jovial Brown Rice Pasta for a gluten-free option)

1 recipe Cauliflower Cream (page 244)*

1 tablespoon olive oil

1 pound ground turkey (dark meat preferred) or chicken, preferably local

Kosher salt and freshly ground pepper

3 shallots, peeled and diced

1 red bell pepper, seeded and diced

3 cloves garlic, peeled and minced or grated

½ teaspoon paprika

2 teaspoons chili powder

1 tablespoon coconut aminos

1 tablespoon unsalted butter

½ cup parsley, chopped fine

INSTRUCTIONS

1. Cook the pasta according to the instructions on the package. Reserve about ½ cup pasta water, then drain and rinse the pasta once it's cooked. You can also make the Cauliflower Cream at this point if you haven't already.

2. Heat the olive oil in a large skillet over medium heat. Add the meat and break apart as it cooks. Season with salt and pepper.

3. When the meat is almost cooked, add the shallots. Cook for a few minutes then add the bell pepper, garlic, and spices. Cook for a few more minutes, stirring every so often.

4. Add the Cauliflower Cream and coconut aminos. Stir until combined. Allow the mixture to thicken slightly for a few minutes.

5. Add the drained pasta, butter, parsley, and ¼ cup reserved pasta water. Turn off heat and adjust seasoning if needed. Add up to another ¼ cup pasta water to reach desired consistency.

Chicken Lettuce Wraps

Growing up my family loved ordering Chinese takeout. While it's tasty, it usually contains excess oil, MSG, and other migraine triggers. These lettuce cups are a delicious, guilt-free alternative and can be served as an appetizer or entrée.

INGREDIENTS

1 recipe Ginger Glaze (page 233), uncooked

2 tablespoons olive oil

1 pound ground chicken, preferably local

Kosher salt and freshly ground pepper

1 (8 oz) container water chestnuts in water, drained and chopped

3 garlic cloves, peeled and grated or minced

4 scallions, trimmed and sliced thin

Butter or Bibb lettuce leaves for serving

Sesame seeds to garnish and brown rice for serving (optional)

INSTRUCTIONS

1. Combine the ingredients for the Ginger Glaze if you haven't already. Set aside.

2. Heat the oil in a large skillet over high heat. Once hot, add the chicken to the pan and season with some salt and pepper. Continue cooking the chicken until it's done, breaking it apart as it cooks.

3. Once the chicken is cooked add the water chestnuts, cooking a few minutes over medium heat.

4. Add the garlic and stir. Then add the Ginger Glaze. Stir to combine and allow the mixture to thicken about 5–8 minutes. Add the scallions and turn off the heat.

5. To serve add some brown rice (if using) to the bottom of a lettuce cup then top with the chicken mixture. Garnish with sesame seeds.

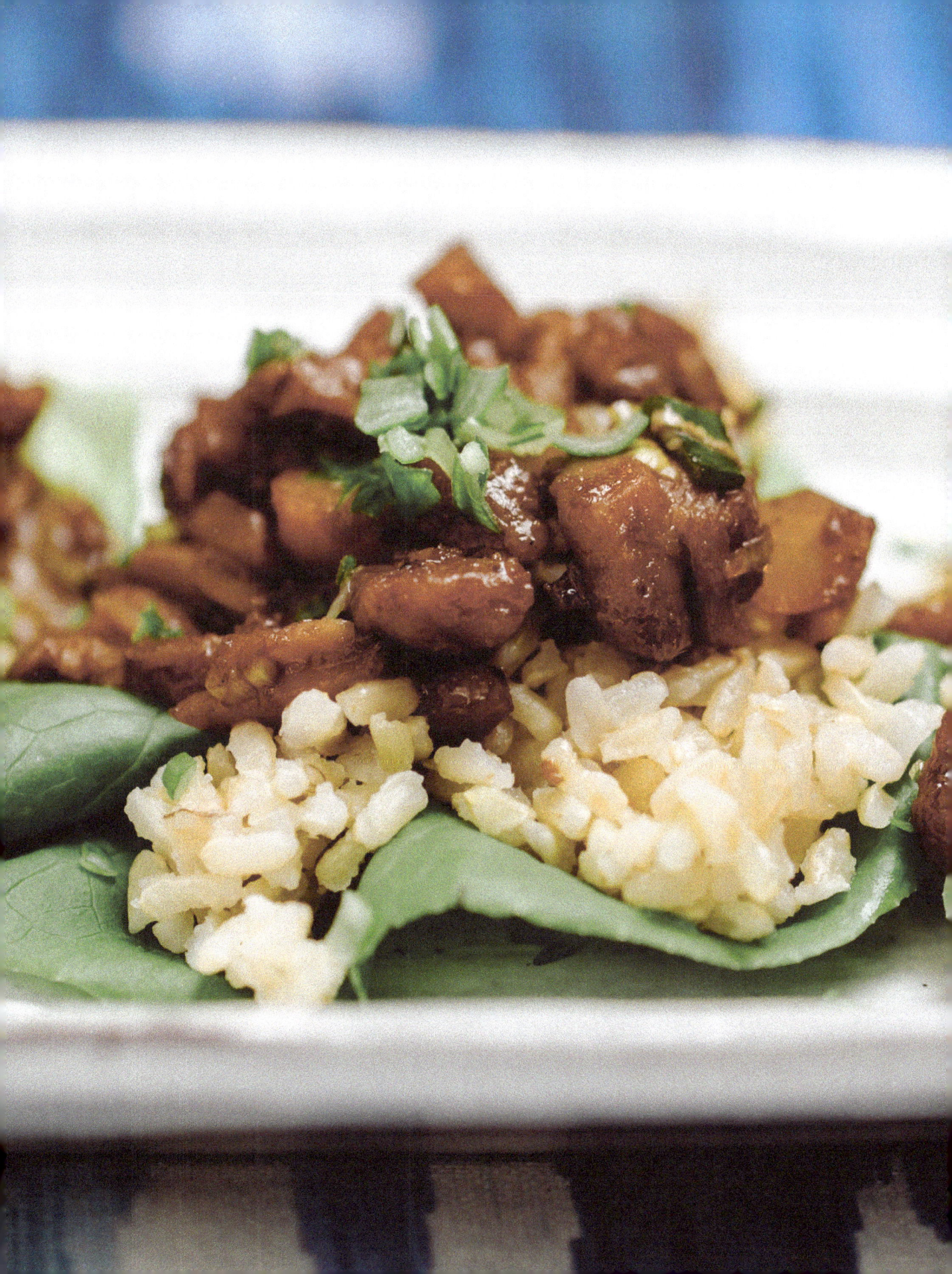

Mama's Chicken and Wild Rice Casserole

This casserole has always been a comfort food for me. When I left for college, my mom wrote down some family recipes she knew I liked. One recipe was similar to this one, and although hers didn't include cauliflower cream, it was still just as tasty.

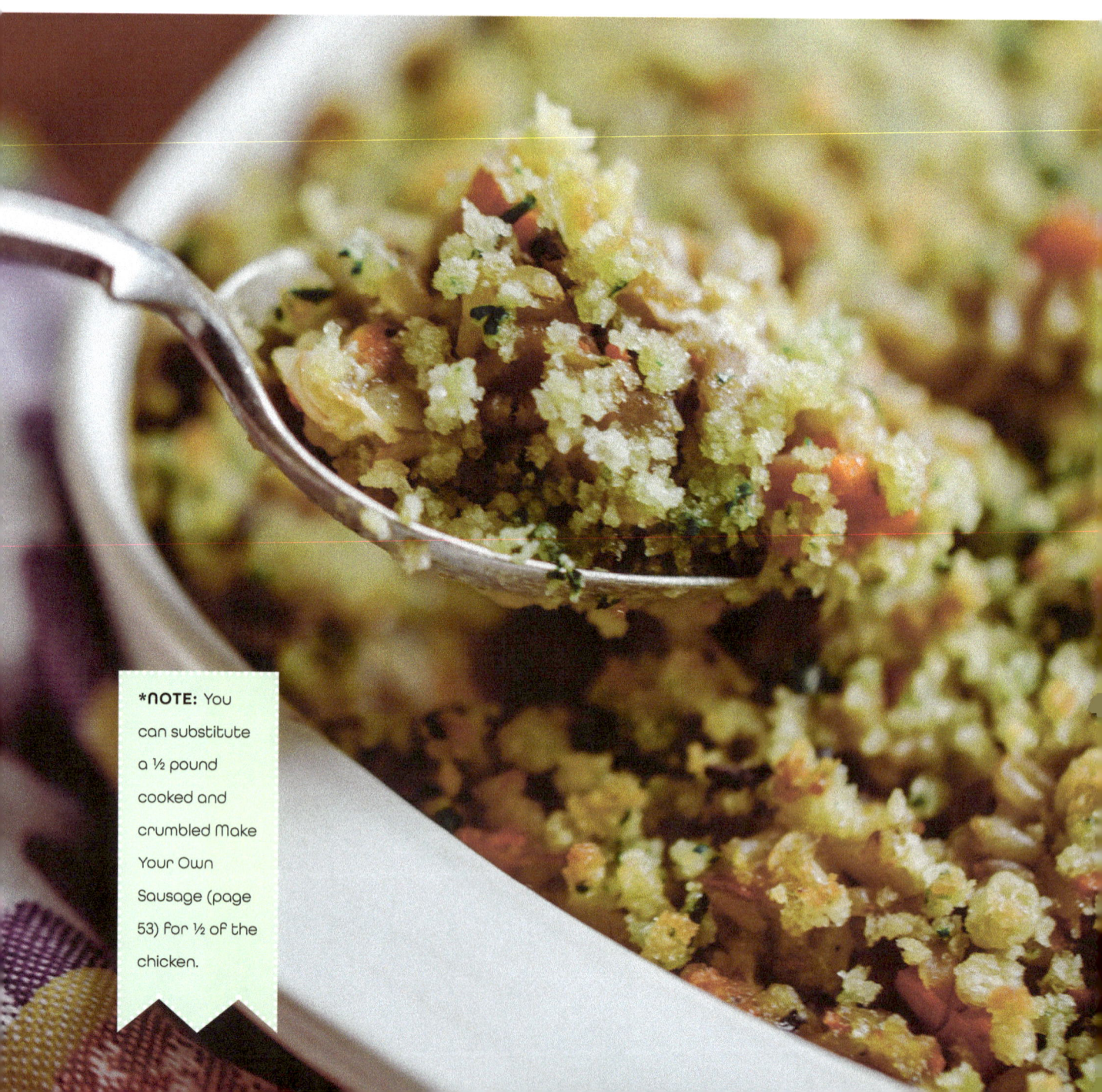

*NOTE: You can substitute a ½ pound cooked and crumbled Make Your Own Sausage (page 53) for ½ of the chicken.

INGREDIENTS

1 cup wild rice blend, such as Lundberg or RiceSelect Royal Blend

2½ cups water

Salt

Olive oil

3 shallots, peeled and diced

2 large carrots, diced

2 stalks celery, diced

2 garlic cloves, peeled and minced or grated

1 tablespoon unsalted butter

1 tablespoon all-purpose or gluten-free flour

2 cups vegetable or chicken stock, preferably homemade (pages 84, 86), or non-MSG stock

1¼ cups Cauliflower Cream (page 244) or 1 (10 oz) can cream of cauliflower soup (such as Pacific)

2 teaspoons Italian seasoning

1 teaspoon garlic granules

½ teaspoon dry dill

Pinch of red pepper flakes (optional)

1 pound chicken, cooked and shredded (thighs preferred)* preferably local

Topping

2 tablespoons unsalted butter, slightly melted

2 tablespoons fresh chopped parsley

⅓ cup panko (or gluten-free breadcrumbs)

INSTRUCTIONS

1. Bring the rice, 2¼ cups water, and a large pinch of salt to a boil. Then turn down the heat and simmer, covered, for about 40 minutes or until the rice is cooked and no water remains.

2. Preheat oven to 400°F.

3. In a large skillet, heat some olive oil and once hot, add the shallots (or all of the vegetables if chopped in a food processor, see Tip) and cook a few minutes over medium heat until soft.

4. Add the carrots and celery and cook until vegetables begin to soften, about 10 minutes. Season with salt and pepper. Add the garlic and cook until fragrant, about 1 minute.

5. Push the vegetables to the side of the pan and with the heat on medium, add 1 tablespoon butter on the empty side of the pan. Once the butter has melted, mix in the flour and stir to make a roux.

6. Continue to cook a few minutes until the roux starts to turn a golden-brown. Then incorporate the vegetables back in.

7. Add the stock, Cauliflower Cream, Italian seasoning, garlic granules, dill, and red pepper flakes (if using).

8. Stir and allow the mixture to thicken slightly for a few minutes. Turn off heat and add the rice and shredded chicken.

9. Adjust seasoning if needed, then spoon into a casserole dish and spread out evenly. An 8" x 8" or slightly larger baking dish works great. To make the topping, mix the remaining butter, parsley, and panko in a small bowl. Spread the mixture over the top of the casserole and bake for about 25 minutes or until the panko begins to brown.

10. Remove from oven and allow to cool slightly before serving.

TIP: To speed prep, you can roughly chop the shallots, carrots, and celery and put them in a food processor along with the garlic cloves and pulse until they are about the size of small dice.

Chicken Empanadas with Zucchini and Corn

I became hooked on empanadas when a friend and I ventured down to Puerto Rico one year for a surfing trip. There were so many roadside stands of the delicious fried doughy goodness with every combination of filling you can imagine. This baked version is a little lighter and can be frozen for easy meal prep.

YIELD: ABOUT 28 SMALLER
EMPANADAS

INGREDIENTS

Dough

2 cups all-purpose flour or gluten-free if necessary

1 tablespoon sugar or coconut sugar

1 teaspoon kosher salt

6 tablespoons unsalted butter, cubed

2 eggs, lightly beaten

1 tablespoon distilled white vinegar

Filling

1 tablespoon olive oil, plus more for brushing

1 cup diced zucchini

3 scallions, trimmed and sliced thin

3 cloves garlic, peeled and minced or grated

1 cup corn kernels

2 teaspoons ground cumin

½ teaspoon dried thyme

2 teaspoons chili powder

8 oz queso fresco cheese, crumbled

1 pound cooked, shredded chicken, preferably local

1 egg, for egg wash

INSTRUCTIONS

Dough

1. Combine the flour, sugar, and salt in a food processor. Pulse twice. Then add the cold butter and pulse a few more times until the butter is in small chunks.

2. Combine the eggs with the white vinegar and 1 tablespoon water. Stir to combine.

3. Add the egg mixture to the food processor and pulse until it comes together to form a ball of dough. Make sure not to overmix at this point.

4. Wrap dough and refrigerate for about 1 hour (at least 30 minutes) while you make the filling. It can also be made a day in advance.

Filling

1. Heat the olive oil in a large sauté pan over medium heat. Sauté the zucchini.

2. After a minute or so add the scallions, garlic, and corn along with a pinch of salt and pepper.

3. Cook a few minutes until the vegetables begin to soften and then add the cumin, thyme, and chili powder.

4. Cook another couple of minutes then turn off heat. Transfer mixture to a bowl and let cool slightly. Stir in the cheese and shredded chicken. At this point you can cover and refrigerate the mixture until ready to make the empanadas.

5. For the egg wash, whisk the egg in a small bowl with 1 tablespoon water. Set aside.

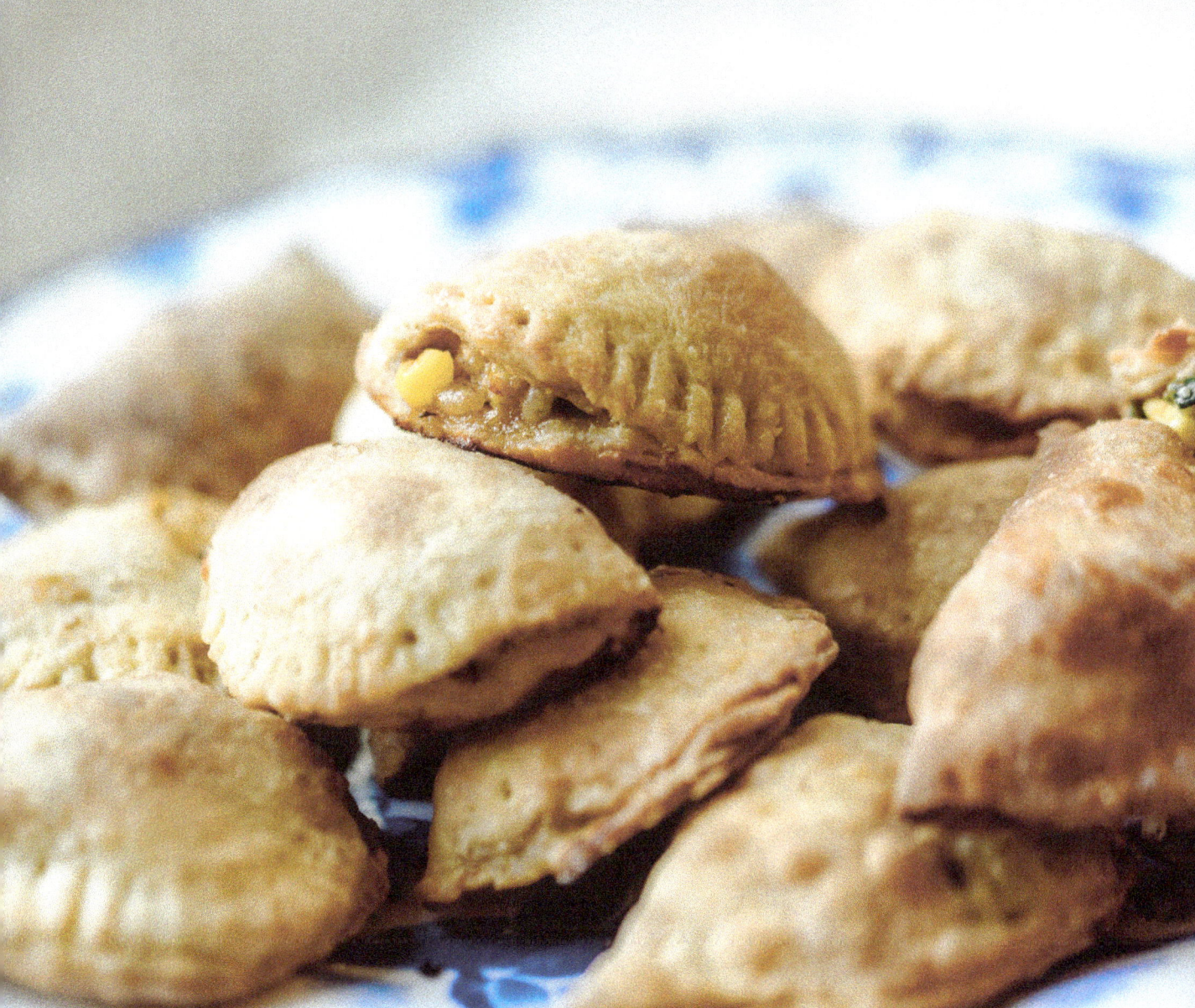

Empanadas

1. Preheat oven to 425°F.
2. Remove half the dough from the fridge and roll out on a lightly floured surface. Use a circular biscuit cutter or glass to cut out circles of dough. I use a large, 5-inch biscuit cutter.
3. Place a heaping tablespoon of the filling in the center of each circle of dough and using your finger, spread a little egg wash around half of the circle along the edge.
4. Fold the empanada over so it is a half-moon and crimp the edges with a fork, pressing down lightly. Continue until all the dough is used.
5. Arrange empanadas on a sheet tray lined with parchment paper or a Silpat mat and brush with olive oil or remaining egg wash. Bake for 20–25 minutes or until golden-brown.

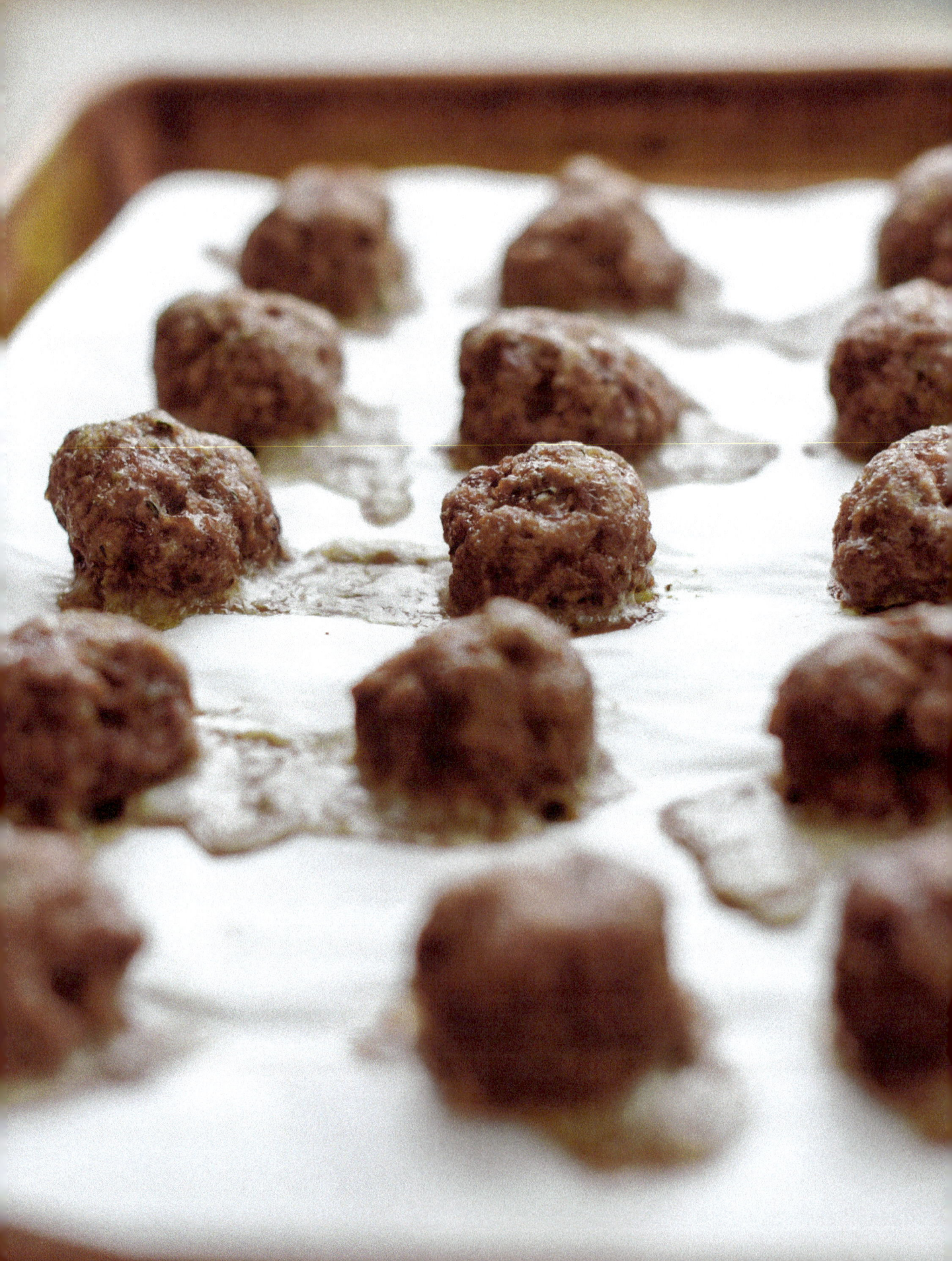

Classic Italian Beef Meatballs

YIELD: 4 SERVINGS OR
12–16 MEATBALLS

INGREDIENTS

1 pound ground beef or bison,
    preferably local

1 egg

2 tablespoons milk or coconut
    milk

¼ cup breadcrumbs or oat
    flour (page 13)

1 teaspoon Italian seasoning

2 garlic cloves, peeled and
    grated

1 teaspoon kosher salt and
    freshly ground pepper

Fresh basil or parsley,
    chopped fine, to top

TIP: These are great with
Instant Pot Marinara (page
224), Roasted Red Pepper
Vodka Sauce (page 241), or
Basil Sunflower Seed Pesto
(page 228).

INSTRUCTIONS

1. Preheat oven to 425°F.

2. In a large bowl combine all the ingredients.

3. Roll into 12–16 meatballs and place on a Silpat mat or parchment-lined sheet tray.

4. Bake for about 17–20 minutes or until cooked through. Serve topped with chopped herbs.

Herby Turkey Meatballs

Who doesn't love homemade meatballs? They can be made ahead, they freeze well, are kid-friendly, and act like a blank canvas for whatever else you want to pair with them. These turkey meatballs can be tossed with Ginger Glaze (page 233) or can be smothered with homemade marinara for a more Italian dish.

YIELD: 4 SERVINGS (12–16 MEATBALLS)

INGREDIENTS

1 pound ground turkey meat, dark meat preferred, preferably local

1 shallot, minced

1 egg

¼ cup breadcrumbs or oat flour (page 13)

2 garlic cloves, peeled and minced or grated

¼ cup chopped fresh cilantro (leaves and stems)

¼ cup chopped fresh parsley (leaves and stems)

1 teaspoon kosher salt

Freshly ground pepper

INSTRUCTIONS

1. Preheat oven to 400°F and line a sheet tray with a Silpat mat or parchment paper.

2. In a large mixing bowl, combine all ingredients.

3. Roll out about 12–16 meatballs and place them on the sheet tray. Bake for about 17–20 minutes or until the meatballs are cooked through. An instant-read thermometer should read 160°F.

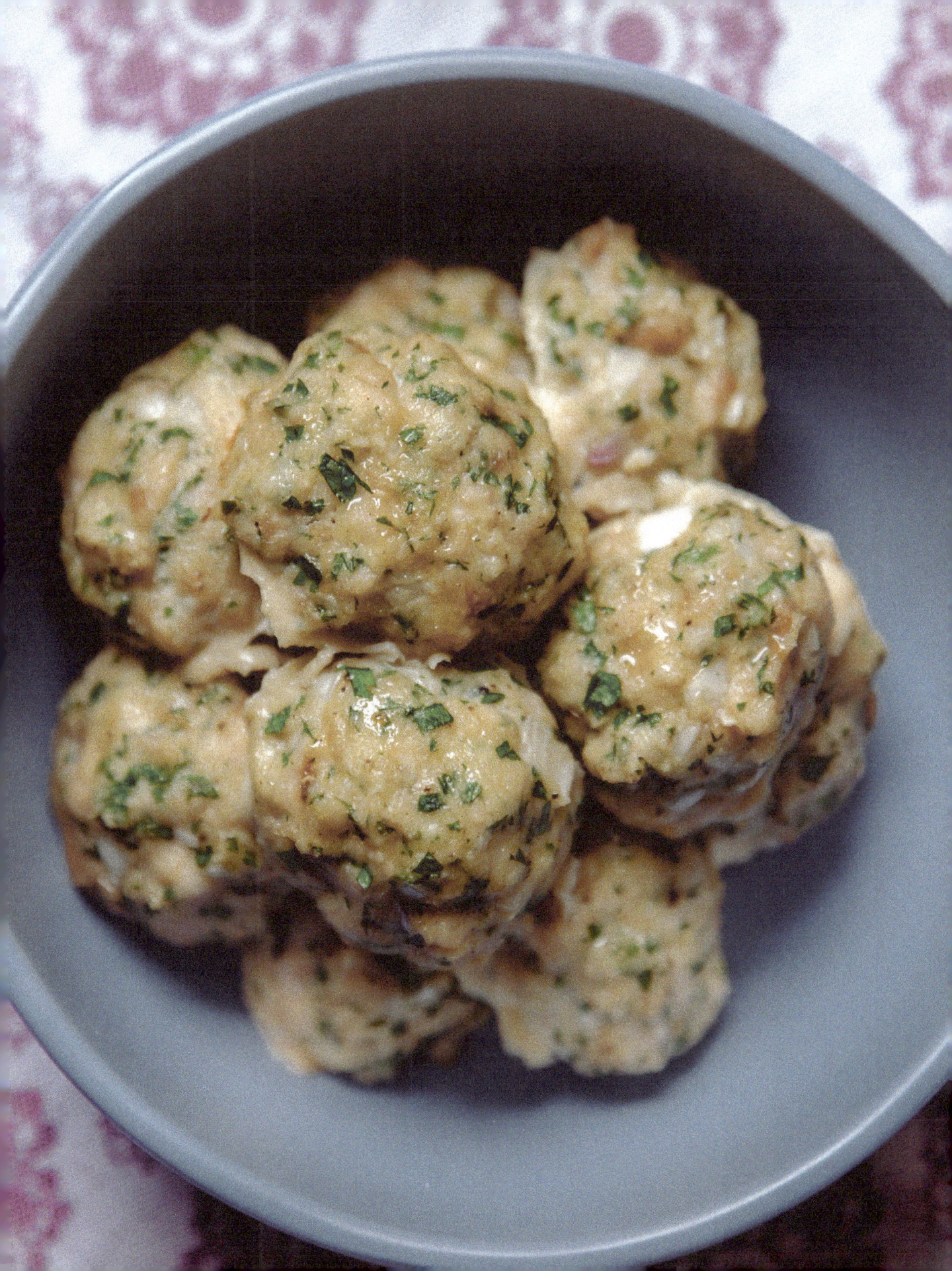

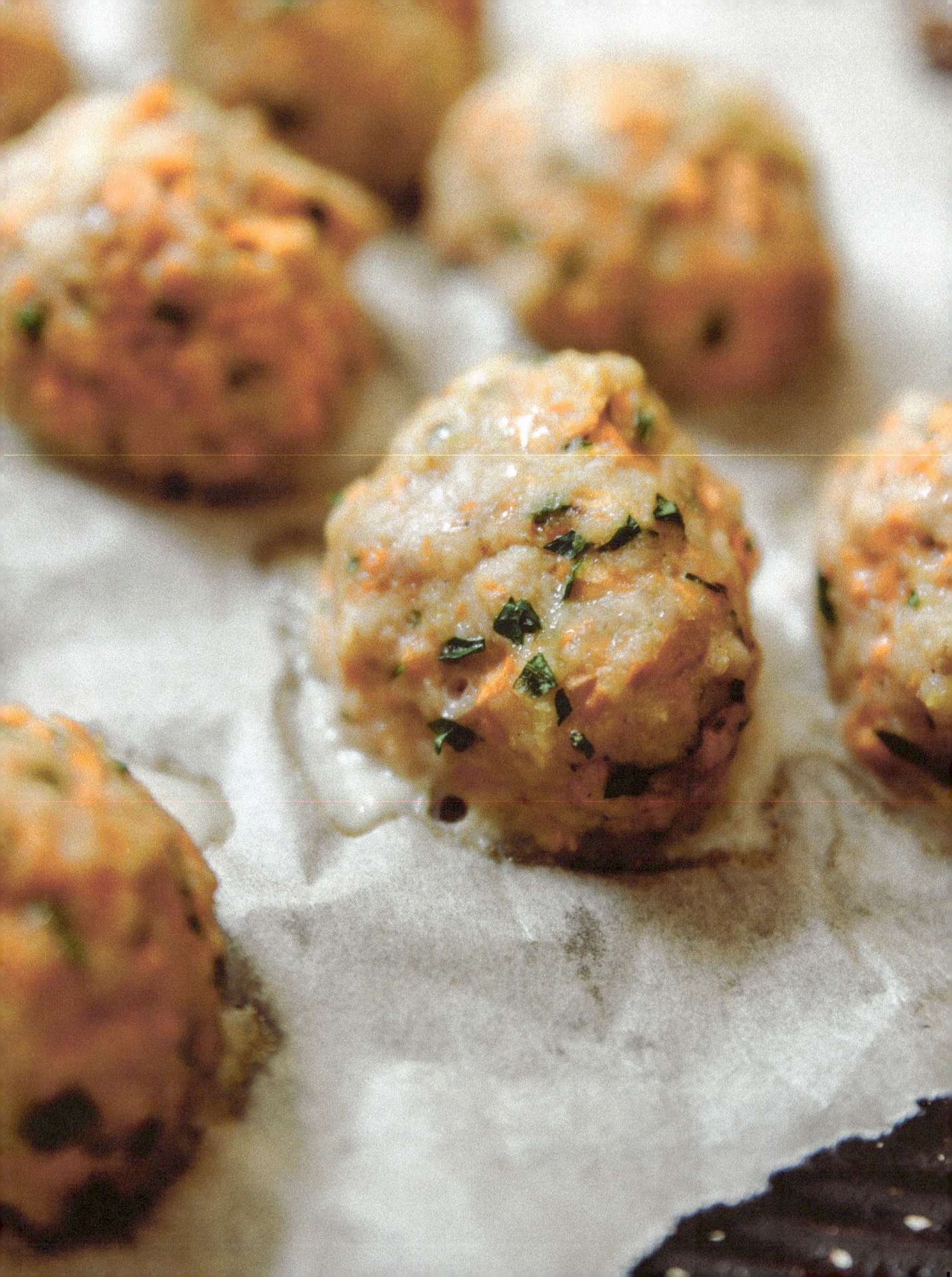

Chicken Sweet Potato Meatballs

For a kid-friendly meatball with hidden vegetables

YIELD: 12–16 MEATBALLS

INGREDIENTS

1 pound chicken (or turkey), light and dark meat, preferably local

1½ cups sweet potato, minced

1 egg

⅓ cup breadcrumbs or oat flour (page 13)

1 teaspoon garlic granules

¼ cup parsley chopped

1 teaspoon Taco Seasoning (page 239)

Splash of milk or canned coconut milk

Salt and freshly ground pepper

1 tablespoon olive oil

INSTRUCTIONS

1. Combine all ingredients except the olive oil in a bowl and season with salt and pepper. Mix thoroughly and form into meatballs.

2. Heat olive oil over medium heat in a large skillet. Add meatballs and sear on all sides, cooking until the internal temperature is 160°F. You can also bake at 400°F for 17–20 minutes or until cooked through.

Ginger Chicken with Lemongrass

This is my rendition of chicken galangal, which I first experienced while traveling in Thailand with some friends. This dish is packed with flavor, and you can be in control of the spice level. Galangal is a tuberous root usually found in Asian markets, and you may use it in place of ginger in this recipe.

YIELD: 4–6 SERVINGS

INGREDIENTS

2 large shallots, peeled and quartered

4 garlic cloves, peeled

2-inch piece of ginger, peeled and chopped, can substitute fresh galangal

¼ cup raw sunflower seeds

1 poblano pepper, seeded and chopped

1 stalk lemongrass, cored, trimmed and sliced

Kosher salt and freshly ground pepper

1 (8 oz) can tomato sauce or Instant Pot Marinara (page 224)

1 tablespoon coconut aminos

¼ teaspoon ground turmeric

¼ teaspoon paprika

⅛ teaspoon ground coriander

2 teaspoons coconut sugar

1 pound chicken thighs, boneless and skinless, preferably local

Juice of ½ lime

¼ cup cilantro

Cooked rice for serving

Scallions, sliced thinly for topping (optional)

INSTRUCTIONS

1. Add the shallots, garlic, ginger, sunflower seeds, poblano, and lemongrass to a food processor. You can also use a high-speed blender, but I prefer a food processor.

2. Blend with 1–2 tablespoons water until it reaches a paste-like consistency. You will probably need to scrape down the sides a couple of times.

3. Heat the olive oil in a sauté pan over medium-high heat. (If you are using an Instant Pot, you can also use the sauté setting instead of a separate pan.)

4. Once hot add the lemongrass mixture along with a pinch of salt and sauté for about 10 minutes, stirring occasionally. If the mixture begins to stick to the bottom of the pan, you can add a tablespoon of water to prevent it from sticking or burning.

5. Add the tomato sauce, coconut aminos, spices, and coconut sugar. Give it a stir and add a little more salt.

6. Add the mixture along with the chicken thighs and ½ cup water to your Instant Pot or slow cooker.

7. Set to the manual setting for 30 minutes on the Instant Pot. If using a slow cooker, cook on high for 4 hours or low for 6–8 hours.

8. If you are using an Instant Pot, allow the mixture to vent naturally. Remove the lid and shred the chicken.

9. Add the lime juice and most of the cilantro, reserving a little to top. Add some freshly ground pepper and adjust seasoning if needed.

10. Serve over rice and top with the rest of the cilantro and scallions (if using).

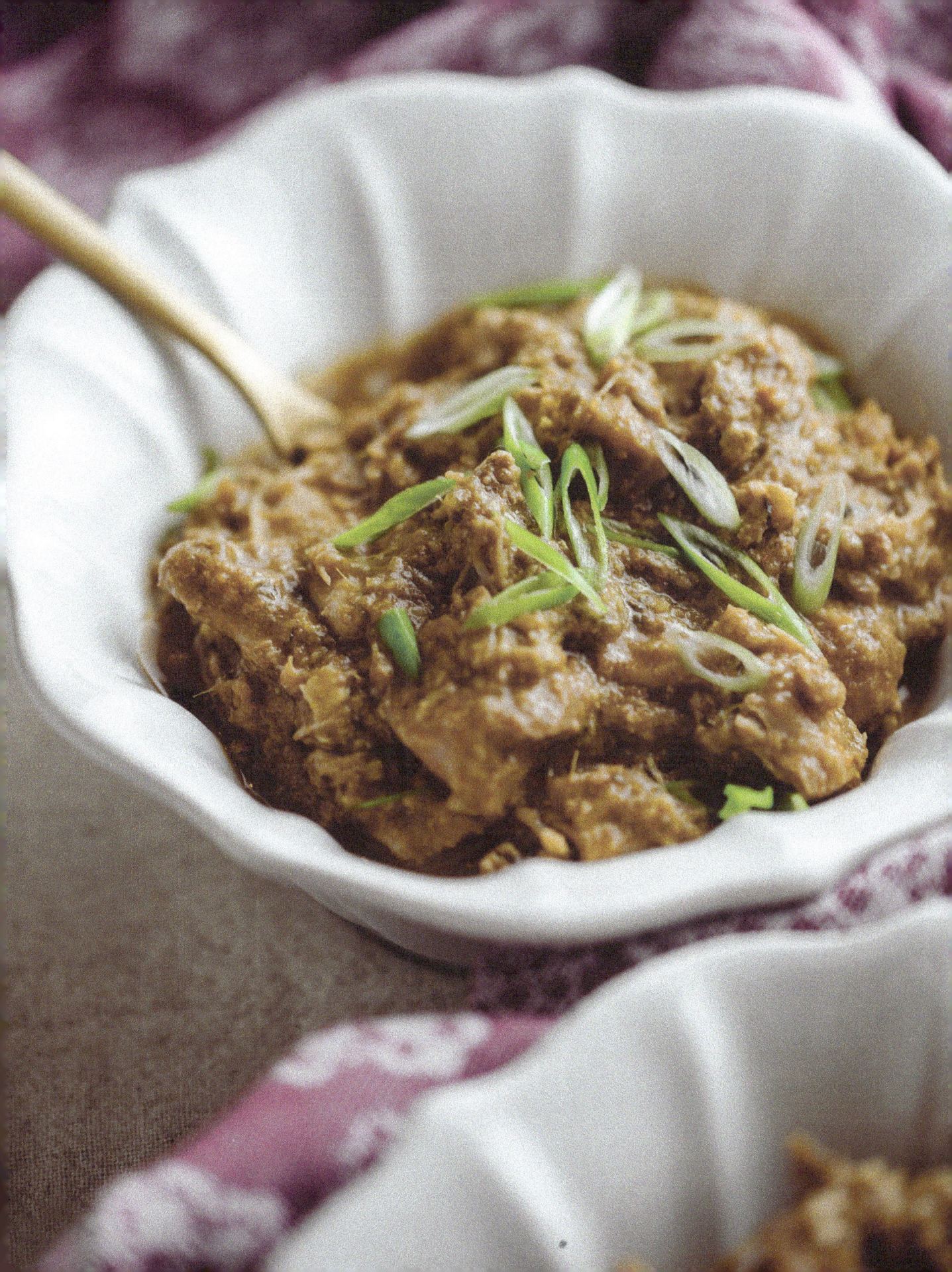

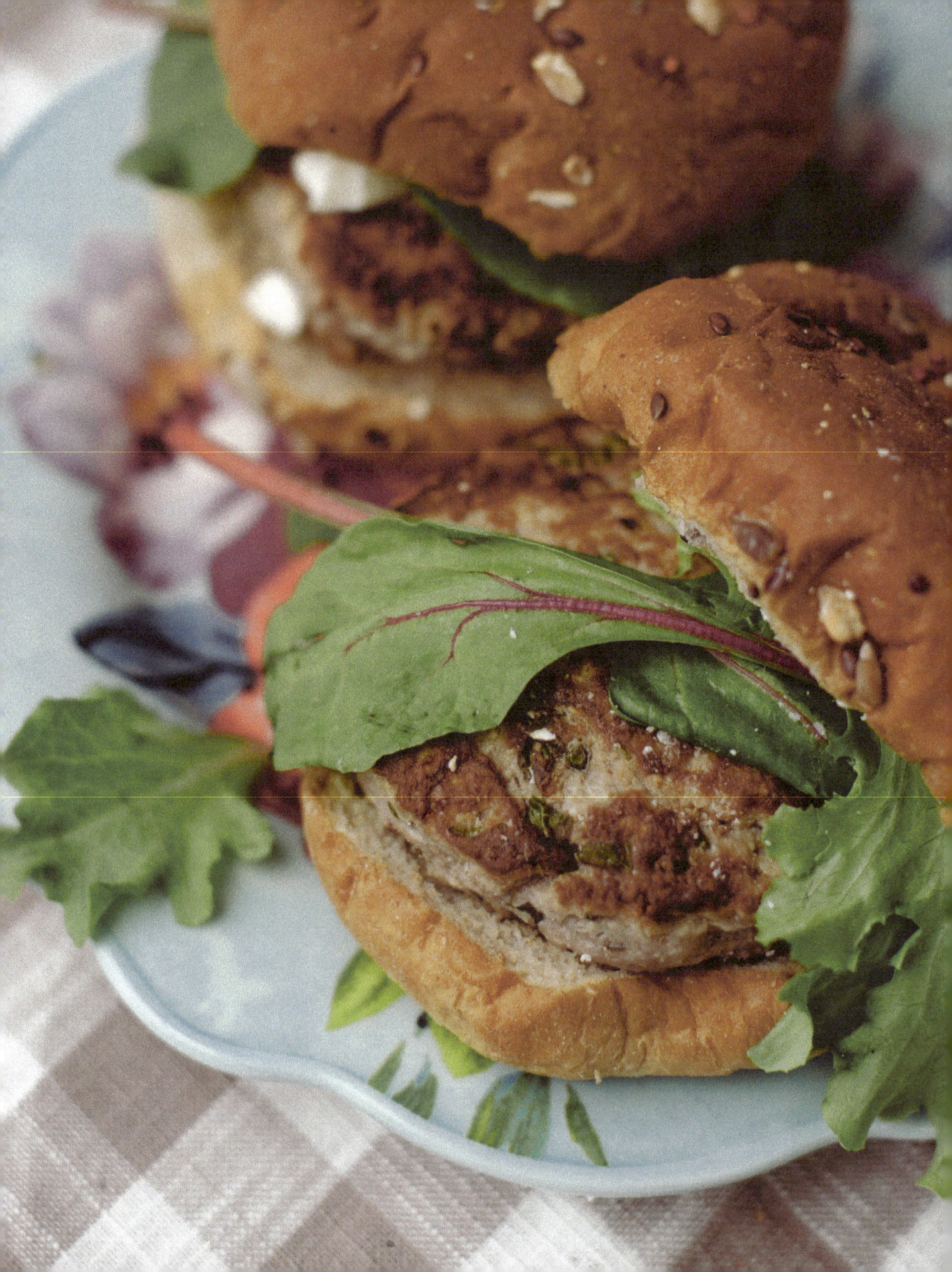

Mediterranean Turkey Burgers

For a flavor-packed turkey burger

INGREDIENTS

1 pound ground turkey, dark and light meat, preferably local

½ cup fresh basil leaves, chopped

4 sun-dried tomatoes, minced (about ¼ cup)

1 garlic clove, peeled and minced or grated

1 teaspoon kosher salt

Freshly ground pepper

Oil for grill or pan

⅓ cup crumbled fresh feta, if not a trigger, if using decrease salt to ½ teaspoon

INSTRUCTIONS

1. In a large bowl, add the first 6 ingredients and feta (if using).
2. Mix until combined then form into 4 equal patties.
3. Heat a little oil in a large skillet over medium-high heat or heat your grill and using a small paper towel add a little oil to the grates.
4. Add the patties and sear (or grill) until halfway cooked. Flip them over and continue cooking until they are fully cooked. Remove and allow to cool slightly.
5. Serve on hamburger buns (preferably heated slightly on the grill or in the pan) with toppings of choice, such as lettuce, aioli, BBQ sauce, or avocado if not a trigger.

Delicious Roasted Chicken with Herb Butter

This recipe is dedicated to my dad, who is always cooking up a delicious bird for special occasions (or just a quiet Tuesday dinner at home). He has prepared them numerous ways over the years, but they always come out juicy and tender on the inside with an extra-crispy skin. And if I'm lucky, he lets me help with the gravy.

YIELD: 6 SERVINGS

INGREDIENTS

1 chicken, 3½–4 pounds, preferably local, giblets removed but saved

1 large shallot, peeled and chopped

1 stalk celery, chopped

1 medium carrot, chopped

2 garlic cloves, peeled and quartered

Half a lemon, quartered

Salt and freshly ground pepper

Herb Butter

3 tablespoons unsalted butter, room temperature

1 tablespoon chopped fresh herbs such as thyme, oregano, sage, and rosemary

½ teaspoon garlic granules

¼ teaspoon onion granules, if not a trigger

INSTRUCTIONS

1. Place oven rack in the center of oven or just below, making sure there is plenty of room for your bird to roast. Preheat oven to 425°F.
2. Place the chicken breast side up on a roasting rack fitted with a pan below or place the chicken in a cast-iron skillet.
3. Combine the shallot, celery, carrot, garlic, and lemon.
4. Pat the bird dry with a paper towel.
5. Salt the inside of the chicken and stuff the inside with the shallot mixture.
6. Tie the legs together with kitchen twine. (This is called trussing the bird and helps to cook the meat evenly as well as make for a nice presentation.) Tuck the wings under the body of the chicken.
7. To make the herb butter, combine all its ingredients and mix together.
8. Take about half the herb butter and stuff under the skin of the chicken breasts. Take the other half and smear it on top and around the sides of the chicken.
9. Season with salt and pepper and roast for 25 minutes.
10. Reduce oven temperature to 350°F and roast about another hour or until the chicken is 165°F internally at the thickest part.
11. Remove from oven and allow to rest about 30 minutes before slicing. This will keep all the juices from running out.

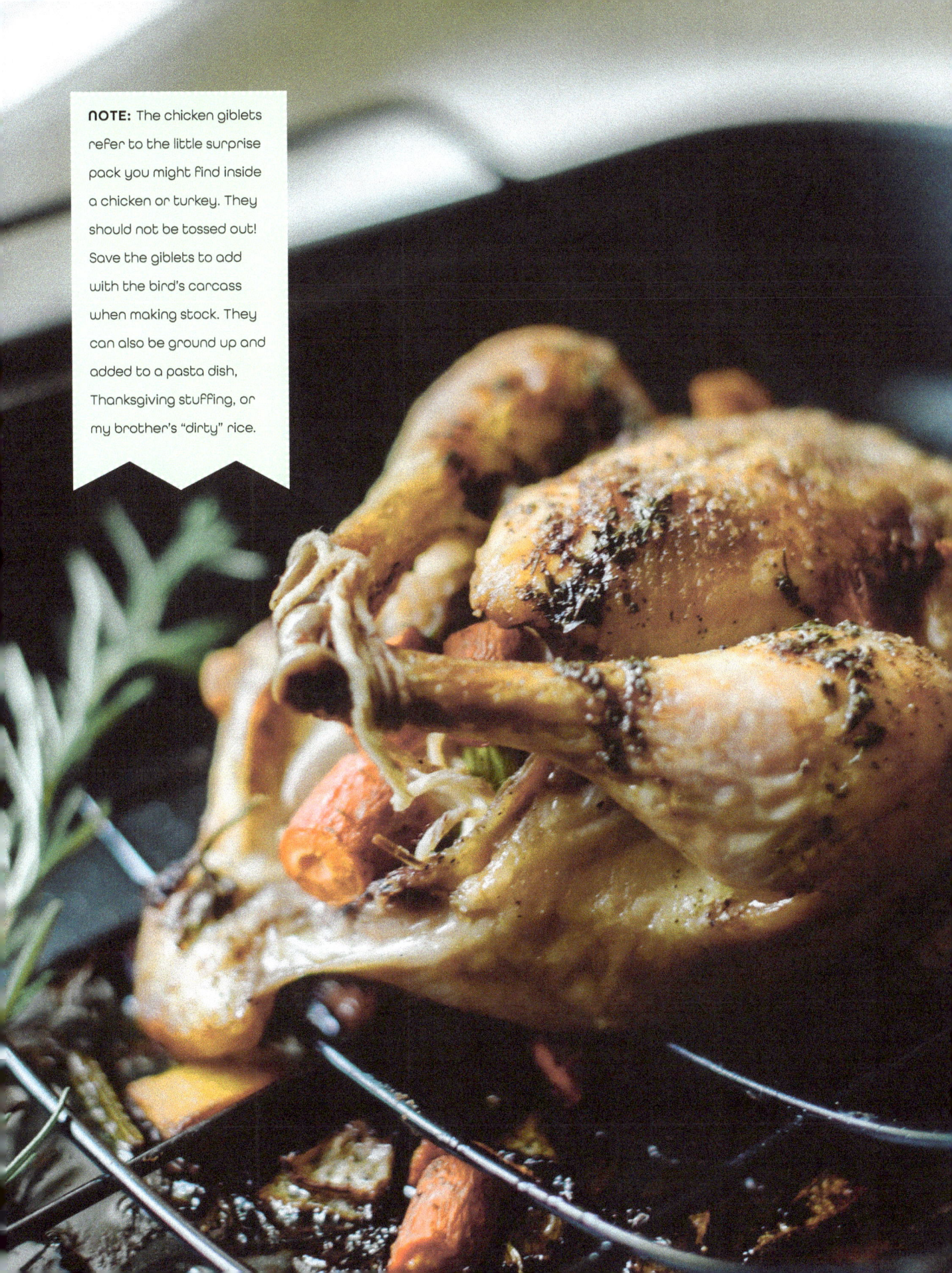

NOTE: The chicken giblets refer to the little surprise pack you might find inside a chicken or turkey. They should not be tossed out! Save the giblets to add with the bird's carcass when making stock. They can also be ground up and added to a pasta dish, Thanksgiving stuffing, or my brother's "dirty" rice.

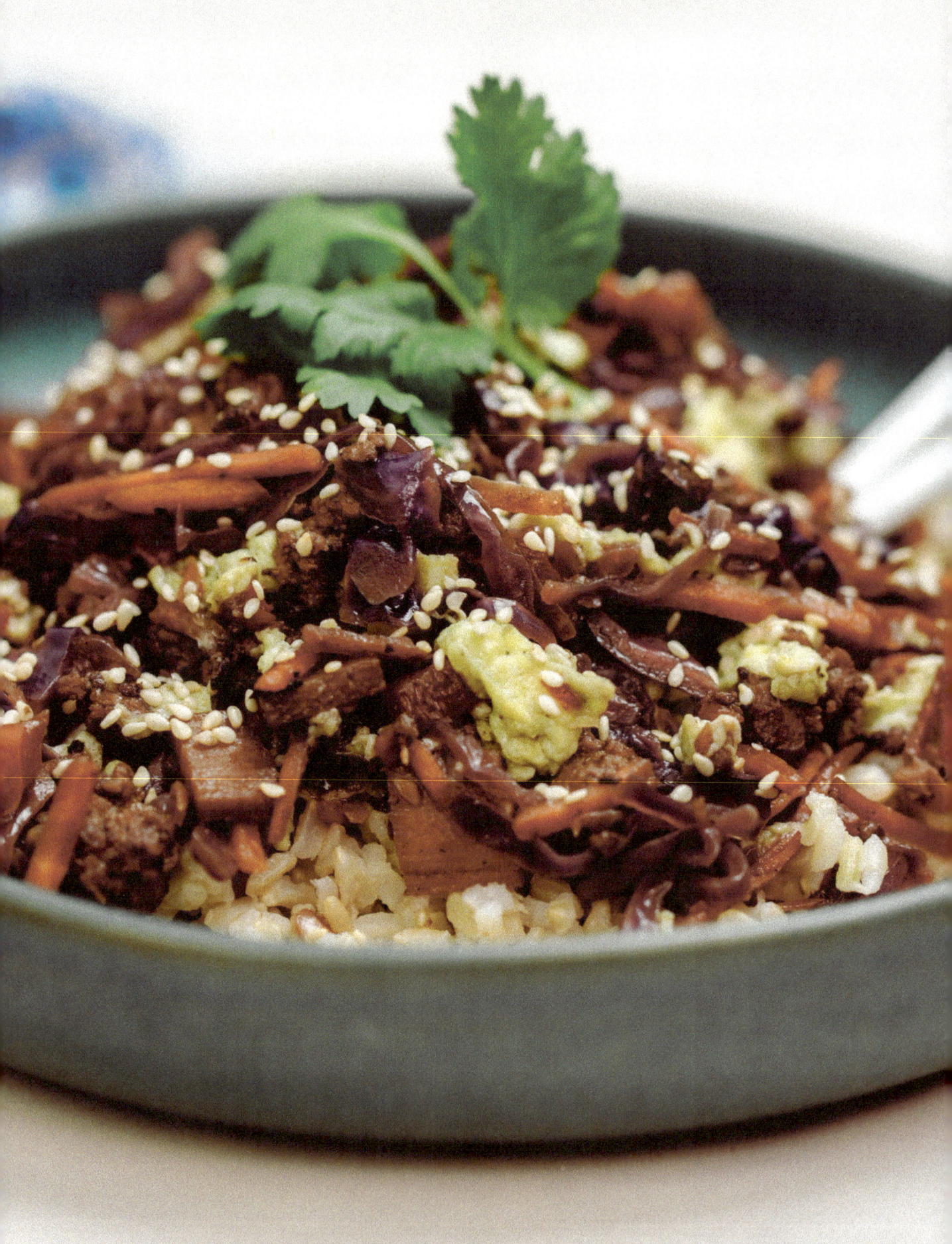

Quick Moo Shu Bowl

This dish is a great weeknight dinner that can come together quickly. I usually have some of the glaze in the freezer and the prep work can be trimmed down, thanks to bags of preshredded carrots and cabbage.

YIELD: 4 SERVINGS

INGREDIENTS

Olive oil

2 eggs, whisked

1 pound ground pork, preferably local

3 shallots, peeled and diced

1 bell pepper, seeded and diced

3 garlic cloves, peeled and minced or grated

12 oz red cabbage, thinly shredded

2 cups shredded carrots

1 (4 oz) can bamboo shoots, drained and chopped

½ teaspoon red pepper flakes (optional)

1 recipe Ginger Glaze (page 233)

Kosher salt and freshly ground pepper

Cooked quinoa or rice for serving

Thinly sliced scallions, chopped cilantro, or sesame seeds for topping

INSTRUCTIONS

1. In a large skillet, heat a little olive oil over low-medium heat.

2. Add the eggs and stir until they are cooked and scrambled. Remove eggs and set aside.

3. In the same skillet, heat a little more olive oil and cook the ground pork over medium heat, breaking it apart with a spatula. Once the pork is almost cooked, add the shallots. Season a little with salt and pepper.

4. Once the shallots have softened, add the bell pepper. Cook 5–8 minutes, stirring occasionally over medium heat.

5. Add the garlic and cook another minute or 2 until fragrant. Add the cabbage, carrots, bamboo shoots, and optional red pepper flakes. Stir. Then add the Ginger Glaze and allow it to cook until slightly thickened.

6. Serve over quinoa or rice. Top with sliced scallions, cilantro, or sesame seeds.

Sausage and Apple Stuffed Acorn Squash

I love everything about acorn squash. It's the perfect size and has a delicate, sweet flavor after it's roasted. Add some sausage, apple, and sage to it, and you've got the perfect fall meal.

YIELD: 6 HALVES OR 6 PORTIONS

INGREDIENTS

3 small–medium acorn squashes

Olive oil

1 pound Make Your Own Sausage (page 53)

2 large leeks, white parts only, rinsed and diced

2 stalks celery, diced

2 garlic cloves, peeled and minced or grated

¼ cup fresh sage leaves, chopped

1 apple, diced

6 oz fresh mozzarella, shredded

Kosher salt and freshly ground pepper

INSTRUCTIONS

1. Preheat oven to 400°F.

2. Slice off the top and bottom ends of each acorn squash. (Not much, just enough so they sit flat.) Then cut each squash crosswise into halves. Remove the seeds and pulp from each half.

3. Place the squash on a Silpat mat or parchment-lined baking sheet, drizzle with olive oil and sprinkle with salt. Rub to coat all sides of the squash and place flesh side down.

4. Roast for 35–40 minutes or until fork-tender. Remove and allow to cool slightly.

5. Meanwhile, cook the sausage over medium heat in a large skillet. Break apart while it's cooking. Once it's cooked, stir in the leeks, celery, and a little salt and pepper. Cook for 6–8 minutes, stirring occasionally.

6. Add the garlic, sage, and apple. Sauté until the apple starts to soften, about 5 minutes, and turn off heat.

7. Once cool enough to handle, scrape out some of the flesh of each half of the squash (making sure to leave some around the edges) and add it to a large bowl. Mash it with a fork or pastry blender.

8. Add the sausage mixture. Stir to combine and adjust seasoning if needed.

9. Stuff the sausage mixture into the acorn squash halves, dividing it evenly between halves. Top with cheese and bake about 20 minutes or until heated through and the cheese has melted.

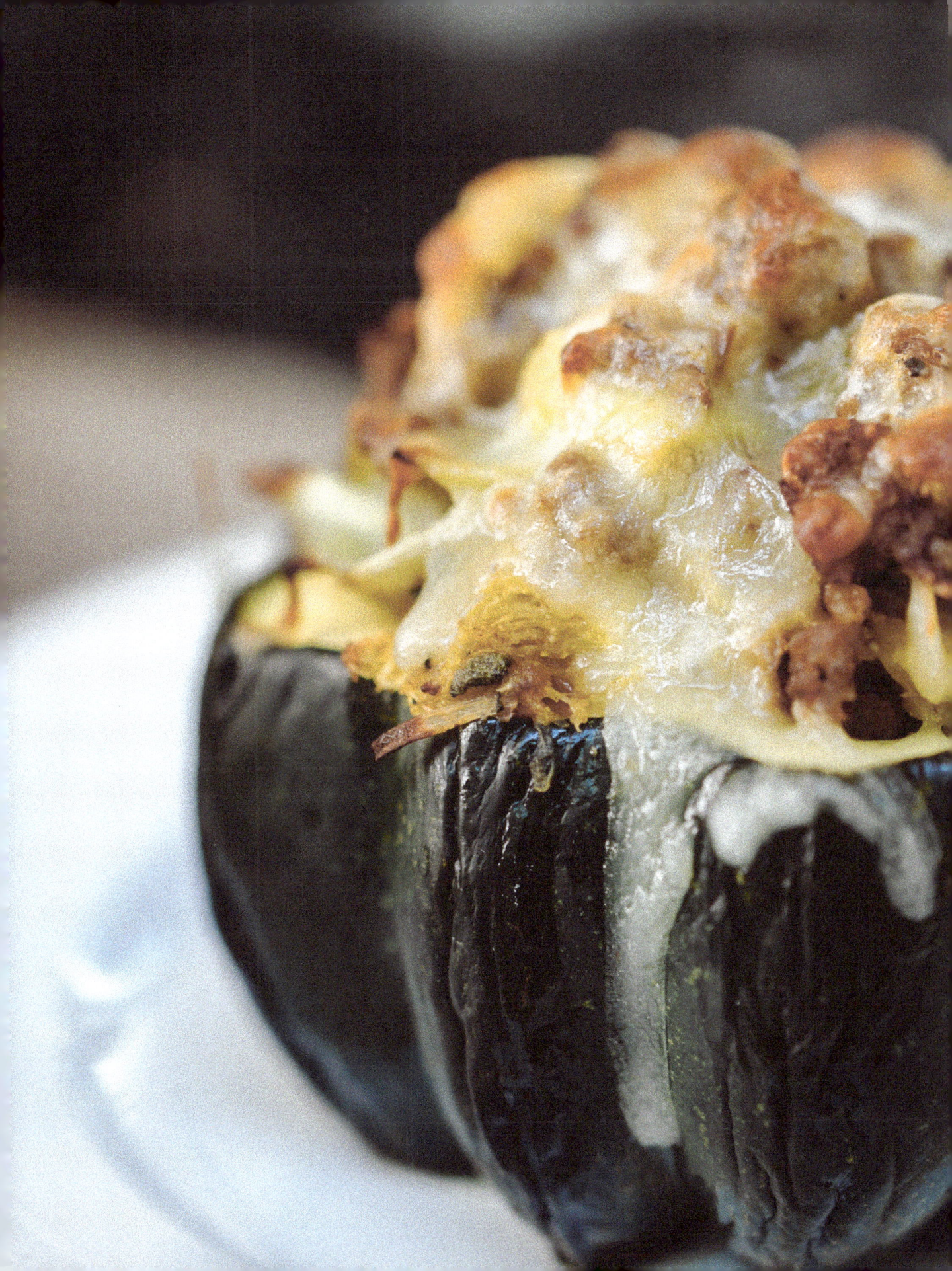

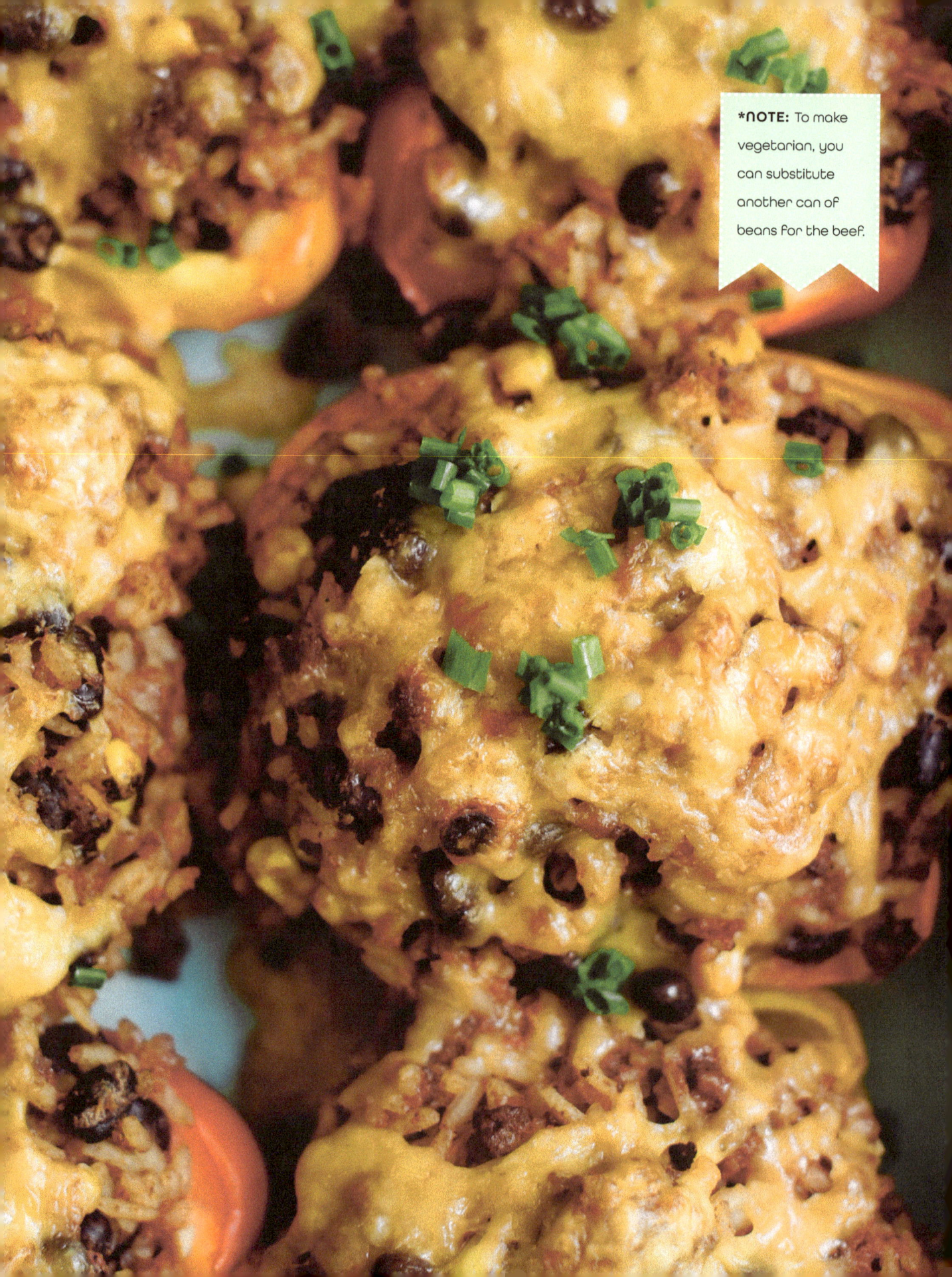

*NOTE: To make vegetarian, you can substitute another can of beans for the beef.

Southwestern Stuffed Bell Peppers

This recipe dates all the way back to my college years and hasn't changed much at all. There are many beans, grains, and different meats you can use here, so don't hesitate to mix it up a little.

YIELD: 10 LARGE PEPPER
HALVES

INGREDIENTS

5 bell peppers, red, orange, or yellow

1 cup basmati (or similar) rice, uncooked

2 cups water

Salt

1 pound ground beef, preferably local*

1 cup shallots, peeled and diced, about 3–4

5 garlic cloves, peeled and grated or minced

1 recipe, or about ¼ cup, Taco Seasoning (page 239)

1 (15 oz) can black beans, drained and rinsed

1 cup corn kernels

4 oz fresh mozzarella, shredded, plus more for topping (optional)

INSTRUCTIONS

1. Preheat oven to 375°F.
2. Cut the peppers in half lengthwise and remove the seeds and ribs. Place the halves cut side up in a baking dish or on a sheet tray and bake for 15 minutes.
3. While the peppers are cooking, prepare the rice by bringing the rice, 2 cups of water, and a large pinch of salt to a boil. Then cover and simmer for 15 minutes. Remove from heat and fluff with a fork.
4. Set the rice and peppers aside when they are done cooking.
5. Heat a large skillet over medium heat and add the beef. Break apart as it cooks and add a large pinch of salt.
6. Once the beef is cooked, add the shallots and allow to soften. Then add the garlic and Taco Seasoning. Cook for another minute until fragrant.
7. Add the beans and corn. Stir to combine and cook a few minutes.
8. Turn off heat and stir together with the rice and the cheese (if using). Taste and adjust seasoning if needed.
9. Divide the filling among the 10 pepper halves. When stuffing them they will be very full, and you will need to gently press the filling in. Top with a little more cheese if desired.
10. Bake for 20 minutes and remove from oven.

Fully Loaded Sweet Potatoes

To take the standard baked potato up a notch

YIELD: 4 SWEET POTATO
HALVES

INGREDIENTS

2 large sweet potatoes

¼ cup Basil Sunflower Seed Pesto (page 228)

1 pound Make Your Own Sausage (page 53)

1 large shallot, peeled and diced

1 green bell pepper, diced

1 tablespoon chopped fresh sage

Salt and freshly ground pepper

¾ cup fresh ricotta or fresh mozzarella (optional)

INSTRUCTIONS

1. Preheat oven to 400°F.
2. Place the sweet potatoes on a parchment-lined baking sheet tray and roast until fork-tender. This will take about 1 hour–1 hour and 15 minutes.
3. While the sweet potatoes cook, make your pesto and set aside.
4. Heat a large skillet over medium heat and add the sausage, breaking it apart as it cooks. Once cooked, add in the shallots. Continue cooking for a few minutes until shallots begin to soften.
5. Add the diced bell pepper, sage, and some salt and pepper. Cook another 5–10 minutes until the vegetables are soft.
6. When the potatoes are cool enough to handle, cut them in half lengthwise and scoop out the center, leaving a little around the edges. Mash the sweet potato in a bowl. Add the sausage mixture, pesto, and ricotta or mozzarella and stir to combine. Taste and adjust seasoning if needed.
7. Divide the mixture evenly among the sweet potato shells.
8. Bake for about 20 minutes. Remove and allow to cool slightly.

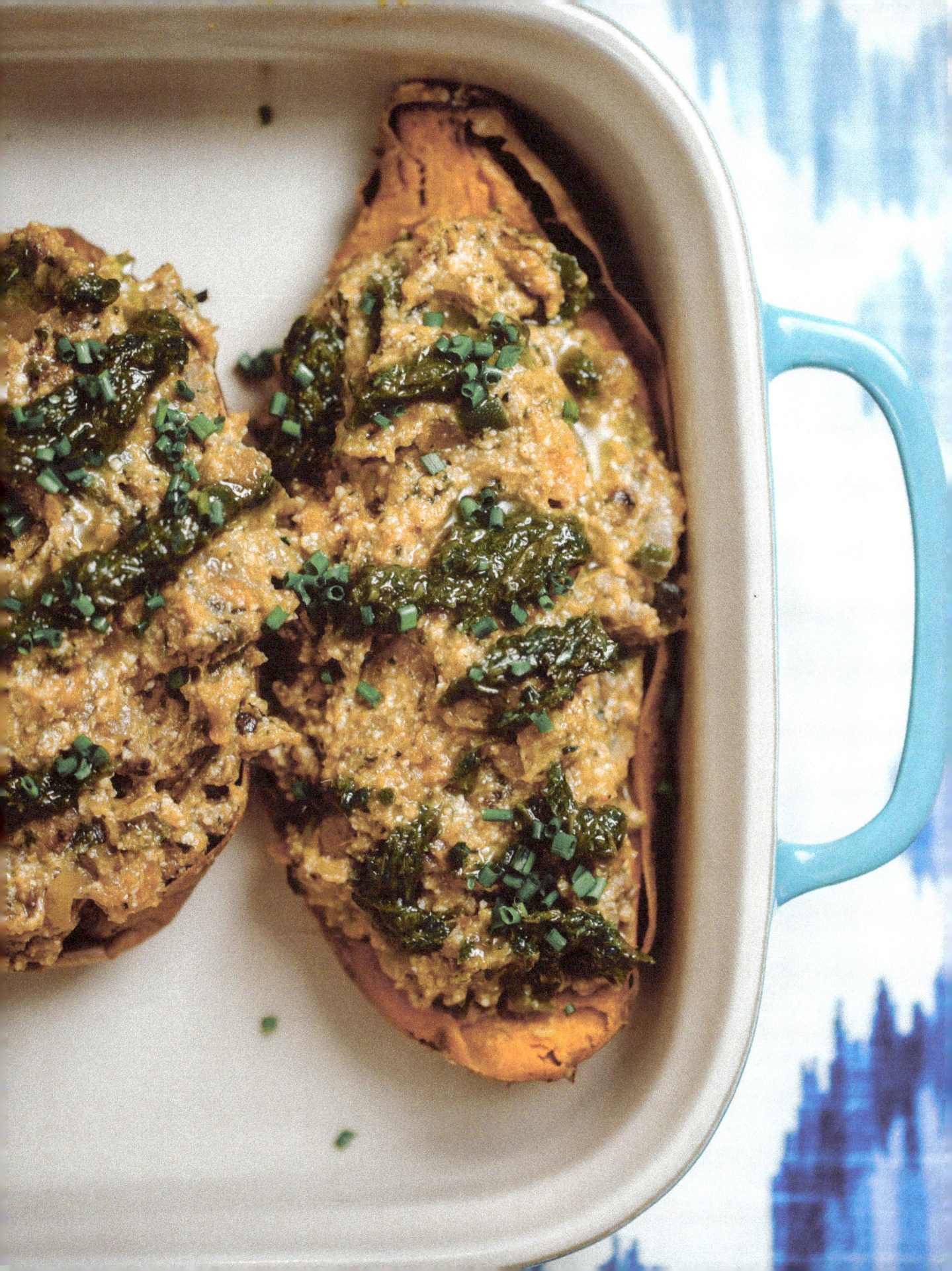

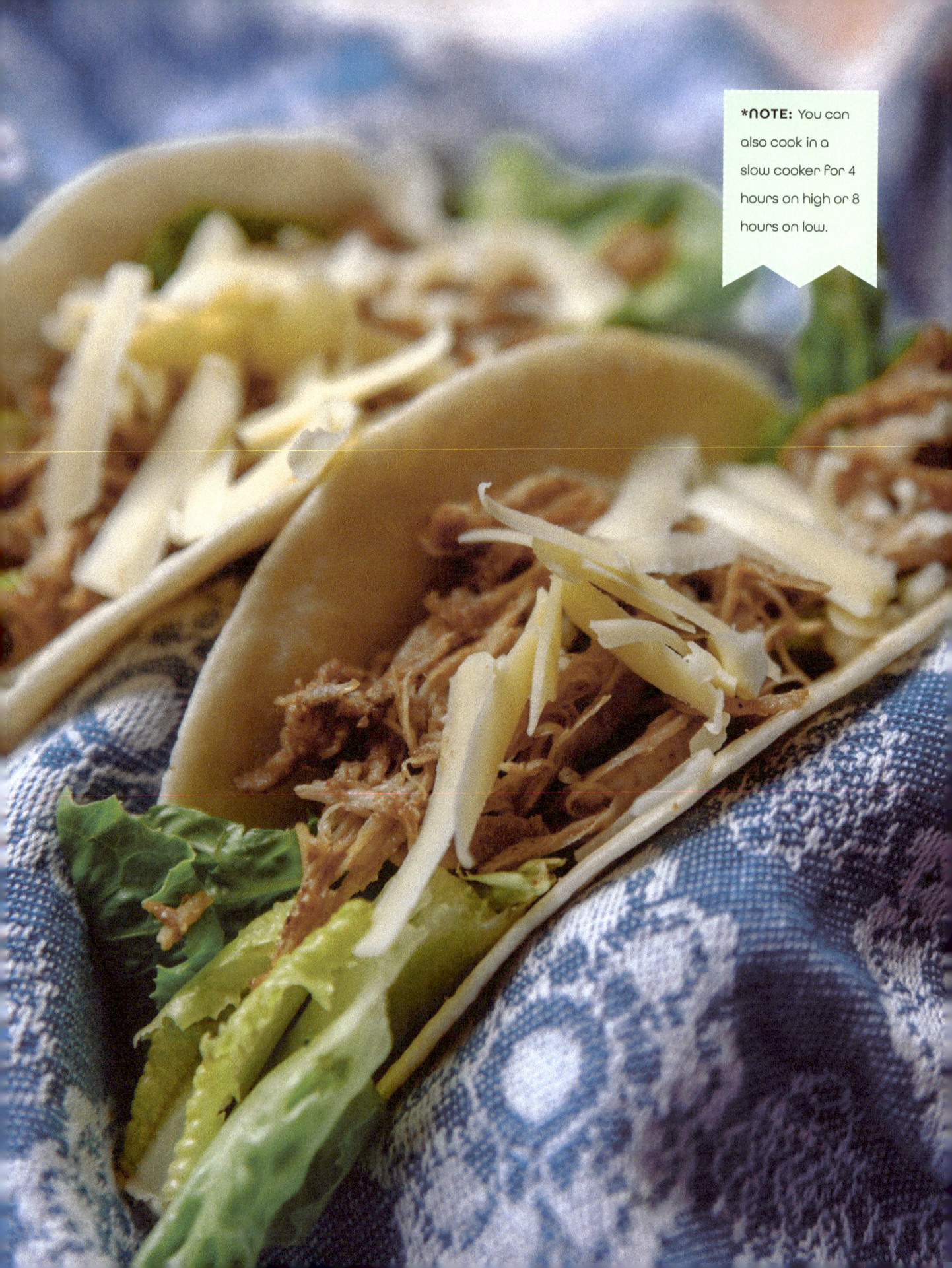

*NOTE: You can also cook in a slow cooker for 4 hours on high or 8 hours on low.

Shredded Taco Chicken

For endless lunch and dinner options

INGREDIENTS

1 pound boneless, skinless chicken thighs, preferably local

¼ cup water

2 tablespoons Taco Seasoning (page 239)

Kosher salt

INSTRUCTIONS

1. Add chicken thighs to an Instant Pot* along with ¼ cup water, Taco Seasoning, and a large sprinkle of salt.

2. Cook on the meat setting for 25 minutes. Once vented, remove lid and allow to cool for a few minutes.

3. Shred the chicken. Adjust seasoning, if needed.

Pork Dumplings

You can find dumpling wrappers in the refrigerated section of some grocery stores and most Asian markets. If you can't find dumpling wrappers, you can substitute wonton wrappers, which are square and a little thicker on the edges, so you will end up with more of a triangle shape when you make the dumplings.

YIELD: 60 DUMPLINGS

INGREDIENTS

1 pound ground pork

2 teaspoons fresh ginger, peeled and grated

6 cloves garlic, peeled and grated

1 bunch scallions, trimmed and finely sliced, about 1 cup

2 tablespoons coconut aminos

2½ cups cabbage, minced

2 eggs, divided

2 teaspoons kosher salt

Freshly ground pepper

60 dumpling wrappers

Sesame oil

INSTRUCTIONS

1. Combine the pork, ginger, garlic, scallions, coconut aminos, cabbage, 1 egg, salt, and some pepper in a bowl and mix well. Set aside.

2. For the egg wash, whisk the other egg in a small bowl with 1 tablespoon water. Set aside.

3. Lay the dumpling wrappers out on a clean work surface.

4. Place a small tablespoon of the pork mixture in the center of each and brush the edges with the egg wash. Fold the dumpling over and press the edges slightly to close in the filling.

5. To pan-sear, heat 1 tablespoon sesame oil in a skillet and once hot add the dumplings. You will have to do this in batches. Sear until golden-brown on one side then flip over.

6. After a minute or so on the other side add some water to the pan and cover with a lid. This will finish cooking the filling and soften the dumplings.

You could also cook the dumplings by *only* steaming them until the filling is fully cooked.

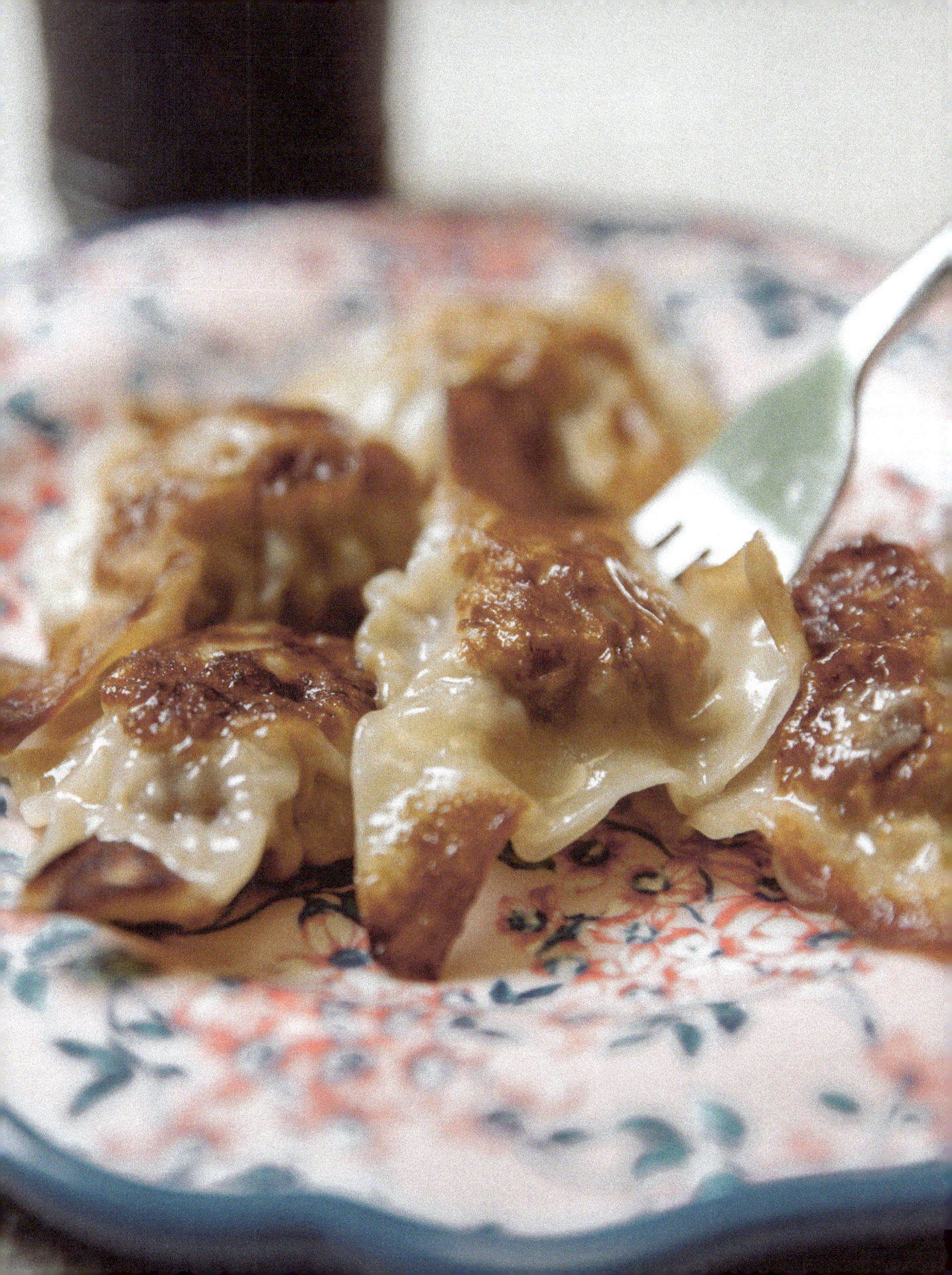

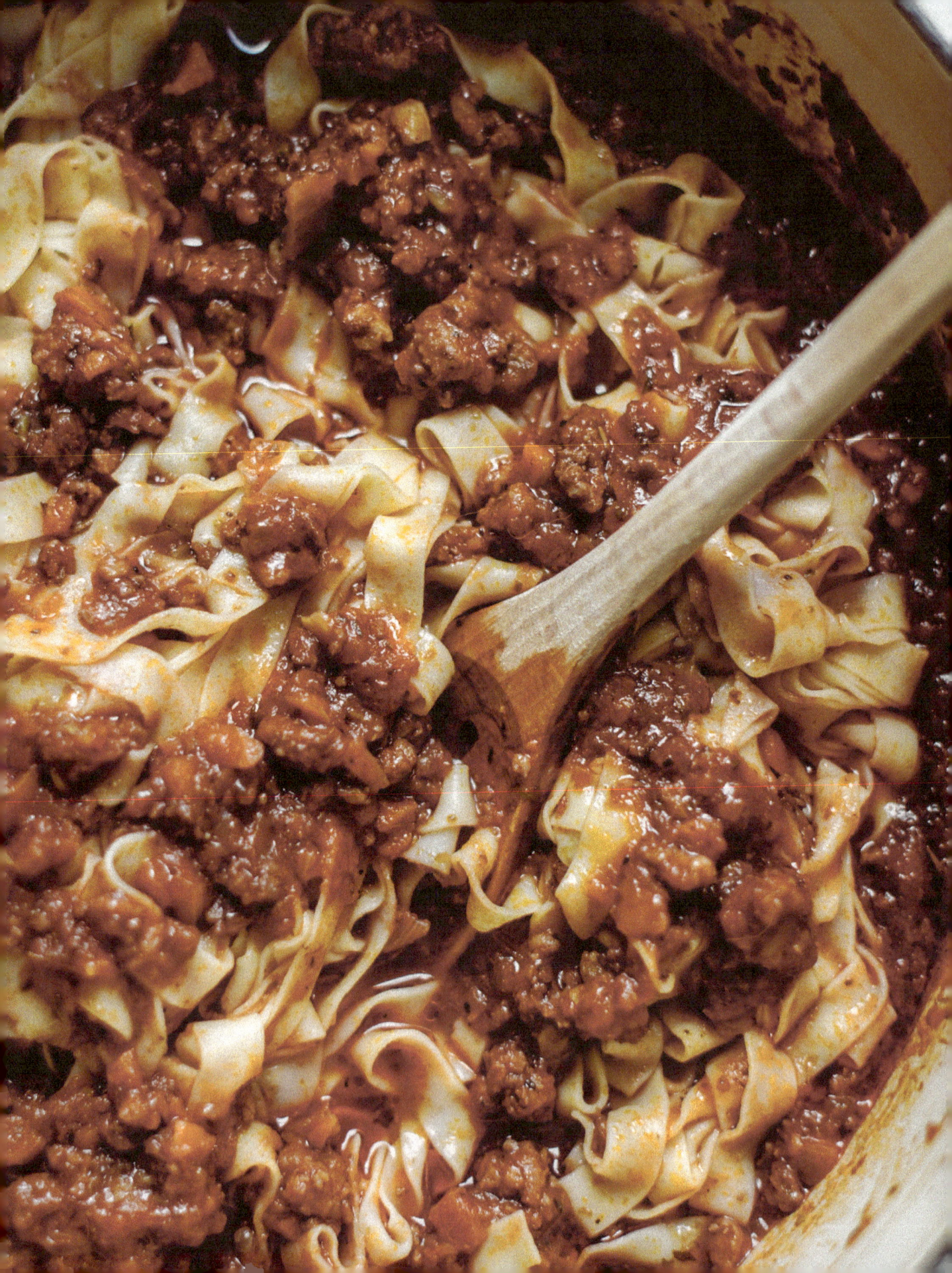

Pasta

Basic Pasta Dough 166

Fettuccine Noodles 167

Grandma Parker's Pasta Bolognese 169

Gnocchi 170

Creamy Gnocchi with Peas and Carrots 173

Pumpkin Gnocchi with Sage Brown Butter Sauce 174

Creamy Beet Pasta.. 177

Butternut Squash Fettuccine Alfredo 178

Spring Pea Ravioli 181

Sweet Corn Ravioli 182

Basic Pasta Dough

This dough recipe is similar to one I learned while working at La Porta dei Parchi, in Abruzzo, Italy. I was lucky enough to spend a few months at this beautiful place, making pasta and cheese and, of course, herding sheep.

YIELD: 4–6 SERVINGS

INGREDIENTS

270 grams 00 flour (approximately 1¾ cups flour)

3 medium eggs, lightly beaten

½ teaspoon olive oil

TIP: You can also place all ingredients in a stand mixer and mix with a dough hook until it forms a smooth ball. Finish kneading on a clean surface before wrapping in plastic wrap. Also, after wrapping the dough in plastic wrap to rest, you can place it in the fridge overnight and roll out the pasta the following day. If you do so, just bring the dough to room temperature for 1 hour before beginning to work with it.

INSTRUCTIONS

1. Place flour in a large mixing bowl. Make a hole in the center and add the eggs and oil. (You can also do this on a clean counter. Just make sure the hole in the center is deep enough so the eggs are contained.) Begin incorporating the flour using a fork to pull it into the center.

2. Once you can't see any raw egg and the mixture is crumbly, scoop the mixture out of the bowl and begin kneading the dough on a clean surface. This may take 10–15 minutes.

3. Continue kneading until the dough is smooth ("like a baby's bottom," as I learned in Italy) and all the crumbs are incorporated into the dough.

4. Wrap the dough in plastic wrap and set aside at room temperature for at least 20 minutes but ideally for 1 hour.

5. Once the dough has rested, you are ready to make your pasta shape of choice!

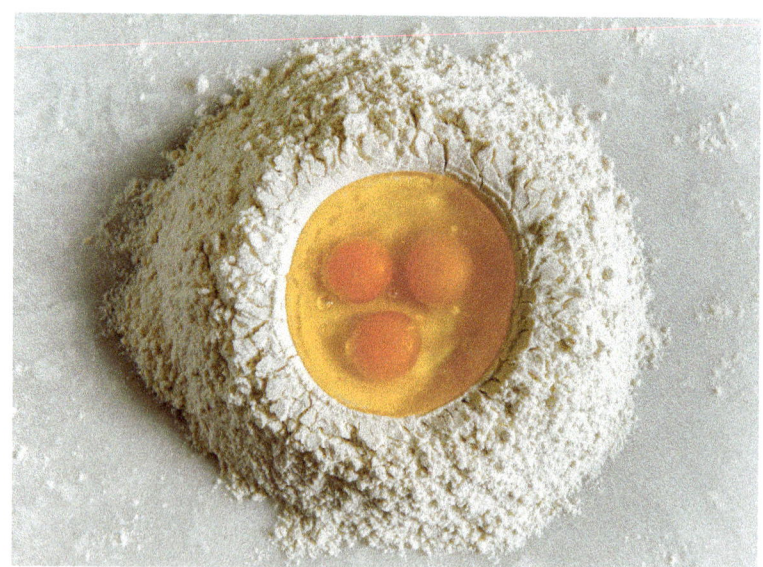

Fettuccine Noodles

The Basic Pasta Dough recipe (at left) makes for great fettuccine, and a pasta machine makes it easy peasy.

INSTRUCTIONS

1. To make fettuccine, take the pasta dough and follow the instructions on the pasta machine. You will only need to start with about ⅙ of the Basic Pasta Dough recipe. Keep the rest wrapped in plastic wrap or under a slightly damp towel until ready to use.

2. Make sure to start at the lowest number on the pasta machine (the widest the machine will go) and work your way up, not skipping any numbers. For the Atlas machine I stop at No. 8 when I am making fettuccine. Then flour the dough on both sides and feed it through the large fettuccini attachment. Dust with flour and make a nest with the noodles on a floured surface until ready to boil. You can also freeze the pasta at this point.

3. Boil noodles in salted water for about 5 minutes or until al dente.

4. Drain and toss with your sauce of choice before serving.

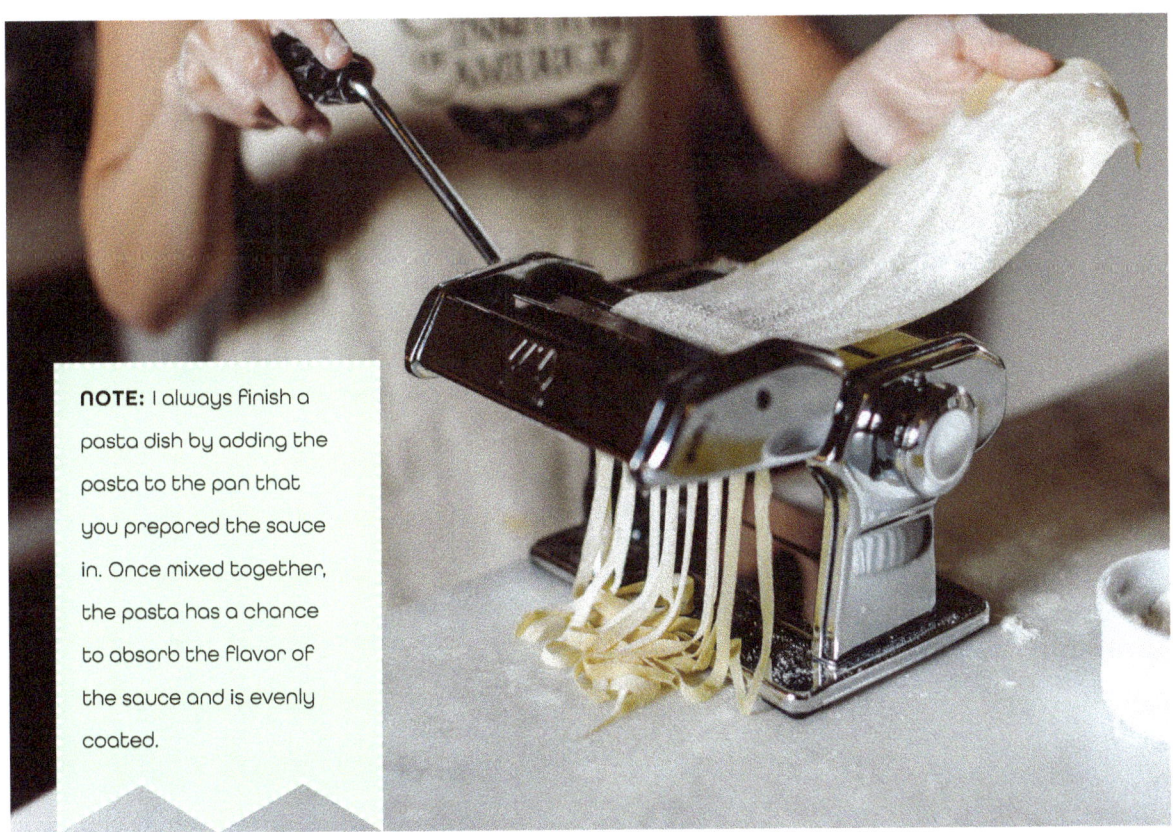

NOTE: I always finish a pasta dish by adding the pasta to the pan that you prepared the sauce in. Once mixed together, the pasta has a chance to absorb the flavor of the sauce and is evenly coated.

*NOTE: You can also cook the meat and vegetables in a large pot on the stove and transfer to a slow cooker to cook on high for 4 hours or low for 7-8 hours.

Bolognese Sauce

1 Onion chopped
2 strips bacon chopped
1 Rib celery chopped
1 carrot chopped
1 TB olive oil
1/2 lb. hot italian sausage (casing removed) or sweet + add cayene
1/2 lb. grd beef
1/2 cup white wine (or red)
1 1/2 cup beef stock
4 tsp tomato paste — 1/8 tsp nutmeg — S&P to taste

1/4 cup cream
3/4 lb. fettuccini or other egg pasta

Grandma Parker's Pasta Bolognese

The ultimate comfort food!

YIELD: 6 SERVINGS

INGREDIENTS

3 shallots, peeled

1 stalk celery

1 medium carrot

3 garlic cloves, peeled

½ pound ground beef, preferably local

½ pound Make Your Own Sausage (page 53) or substitute another ½ pound beef

Salt

2 tablespoons tomato paste

1 (15 oz) can crushed tomatoes

1 cup stock such as beef, turkey, or chicken, more if needed, preferably homemade (page 86), or non-MSG stock

1 tablespoon Italian seasoning

½ teaspoon dry sage or a couple teaspoons fresh sage minced

1 pound pasta, for serving

INSTRUCTIONS

1. Small-dice the shallots, celery, and carrot. Mince the garlic and set aside. Alternatively, you can rough-chop the shallots, celery, and carrot and pulse them in a food processor along with the garlic until almost minced. Set aside.

2. Using the sauté setting on the Instant Pot,* cook the ground beef and sausage. As it cooks, break it apart. Season with some salt. Continue cooking until the meat is cooked through and crumbly.

3. Add the vegetables and cook a few minutes until they start to soften, stirring occasionally.

4. Add the tomato paste and stir. Cook for a few minutes until the bottom of the pot starts to brown slightly.

5. Add the tomatoes and scrape the bottom of the pot, pulling up all the fond (brown bits) stuck to the bottom.

6. Add the stock, Italian seasoning, and sage. Stir to combine and adjust seasoning if needed.

7. Close the lid. Set to chili mode or manual for 30 minutes. Once done, allow to vent and remove lid. Adjust seasoning if needed.

8. Cook pasta according to package instructions and drain.

9. Toss Bolognese with pasta.

> **TIP:** To many people tomatoes may be a trigger, and they should not try this recipe. For some people, pressurized tomatoes in an Instant Pot will prevent tomatoes from being a headache trigger.

Gnocchi

These little fluffy Italian dumplings are some of my favorites. They pair well with most any sauce or can be used as a side to meat and vegetables. I have made gnocchi too many times to count. I encourage using a ricer or food mill so you don't overwork the potato.

YIELD: 4–6 SERVINGS

INGREDIENTS

4 medium or 3 large Russet potatoes

300 grams all-purpose flour (approximately 2 cups)

1 egg

TIP: Make sure you cook the potatoes until they are soft and fork-tender; otherwise, they will be hard to rice.

INSTRUCTIONS

1. Preheat oven to 400°F. Place potatoes on a sheet tray and pierce with a fork in a couple different places. Bake until fork-tender, 1 hour–1 hour 30 minutes, depending on their size. Remove and allow to cool slightly.

2. Cut the potatoes in half and pass through a ricer or food mill. Weigh 700 grams (or just under 5 cups) of the riced potato and cool completely. You can put the bowl of riced potato in the refrigerator to speed the process.

3. Add the flour and egg to the bowl with the cooled riced potato. Stir by hand until the ingredients come together and dump out on the counter. Or, you can place the ingredients in a stand mixer fitted with a paddle attachment and mix on low until the mixture comes together.

4. Knead the dough on a clean work surface, just until it forms a ball (you don't want to overknead the dough). It's OK if it sticks to your hands a little, but it should not stick to the counter. If it does, add a large pinch of flour.

5. Set the dough aside and cut off one piece, about ⅙ of the entire ball.

6. Begin rolling out into a ½-inch-wide rope. Make sure to NOT flour the surface at this point, or you won't have enough traction to stretch the rope. Once the rope of gnocchi is made, flour it and cut it into ¾-inch pieces with a bench scraper.

7. Place the pieces on a floured tray and either freeze or set off to the side to boil. Continue until all the gnocchi is formed.

8. To cook the gnocchi, place in a large pot of salted, lightly boiling water until they float to the top.

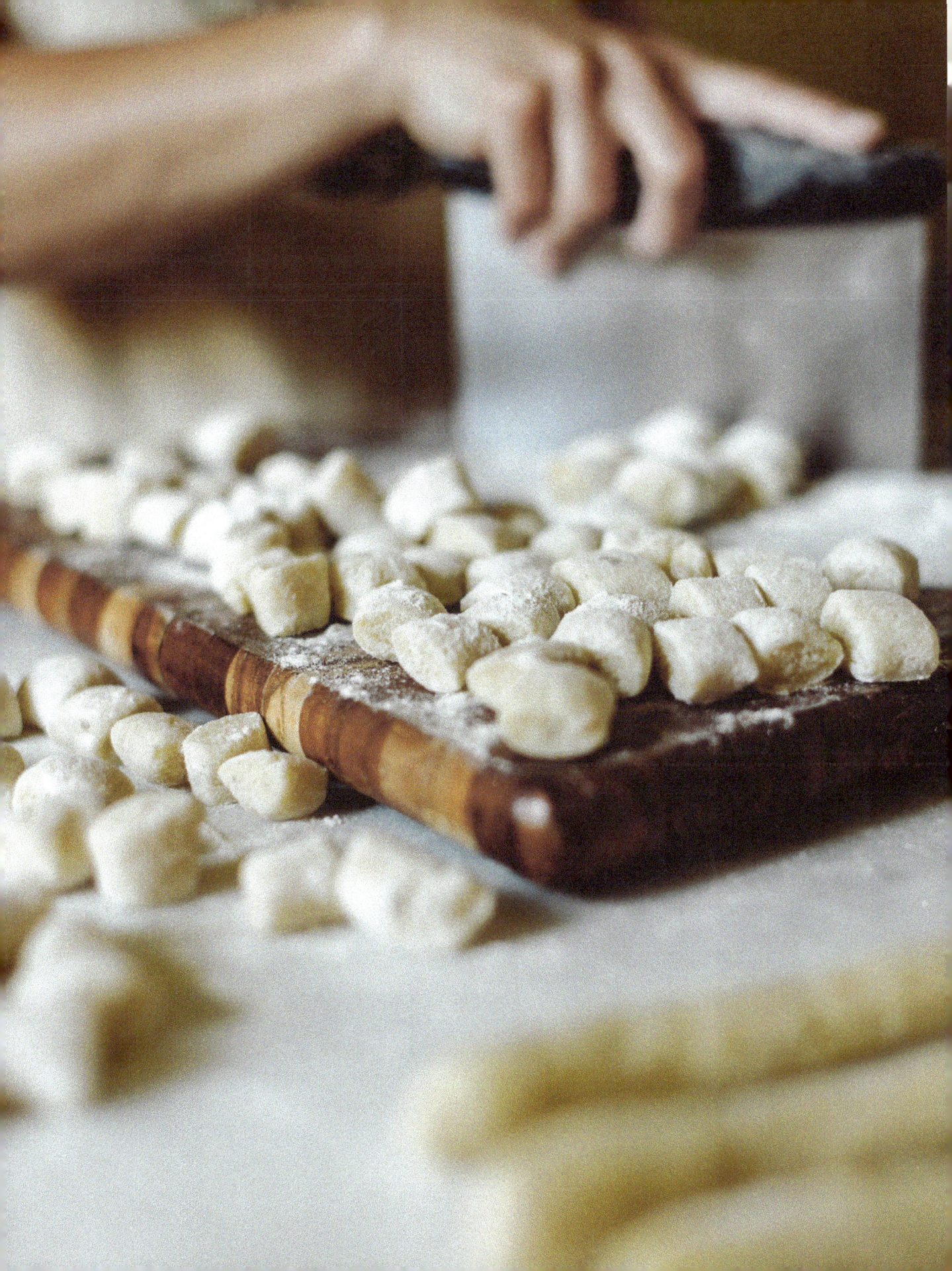

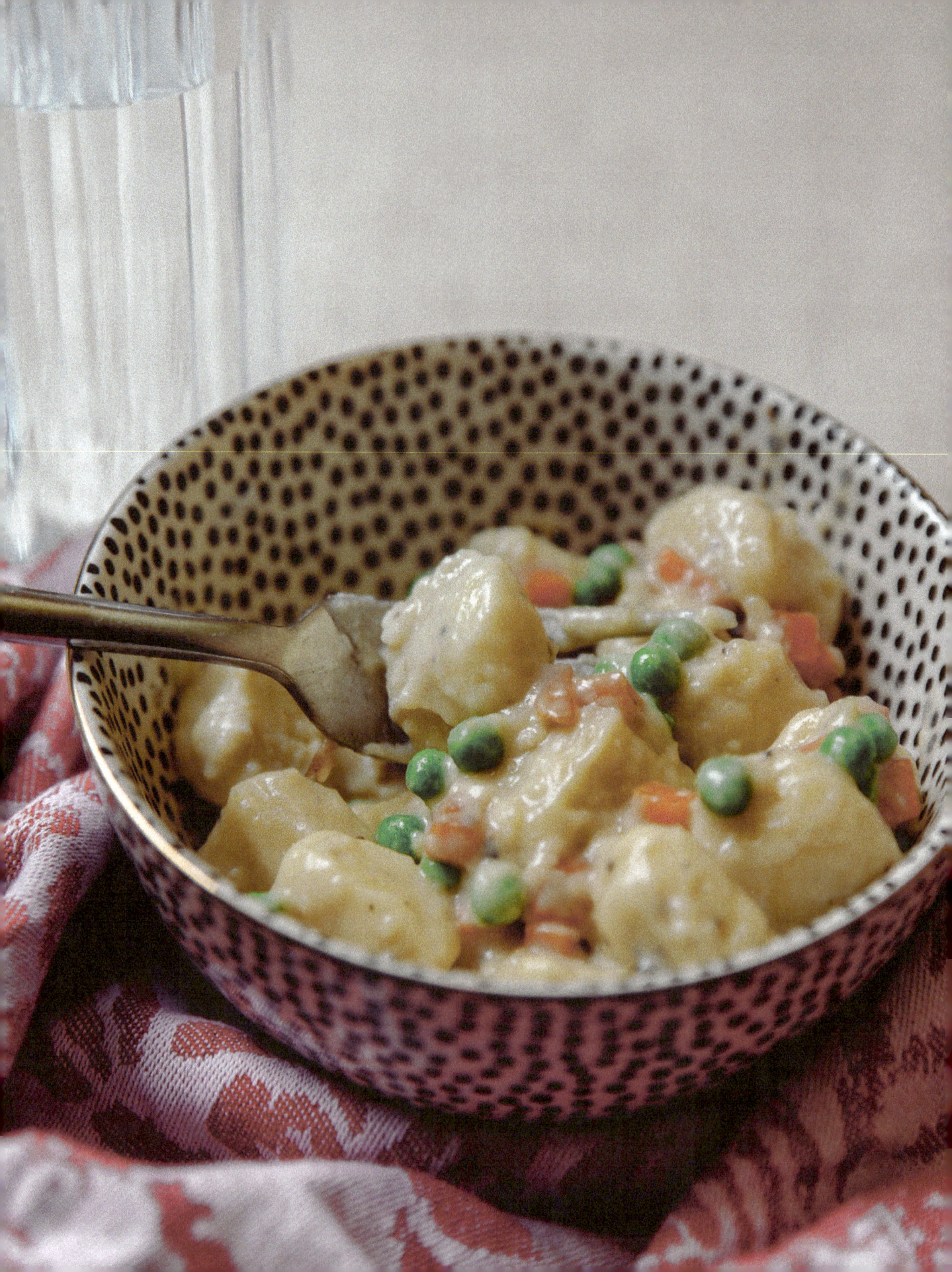

Creamy Gnocchi with Peas and Carrots

If you have gnocchi in the freezer, this dish can come together in about 20 minutes!

YIELD: 4–6 SERVINGS

INGREDIENTS

3 tablespoons butter, unsalted

3 cloves garlic, peeled and grated or minced

2 cups frozen peas and carrots

1 (8 oz) container mascarpone

1 tablespoon lemon juice (optional)

Kosher salt and freshly ground pepper

1 recipe Gnocchi (page 170)

INSTRUCTIONS

1. Place the butter in a large pan and melt over medium heat. Continue cooking until it starts to turn golden-brown. Add the garlic and cook for about 30 seconds, until fragrant.

2. Add the peas and carrots and cook for a couple minutes then turn off heat.

3. Add the mascarpone and lemon juice (if using) and season with salt and pepper. Stir to incorporate and soften the mascarpone.

4. Bring a large pot of water to a boil. Generously salt the water and drop gnocchi in. They will take a few minutes to cook and will slowly float to the top. Remove the gnocchi with a slotted spoon. You might have to gently scrape the bottom of the pot to make sure they don't stick. Reserve 1 cup pasta water for the sauce.

5. Add the cooked gnocchi to the sauce and stir. To thin the sauce, add pasta water ¼ cup at a time until you have reached the desired consistency. Adjust seasoning if needed.

Pumpkin Gnocchi with Sage Brown Butter Sauce

Always a crowd-pleasing dish

YIELD: 4–6 SERVINGS

INGREDIENTS

Gnocchi

3–4 medium–large Russet potatoes or 5 small–medium

¾ cup mashed pumpkin or pumpkin purée

300 grams all-purpose flour (about 2 cups)

1 egg

¼ teaspoon ground nutmeg

Sage Brown Butter Sauce

6 tablespoons butter, unsalted

1 bunch sage leaves (about 15 leaves), chopped

½ teaspoon red pepper flakes (optional)

Kosher salt and freshly ground pepper

TIP: You can compost the potato skins, or you can cook them in a little olive oil with salt and pepper over high heat until crispy on both sides for a snack.

INSTRUCTIONS

1. Preheat oven to 400°F. Place the potatoes on a sheet tray and pierce with a fork in a couple different places. Bake until fork-tender, 1 hour–1 hour 30 minutes, depending on their size. Remove and allow to cool slightly.

2. Cut the potatoes in half and pass through a ricer or food mill.

3. Weigh 500 grams (or approximately 3¾ cups) of the riced potato and cool completely. You can put the bowl of riced potatoes in the refrigerator to speed the process.

4. Place the riced potato in a large bowl along with the pumpkin, flour, egg, and nutmeg. Stir until the ingredients have come together and dump out on the counter.

5. Knead the dough on a clean work surface, just until it forms a ball, and all the crumbs are off the counter (you don't want to over-knead). It's OK if it sticks to your hands a little, but it should not stick to the counter. If it does, add a large pinch of flour.

6. Set the dough aside and cut off one piece, about ⅙ of the entire ball.

7. Begin rolling out into a ½-inch-wide rope. Make sure to NOT flour the surface at this point, or you won't have enough traction to stretch the rope. Once the rope of gnocchi is made, flour it and cut it into ¾-inch pieces with a bench scraper.

8. Place the pieces on a floured tray and either freeze or set off to the side to boil. Continue until all the gnocchi is formed.

9. Bring a large pot of water to a boil. Generously salt the water and drop gnocchi in. They will take a few minutes to cook and will slowly float to the top. Remove the gnocchi with a slotted spoon. You might have to gently scrape the bottom of the pot to make sure they don't stick. Reserve some pasta water for the sauce.

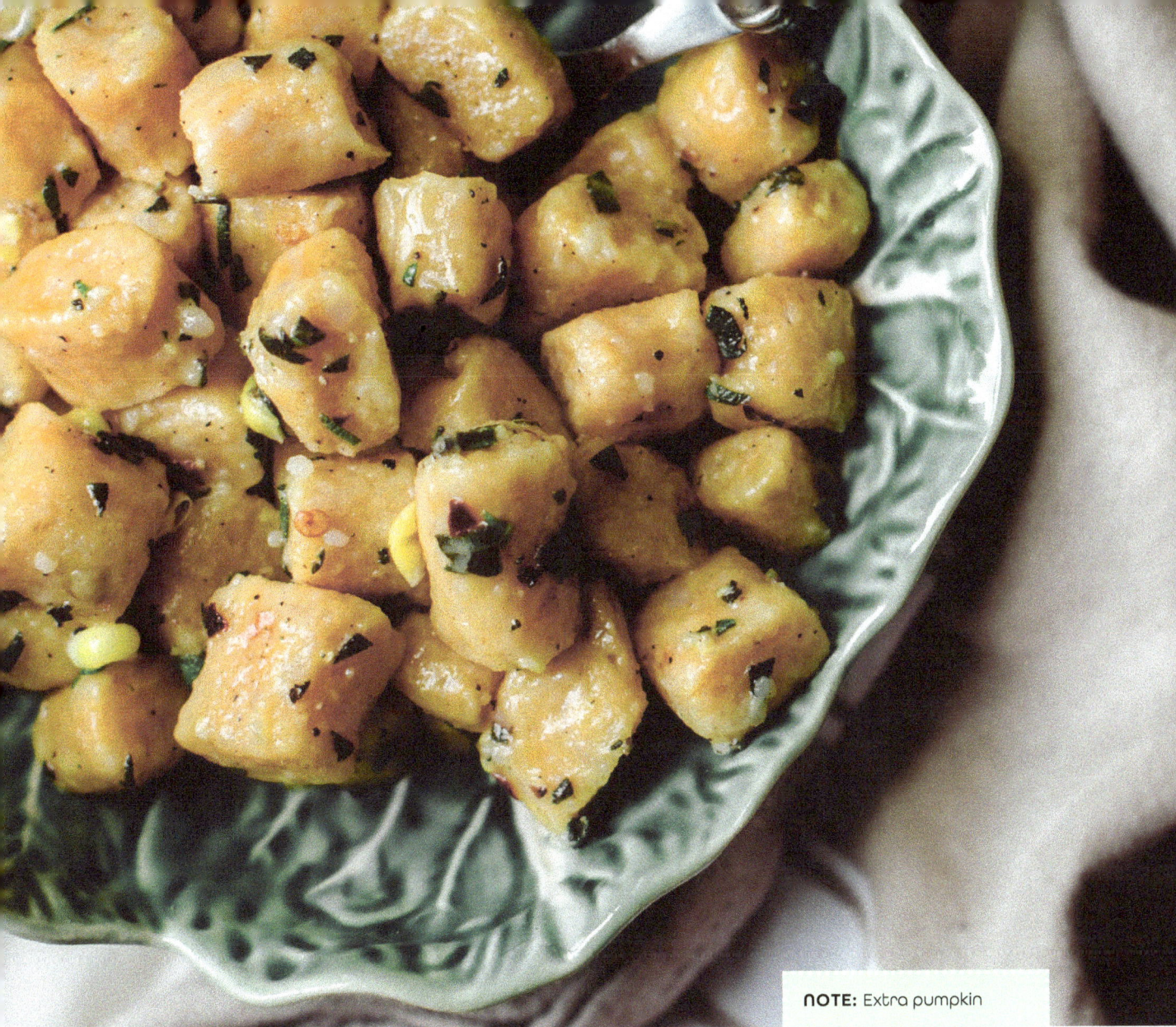

NOTE: Extra pumpkin purée can be used in a smoothie, muffins, pasta sauce, or frozen.

10. Meanwhile, make the sage brown butter sauce by placing the butter in a large pan and melt over medium heat. Continue cooking until it starts to brown, then turn heat off.

11. Add the chopped sage and red pepper flakes (if using) along with some salt and pepper.

12. Add the cooked gnocchi to the sauce and stir, adjusting the seasoning if needed. (I like to add ¼ cup pasta water to the gnocchi before serving.)

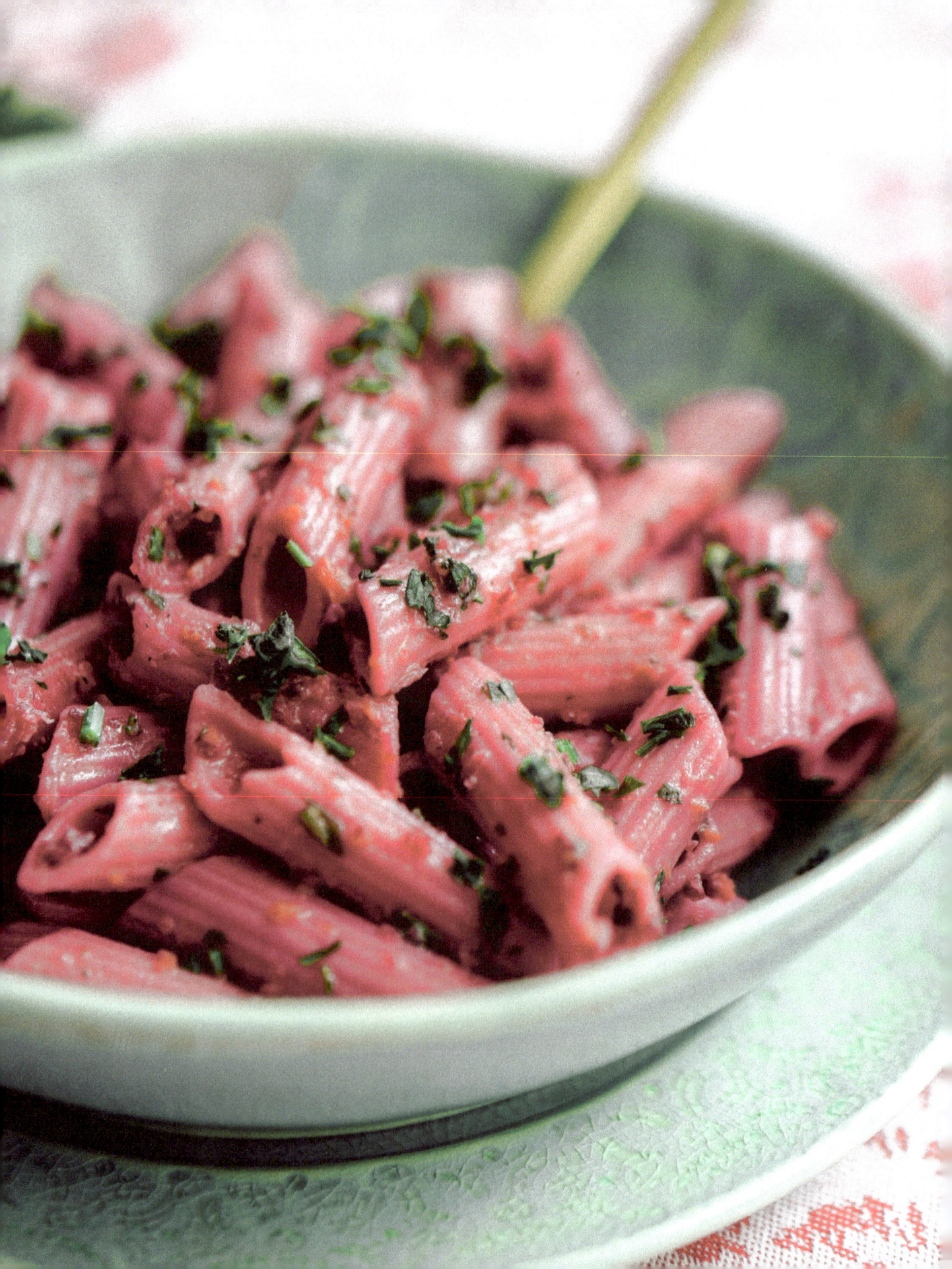

Creamy Beet Pasta

Beets are a superfood for good reason. They are loaded with vitamins and minerals, have a delicious earthy yet sweet flavor, and add a beautiful color to any dish.

YIELD: 4 SERVINGS

INGREDIENTS

1 pound pasta, uncooked, such as bow tie or penne

1 medium beet, raw, peeled and chopped

1 carrot, chopped

1 (5.3 oz) package Boursin cheese

Handful fresh parsley, finely chopped

Kosher salt and freshly ground pepper

INSTRUCTIONS

1. Preheat oven to 400°F. Place the chopped beet and carrot in an oven-safe dish such as a loaf pan along with ½ cup water. Cover with foil and bake for around 35 minutes or until the vegetables are fork-tender. (It may take longer depending on how big the chunks are.)

2. Meanwhile, cook the pasta according to the package instructions, reserving 1 cup pasta water.

3. Allow the vegetables to cool once removed from the oven and add to a high-speed blender along with the cheese, some salt and pepper, and ½ cup of the beet juice left over from baking. Blend until smooth.

4. In a large bowl combine the pasta, beet mixture, chopped parsley, and ½ cup reserved pasta water. Stir to combine. Adjust seasoning if needed and add up to ½ cup more pasta water depending on desired consistency.

Butternut Squash Fettuccine Alfredo

This is one of my favorite dishes for the fall and winter. I love the sweet and slightly nutty taste you get from incorporating butternut squash into this sauce.

YIELD: 4–6 SERVINGS
(MAKES 2½ CUPS
SAUCE)

INGREDIENTS

2 cups of 1-inch peeled and cubed butternut squash

Olive oil

Kosher salt and freshly ground pepper

1 pound pasta, such as fettuccini or pappardelle

¾ cup ricotta cheese

½ cup vegetable or chicken stock, preferably homemade (pages 84, 86), or non-MSG stock

Dash of ground nutmeg

2 tablespoons chopped fresh sage leaves, chopped

2 tablespoons parsley, chopped

2 tablespoons chives, sliced thin

INSTRUCTIONS

1. Preheat oven to 400°F and line a baking tray with a Silpat mat or parchment paper.

2. Place the butternut squash on the baking tray and drizzle with some olive oil. Toss with salt and pepper and spread out on the sheet tray. Bake for 20–25 minutes or until the squash is fork-tender. Remove from oven and allow to cool slightly.

3. Cook the pasta according to the directions, reserving 1 cup of pasta water when you drain the noodles.

4. Meanwhile, place the cooled squash in a high-speed blender along with the ricotta, stock, nutmeg, and some salt and pepper. Blend until smooth.

5. Once the pasta is drained, add it along with the squash purée, sage, parsley, and half the chives to a skillet or pot and toss. I usually use the same pot I cooked the pasta in.

6. Adjust seasoning and reheat gently if needed. Top with the remaining chives and serve.

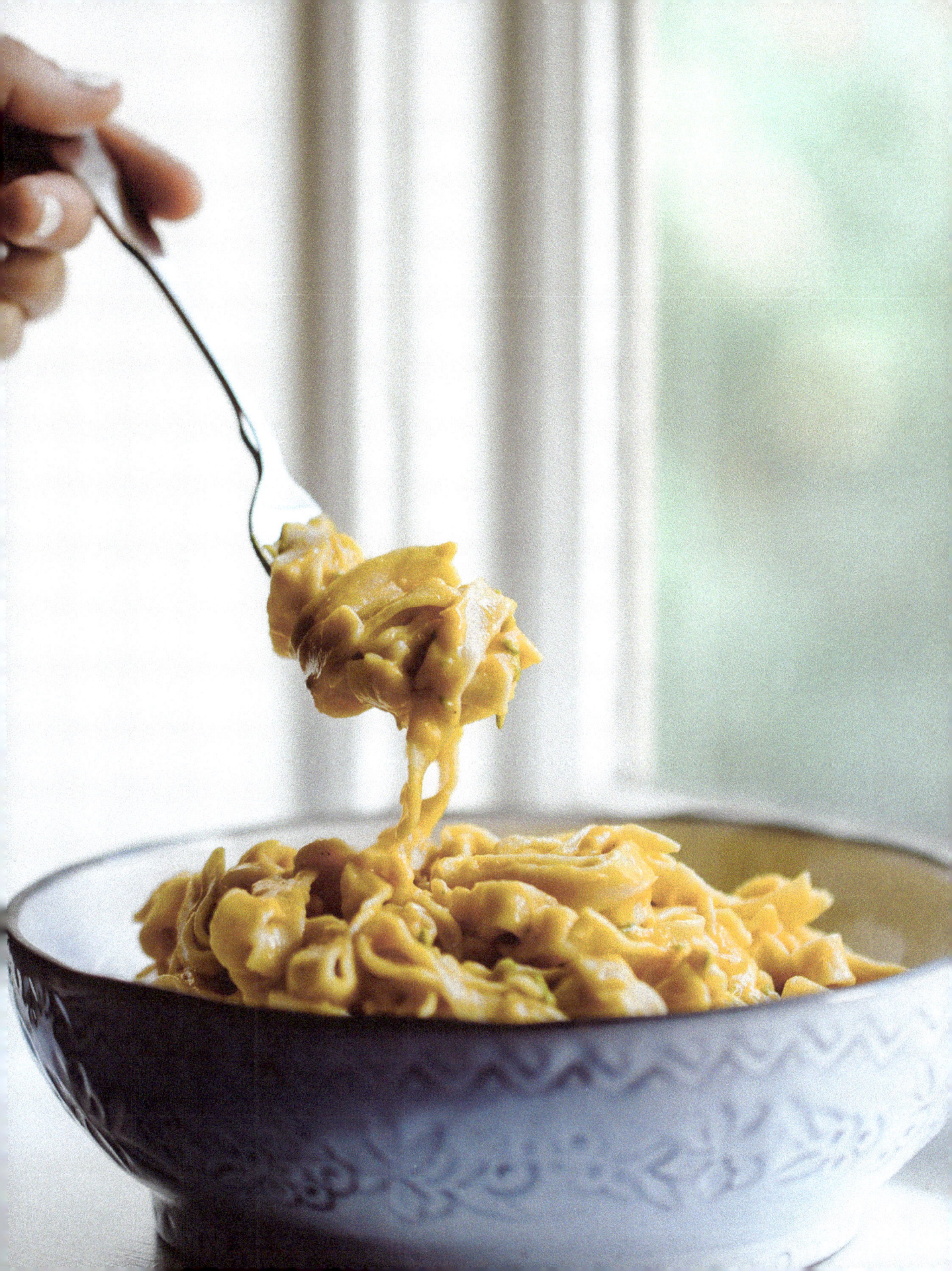

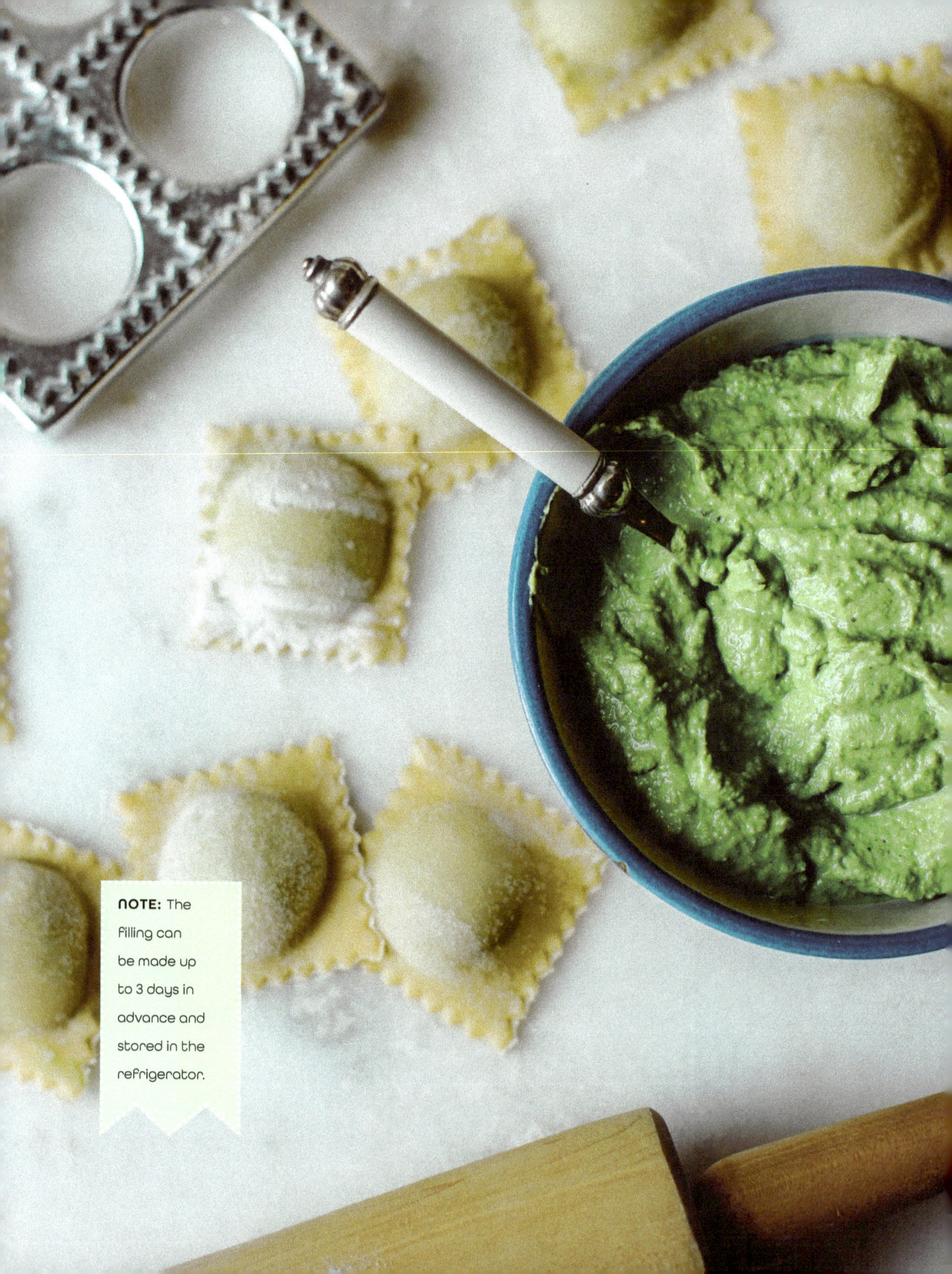

NOTE: The filling can be made up to 3 days in advance and stored in the refrigerator.

Spring Pea Ravioli

For a beautiful ravioli filling

YIELD: 4–6 SERVINGS

INGREDIENTS

Filling

2 cups shelled fresh peas

1 cup fresh ricotta cheese

½ cup basil leaves, packed

⅛ teaspoon grated nutmeg

½ teaspoon kosher salt and
   some freshly ground pepper

Pasta Dough

1 recipe Pasta Dough
   (page 166)

1 egg, lightly beaten for egg
   wash

INSTRUCTIONS

Filling

1. Bring water to a boil in a medium pot.
2. Add the peas and cook (only about 2 minutes).
3. Drain and transfer the peas directly to an ice bath to stop the cooking. Drain when cooled.
4. In a food processor combine the peas, ricotta, basil, nutmeg, salt, and some pepper. Purée until almost smooth but still a little chunky.
5. Set it aside until you are ready to fill ravioli.

Pasta Dough

1. Roll out the ravioli, following the instructions on the pasta machine.
2. Once you get to the desired thickness, place the sheet of pasta on a lightly floured surface.
3. Place 1 tablespoon of filling in the center of the pasta, leaving at least 1 inch between tablespoons.
4. Brush edges with egg wash and top with another layer of pasta. Or you can fold the top half of the ravioli sheet over the filling, then press down on the edges, trying to get all the air out around the filling.
5. Cut and set aside. You have the option to freeze the ravioli at this point.
6. Cook in boiling salted water until al dente, or about 5 minutes. Drain and toss with your favorite sauce, or simply drizzle with extra virgin olive oil and sprinkle with salt and pepper.

Sweet Corn Ravioli

Because, when it's in season, I always seem to buy a big bundle of corn at the farmers market, when I need only 4–6 ears.

YIELD: 4–6 SERVINGS

INGREDIENTS

Filling

1 tablespoon olive oil

3 ears of sweet corn, shucked and taken off cob (about 2½ cups)

1 large shallot, peeled and small-diced

¼ cup fresh basil leaves, packed

1 cup fresh ricotta cheese

Kosher salt and freshly ground pepper

Pasta Dough

1 recipe Pasta Dough (page 166)

1 egg, lightly beaten for egg wash

INSTRUCTIONS

Filling

1. Heat olive oil over medium heat in a sauté pan. Add the corn and shallot.
2. Continue cooking 5–10 minutes until corn is cooked. Turn off heat.
3. Add half the basil and ricotta. Season with salt and pepper.
4. Place the filling in a food processor and pulse for about 20 seconds until almost smooth. Set aside until ready to fill raviolis.

Pasta Dough

1. Roll out the ravioli, following the instructions on the pasta machine.
2. Once you get to the desired thickness, place the sheet of pasta on a lightly floured surface.
3. Place 1 tablespoon of filling in the center of the pasta, leaving at least 1 inch between tablespoons.
4. Brush edges with egg wash and top with another layer of pasta. Or you can fold the top half of the ravioli sheet over the filling then press down on the edges, trying to get all the air out around the filling.
5. Cut and set aside. You have the option to freeze the ravioli at this point.
6. Cook in a large pot of salted boiling water until al dente, or approximately 5–6 minutes. The ravioli is great tossed with the Sage Brown Butter Sauce (page 174) or Mascarpone Herb Sauce (page 226).

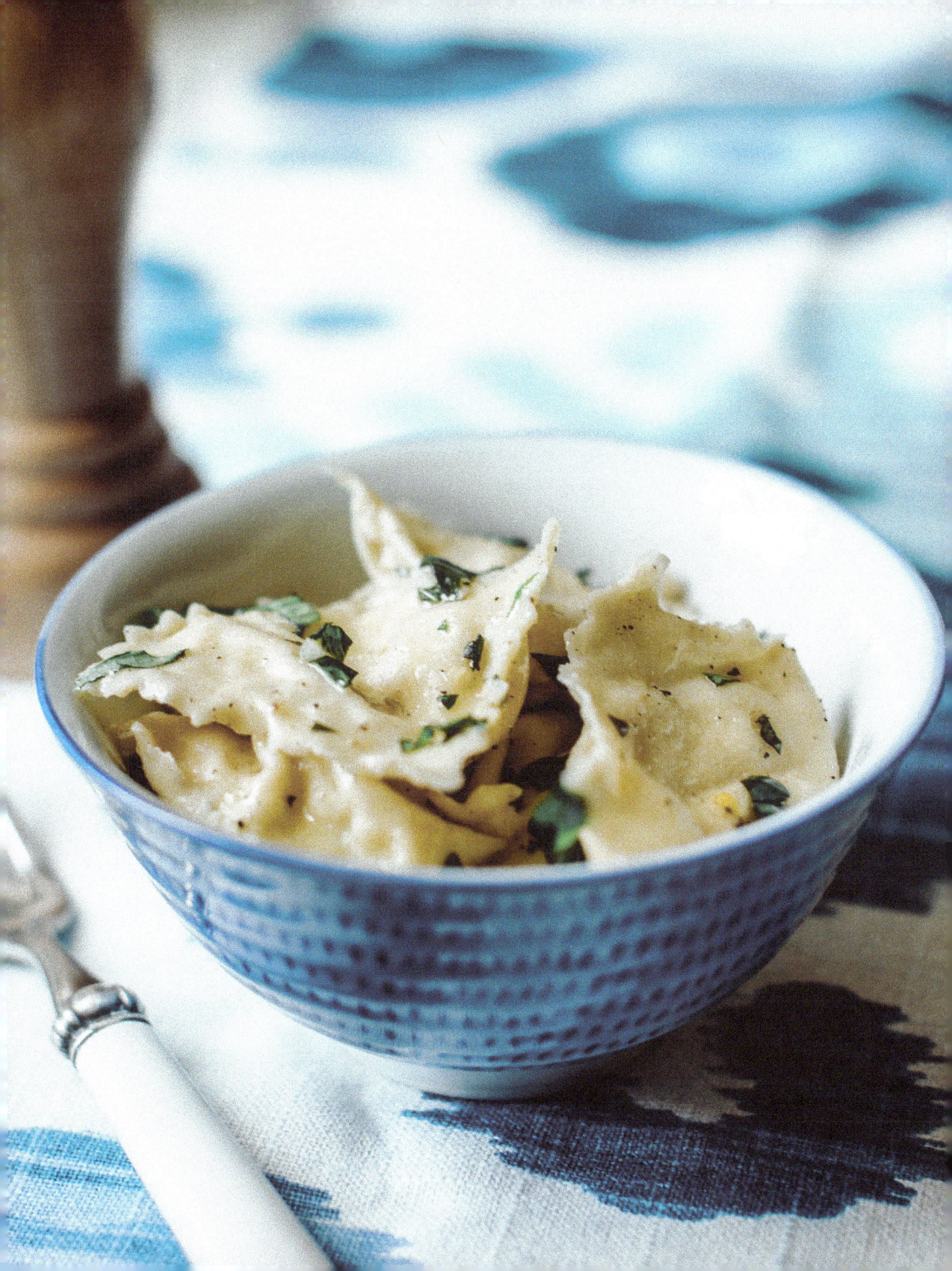

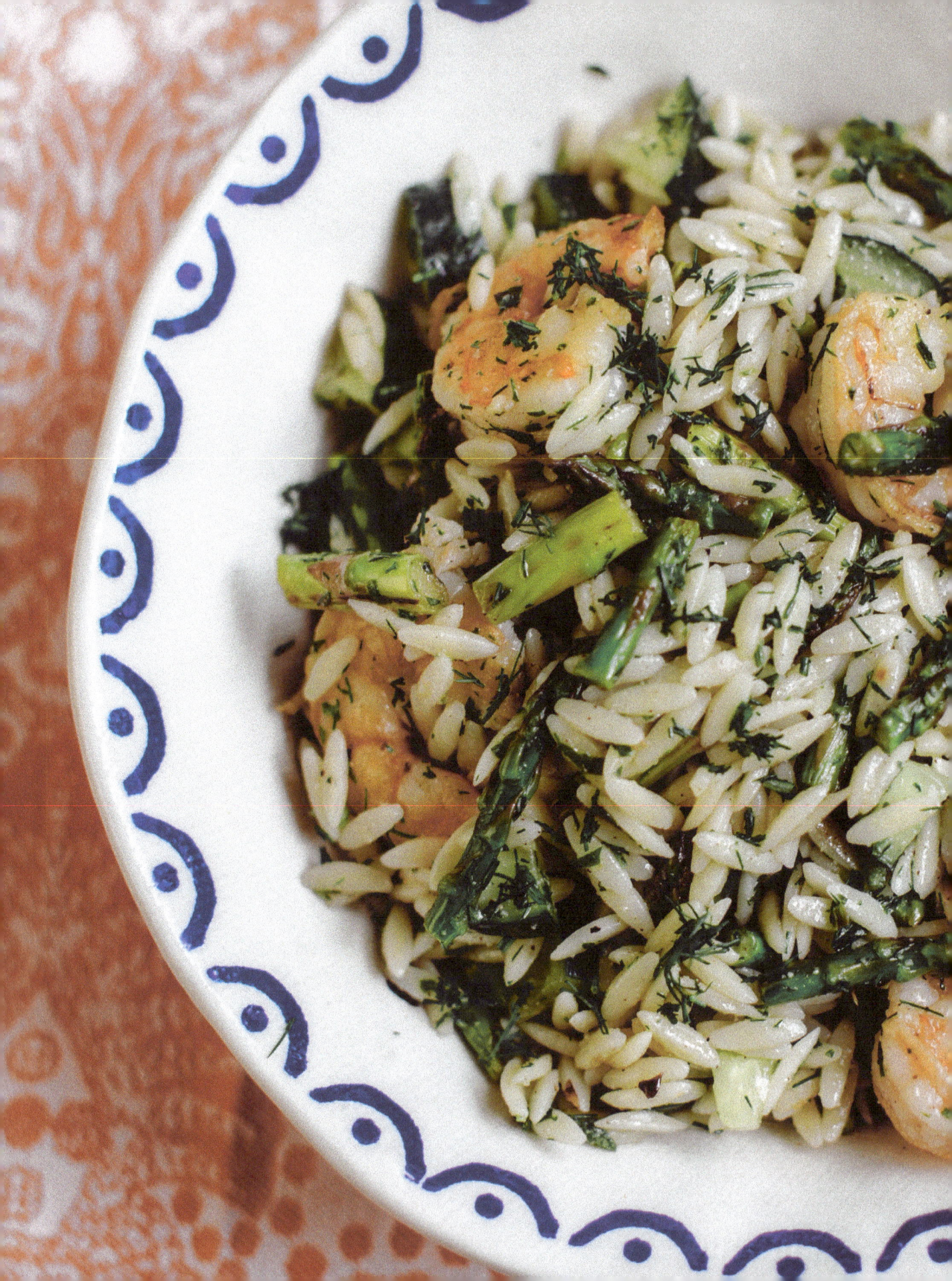

Seafood

Glazed Salmon Quinoa Bowl 186

Coconut-Crusted Fish Tacos with Mango Salsa 189

Ultimate Salmon Burgers...190

Fish en Papillote...193

Grilled Shrimp and Asparagus Salad 194

Glazed Salmon Quinoa Bowl

Because store-bought preglazed anything is typically not migraine-friendly

INGREDIENTS

1 recipe Ginger Glaze, uncooked (page 233)

4 wild-caught salmon fillets, about 6 oz each

Quinoa, to serve

Roasted vegetables to serve, such as asparagus or broccoli (page 202)

2 tablespoons sesame oil or olive oil

Salt and freshly ground pepper

Sesame seeds, to serve (optional)

INSTRUCTIONS

1. Add the Ginger Glaze to a shallow dish and add the salmon, flesh side down. Marinate for 20 minutes.

2. Meanwhile, cook the quinoa and roast your vegetables.

3. Remove the salmon from the marinade and pat with a paper towel.

4. Heat the oil in a large skillet and season the salmon lightly with salt and pepper. Once oil is heated add salmon flesh side down. Cook for a couple of minutes over medium heat, then flip over and cook until the salmon is cooked through. Set salmon aside to rest. Cook the ginger glaze in the same skillet until slightly thickened, stirring occasionally.

5. Place the quinoa, vegetables, and salmon into a bowl. Drizzle with ginger glaze and top with sesame seeds (if using) to serve.

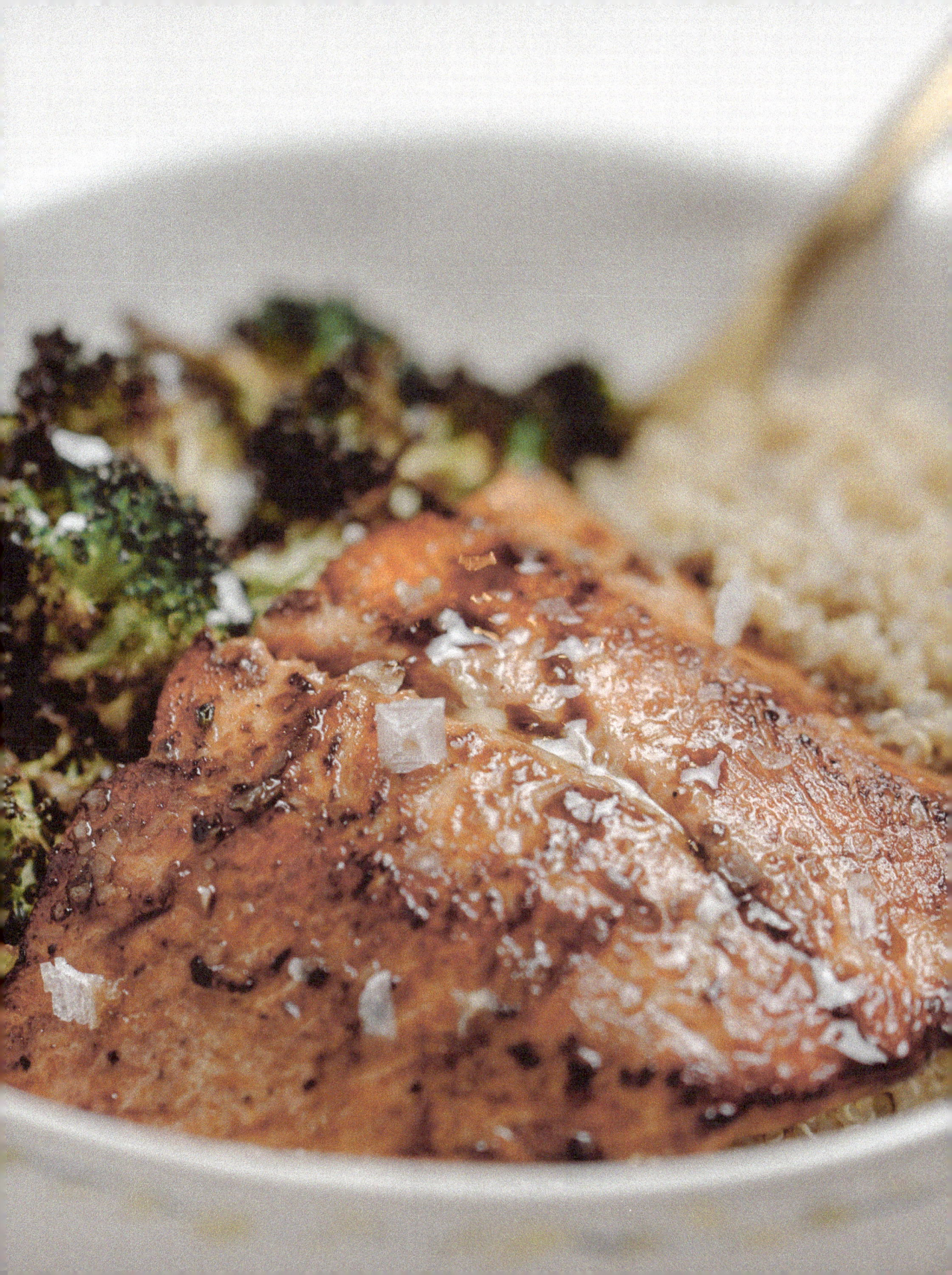

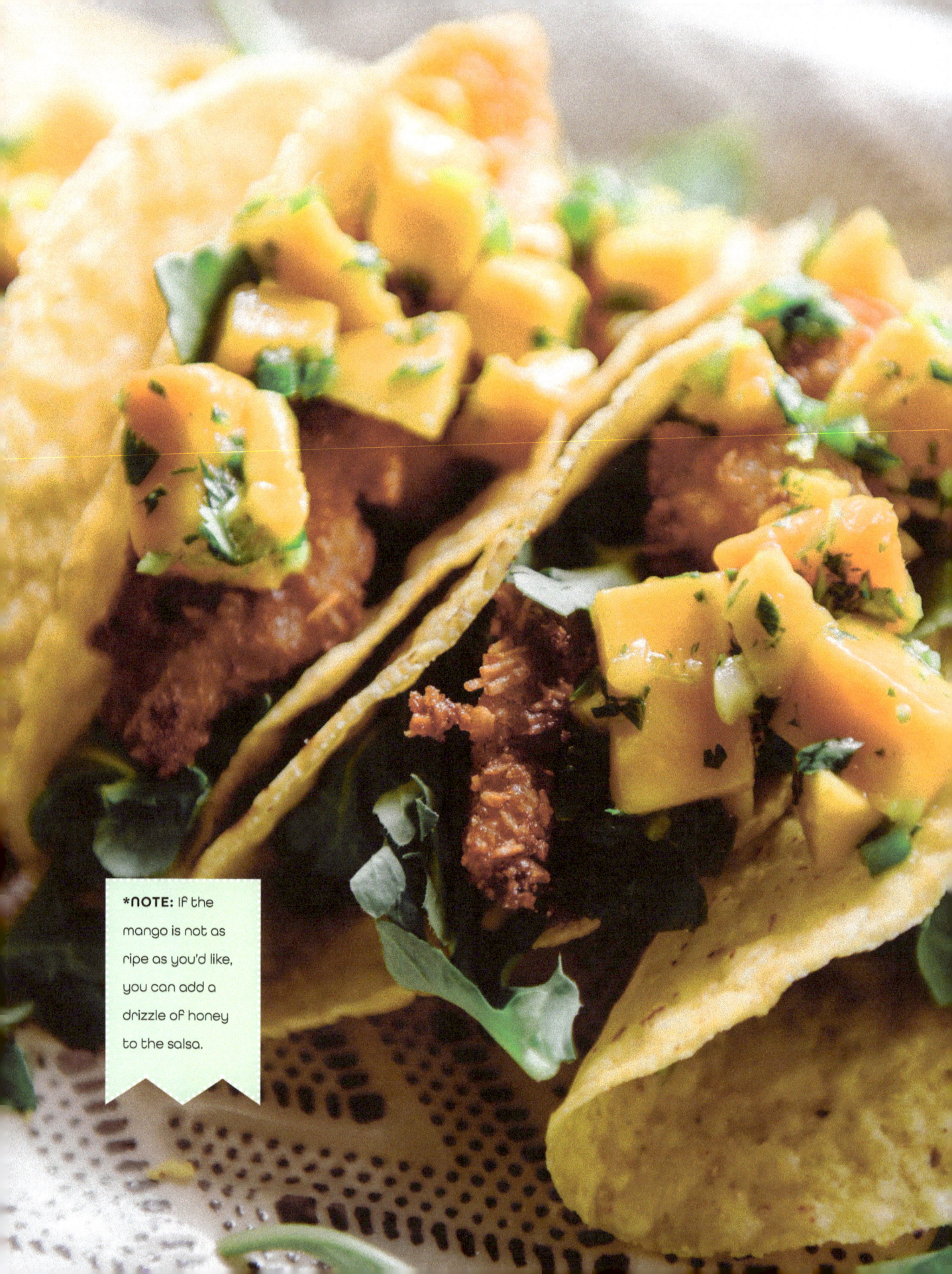

*NOTE: If the mango is not as ripe as you'd like, you can add a drizzle of honey to the salsa.

Coconut-Crusted Fish Tacos with Mango Salsa

I could eat (fresh) fish tacos every day and never get tired of them. Bonus points if they are served outside with a cold beer on a warm day near a large body of water!

YIELD: 4 SERVINGS

INGREDIENTS

Mango Salsa

1 cup fresh ripe mango, diced*

½–1 jalapeño (depending on heat preference), minced

1 tablespoon cilantro, chopped

1 tablespoon parsley, chopped

1 scallion, trimmed and finely diced

Salt and pepper

Fish

1 pound fresh fish such as mahi, wahoo, or halibut, skin off

Kosher salt and freshly ground pepper

1 egg, lightly beaten

1 tablespoon coconut sugar

⅔ cup finely shredded coconut

¼ cup panko breadcrumbs

About ¼ cup high-heat oil such as avocado oil

Assembly

Mixed greens or shredded iceberg lettuce

Corn or flour tortillas or taco shells

INSTRUCTIONS

1. For the salsa, combine all ingredients in a bowl and season to taste with salt and pepper. Set aside until ready to use or refrigerate for up to 3 days.

2. Check for any pin bones in the fish and cut into 1-inch pieces. Place in a bowl and season with salt and pepper.

3. Add the egg to the fish and mix.

4. In a separate bowl, combine the sugar, coconut, and panko. Mix thoroughly.

5. Transfer the egg-coated pieces of fish to the coconut mixture and coat. Make sure most of the fish is coated.

6. In a shallow pan, heat the oil. Once hot, place fish pieces in a single layer (not crowding the pan) and cook until brown. Flip over and cook on the other side until the fish is cooked through.

7. Allow to cool slightly on a wire rack.

8. To assemble tacos, place greens in the tortillas or taco shells, then the fish, and top with salsa.

Ultimate Salmon Burgers

Pescatarians, this burger is for you!

YIELD: 4 PATTIES

INGREDIENTS

1 pound wild-caught salmon, skin on and pin bones removed

1 large egg

⅓ cup breadcrumbs or gluten-free breadcrumbs

1 shallot, peeled and minced

1 tablespoon chopped fresh dill

¼ cup chopped fresh parsley

1 teaspoon Dijon mustard

½ lemon, juiced (optional)

1 large clove garlic, peeled and grated or minced

1 teaspoon kosher salt and freshly ground pepper

1 tablespoon olive oil

Assembly

1 cup greens, such as spinach or arugula (optional)

Sriracha mayo (1 tablespoon sriracha mixed with 4 tablespoons mayonnaise)

4 hamburger buns

INSTRUCTIONS

1. Dice the salmon in half-inch pieces and add to a medium–large mixing bowl.

2. Add the egg, breadcrumbs, shallot, herbs, Dijon, lemon juice (if using), and garlic to the bowl and season with salt and pepper. Stir to combine, form into 4 patties, and place in the fridge for about 15 minutes.

3. Heat 1 tablespoon olive oil over high heat in a skillet and once hot add the patties.

4. Sear the patties until golden-brown and flip to do the same on the other side until cooked through.

5. Serve with toppings and buns of choice.

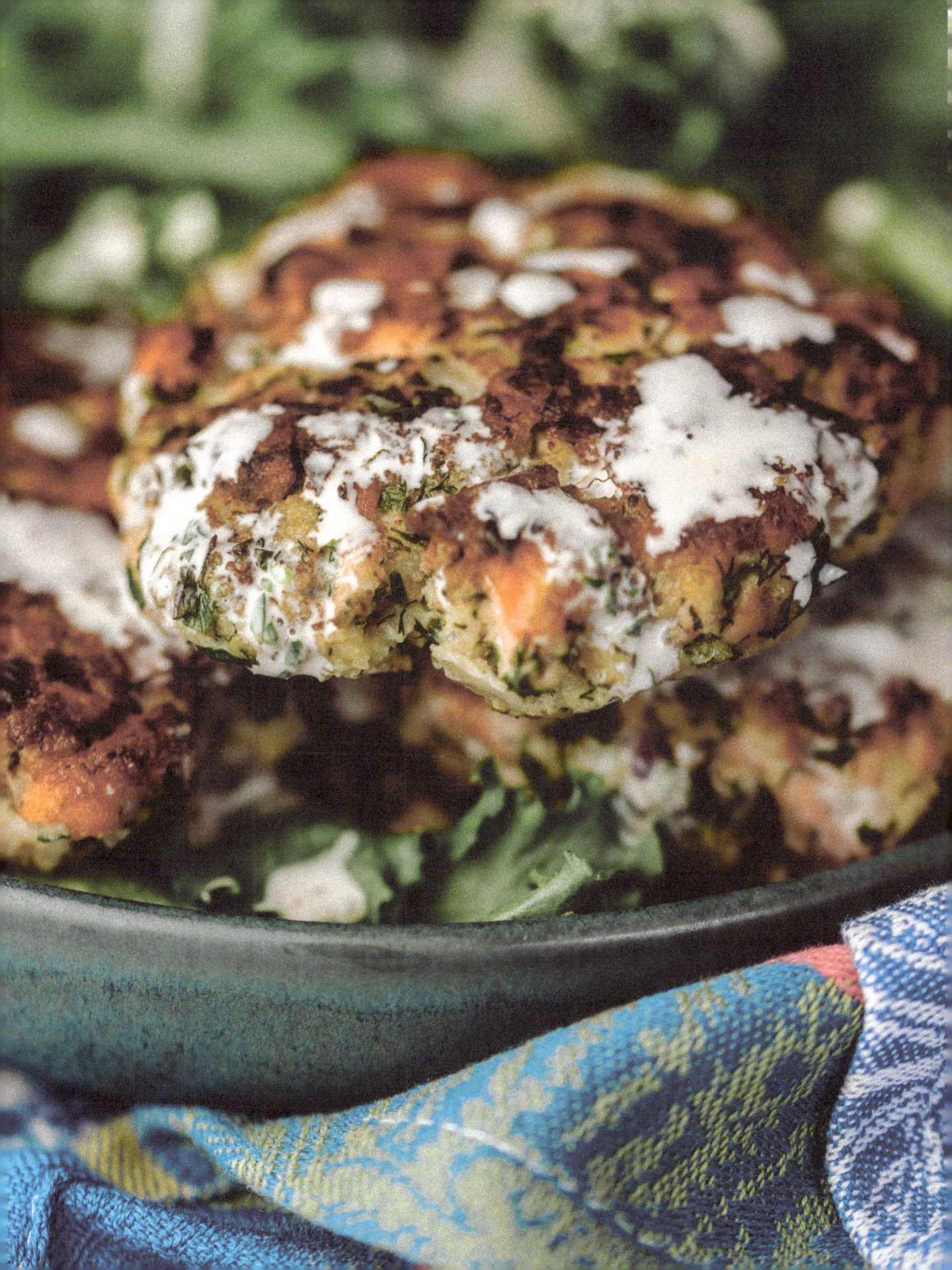

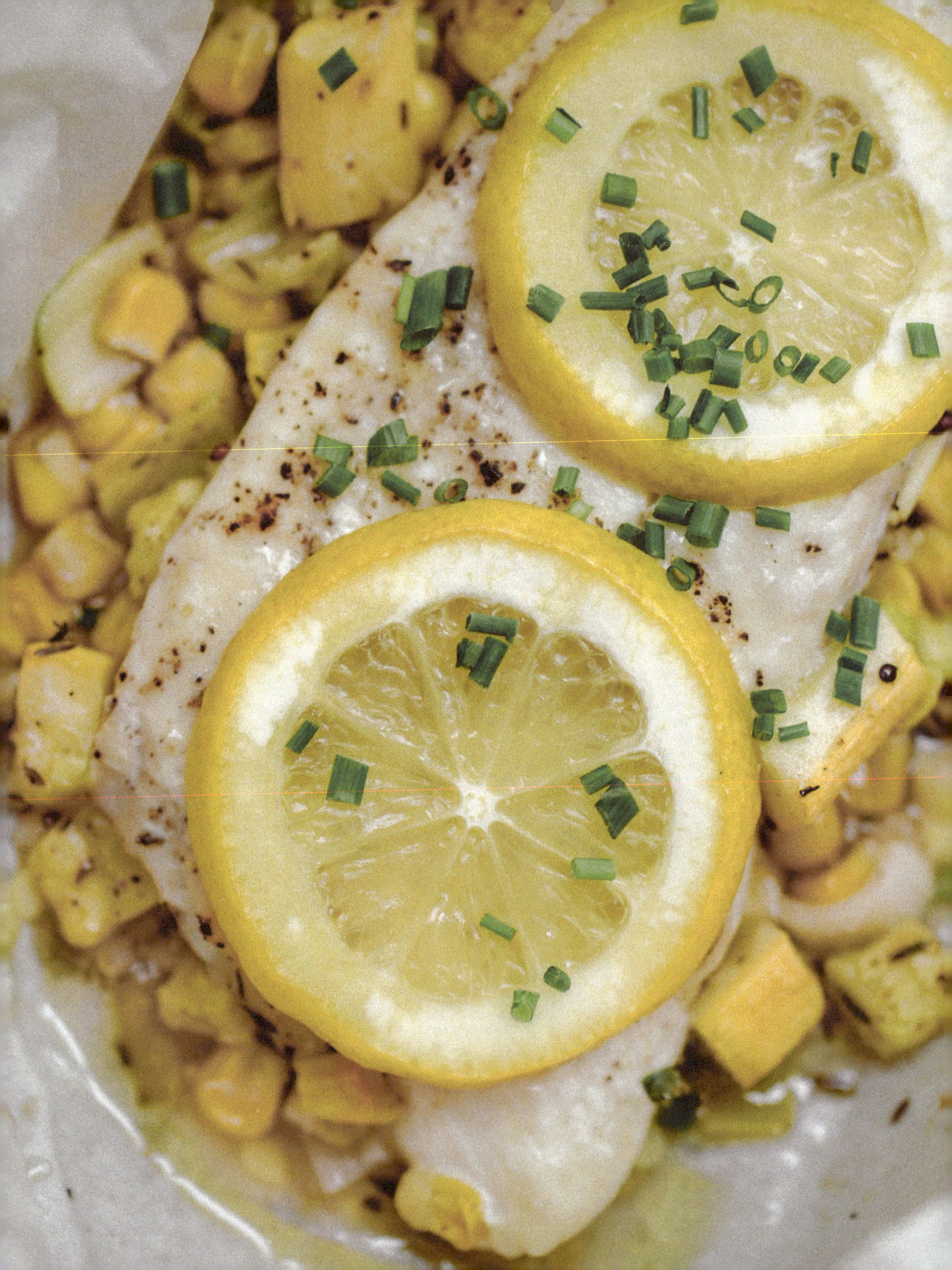

Fish en Papillote

"En papillote" is a French technique for cooking within a packet of parchment paper. Foil works as well.

YIELD: 4 SERVINGS

INGREDIENTS

2 small summer squash, cut into half-moons

2 ears of corn, shucked and corn cut off the cob

1 leek, washed, white part only, diced

4 garlic cloves, peeled and minced

1 teaspoon fresh thyme, divided

1 tablespoon olive oil

Salt and freshly ground pepper

About 2 tablespoons unsalted butter, sliced into 8 pieces

4 fillets of fish such as halibut, flounder, trout, or cod

4 slices of lemon

Chives, thinly sliced, for topping (optional)

TIP: Feel free to mix up the vegetables in this recipe. Shallots, spinach, green beans, fennel, cabbage, and asparagus all work well.

INSTRUCTIONS

1. Preheat oven to 400°F.

2. In a large bowl combine the squash, corn, leek, garlic, ½ teaspoon thyme, and olive oil. Season with salt and pepper and stir.

3. Lay out 4 pieces of parchment paper (can also use foil), each at least 12 inches long. Spoon the vegetable mixture into the center of the 4 pieces, dividing it evenly.

4. Place a piece of fish on top of each of the mounds of vegetables. Season the fish with salt, pepper, and the remaining thyme.

5. Place 2 slices of butter on top of each piece of fish followed by a slice of lemon.

6. Fold one long end of parchment over the fish so it connects to the other end. Start folding and tucking all the way around. With foil packets you can just bring the ends to meet in the center and crimp the edges at the top and on the sides.

7. Place the packets on a sheet tray and bake for 18–25 minutes or until the fish is cooked through. It will depend on the thickness of fish, but fish should fluke apart easily and no longer be opaque in the center. Top with optional chives for serving.

Grilled Shrimp and Asparagus Salad

For a light meal in the spring and summer

YIELD: 4 SERVINGS

INGREDIENTS

1 pound asparagus, trimmed

1 pound shrimp, peeled and deveined

2 tablespoons olive oil

Kosher salt and freshly ground pepper

8 ounces orzo

1 medium–large cucumber, diced

¼ cup fresh dill, chopped (basil works well, too)

¼ cup fresh parsley, chopped

1 recipe Lemon Dijon Vinaigrette (page 233)

INSTRUCTIONS

1. Heat the grill.
2. Drizzle the asparagus and shrimp with olive oil and sprinkle with salt and pepper.
3. Grill the shrimp on both sides just until cooked through. At the same time, grill the asparagus, cooking only a few minutes until they begin to soften.
4. Remove the shrimp and asparagus from the grill and allow to cool slightly.
5. Meanwhile, bring a pot of salted water to a boil and cook the orzo according to the instructions on the package. Drain the orzo and rinse briefly with cool water. Add to a large bowl.
6. Cut the asparagus diagonally into 1-inch pieces. If the shrimp are large, you can cut them in half.
7. Add the shrimp, asparagus, cucumber, herbs, and vinaigrette to the bowl with the orzo and toss. Season to taste with salt and pepper.

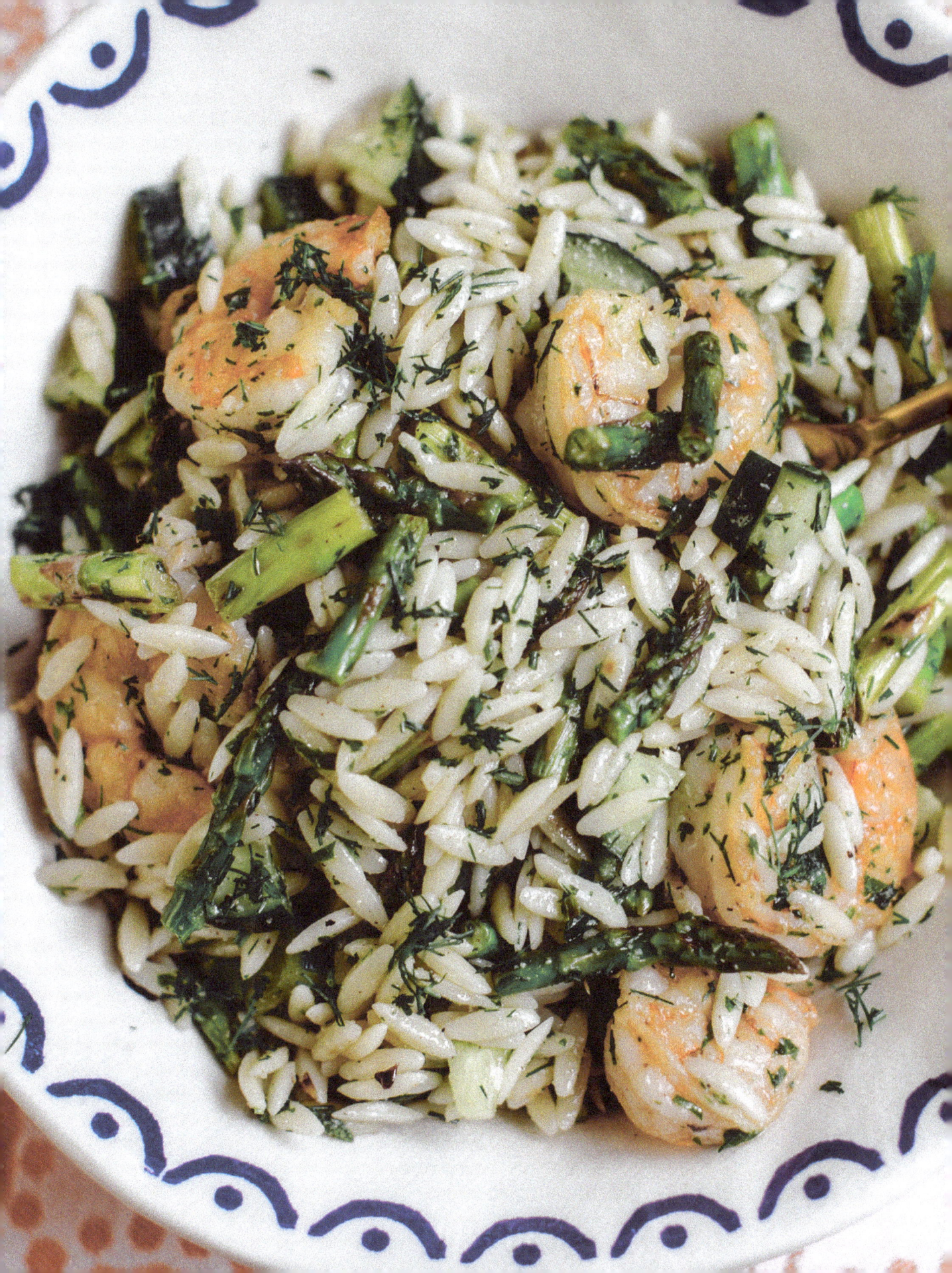

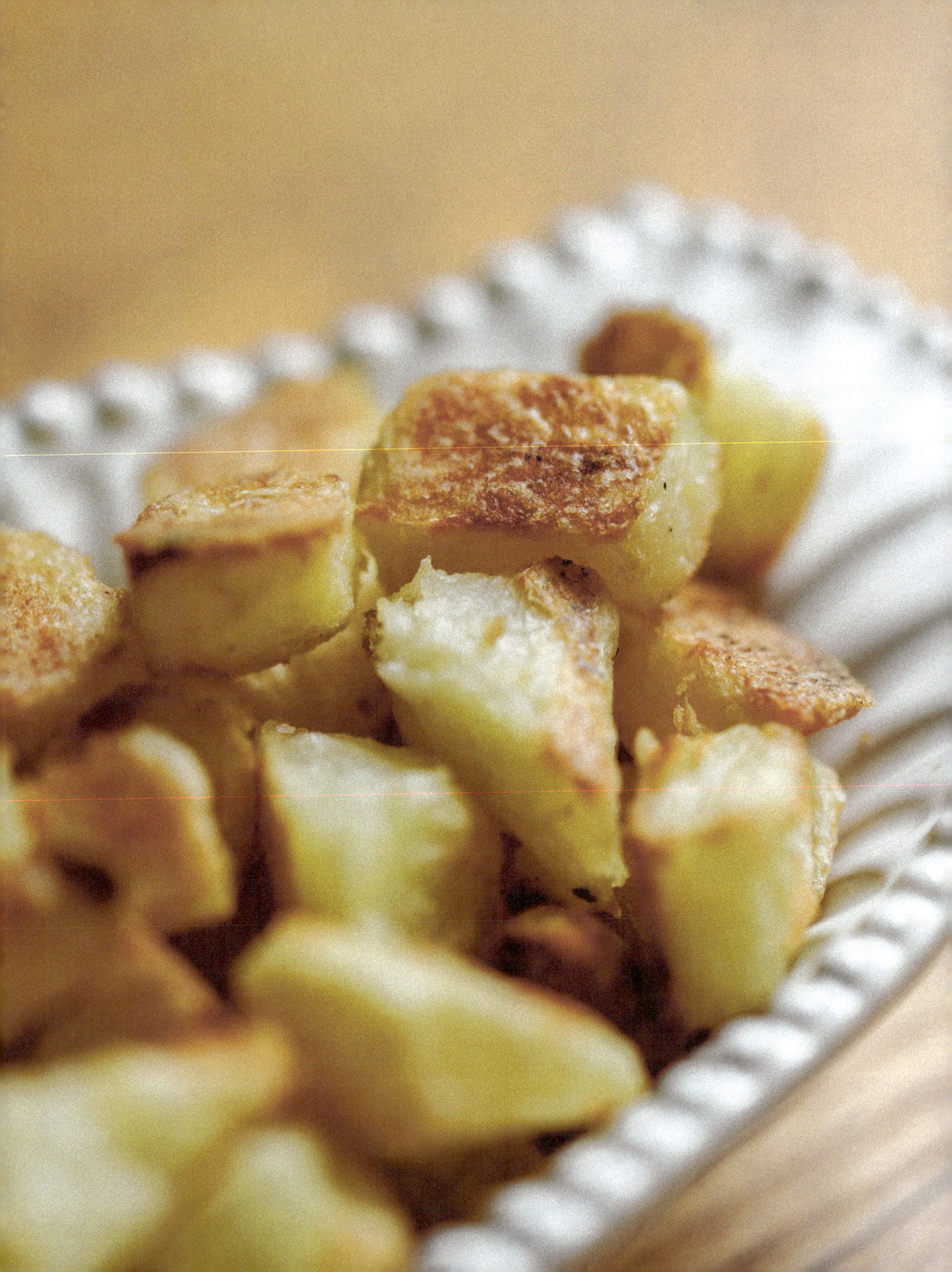

Sides

Cauliflower Fried Rice..198

Snap Pea Brown Butter Rice....................................201

Roasted Broccoli 202

Root Vegetable Latkes..205

Creamy Sweet Potatoes 206

Parsnip and Turnip Purée...209

Crispy Smashed Potatoes 210

Rainbow Slaw 213

Twice-Baked Cheese and Chive Potatoes................214

Roasted Garlic Potatoes...217

Skillet Green Beans 218

Summer Corn Sauté...221

Cauliflower Fried Rice

For a grain-free fried rice

INGREDIENTS

Olive oil

2 eggs, lightly beaten

2 shallots, peeled and diced

2 cloves garlic, minced or grated

1 (16 oz) bag of riced cauliflower

¼ teaspoon ground ginger

1 cup frozen peas and carrots (or fresh, diced and blanched)

1 tablespoon coconut aminos, plus more to taste

Kosher salt and freshly ground pepper

INSTRUCTIONS

1. Heat a little oil in a large skillet. Once the oil is hot add the lightly beaten eggs with a pinch of salt and scramble just until cooked. Remove and set aside. Wipe the pan clean if needed.

2. Add a little more olive oil over medium heat and once hot add the shallots. Stir and cook a couple of minutes until the shallots begin to soften then add in the garlic.

3. Give the garlic a stir and after a minute or 2 add the riced cauliflower, ground ginger, and a pinch of salt. Stir to combine and cook for a few minutes, only stirring occasionally. You want the bottom to become golden-brown.

4. After about 5 minutes add the peas and carrots and cook another couple of minutes. Once cooked, turn off heat and add the coconut aminos and cooked egg. Stir and season to taste with salt and pepper.

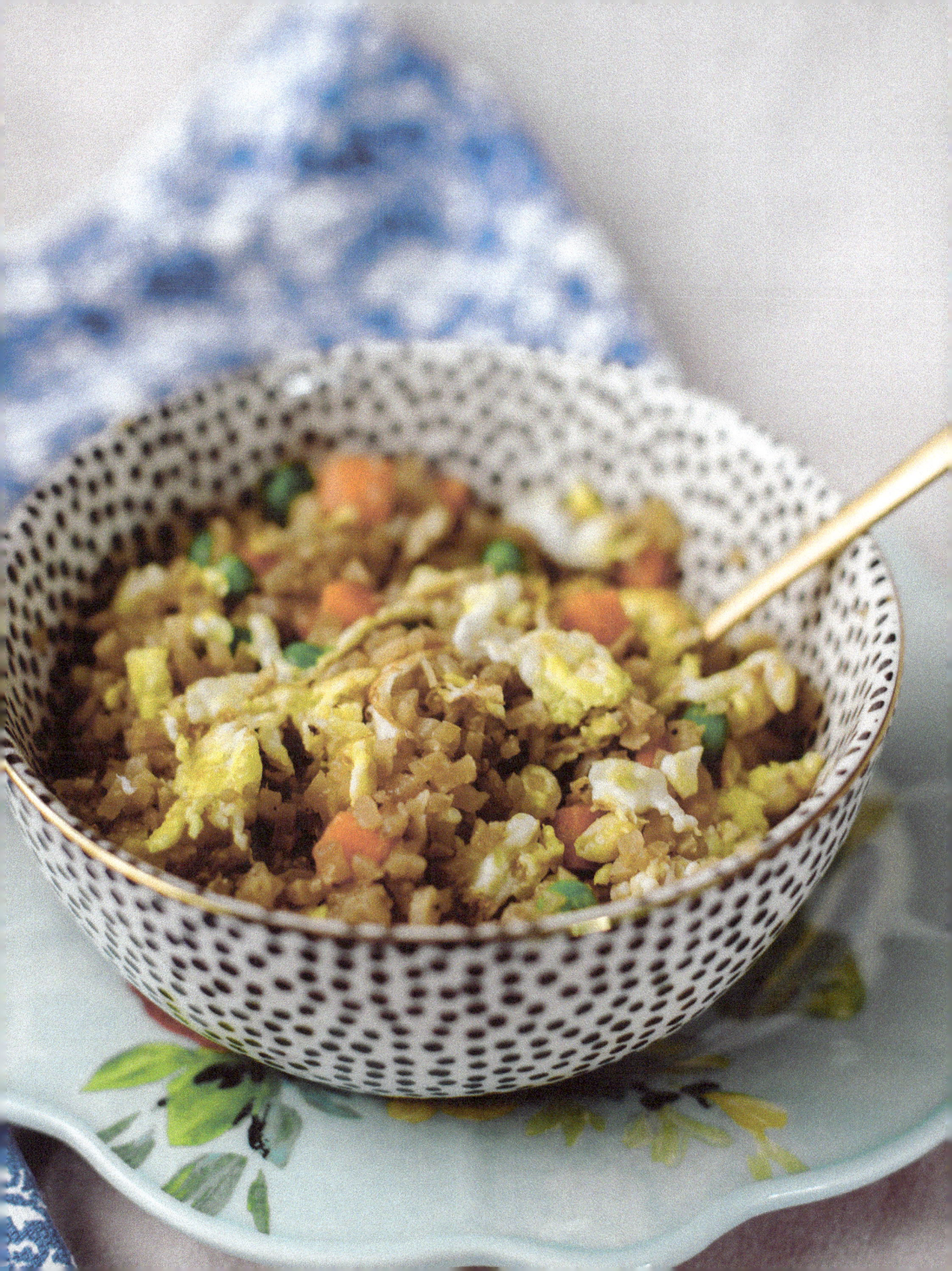

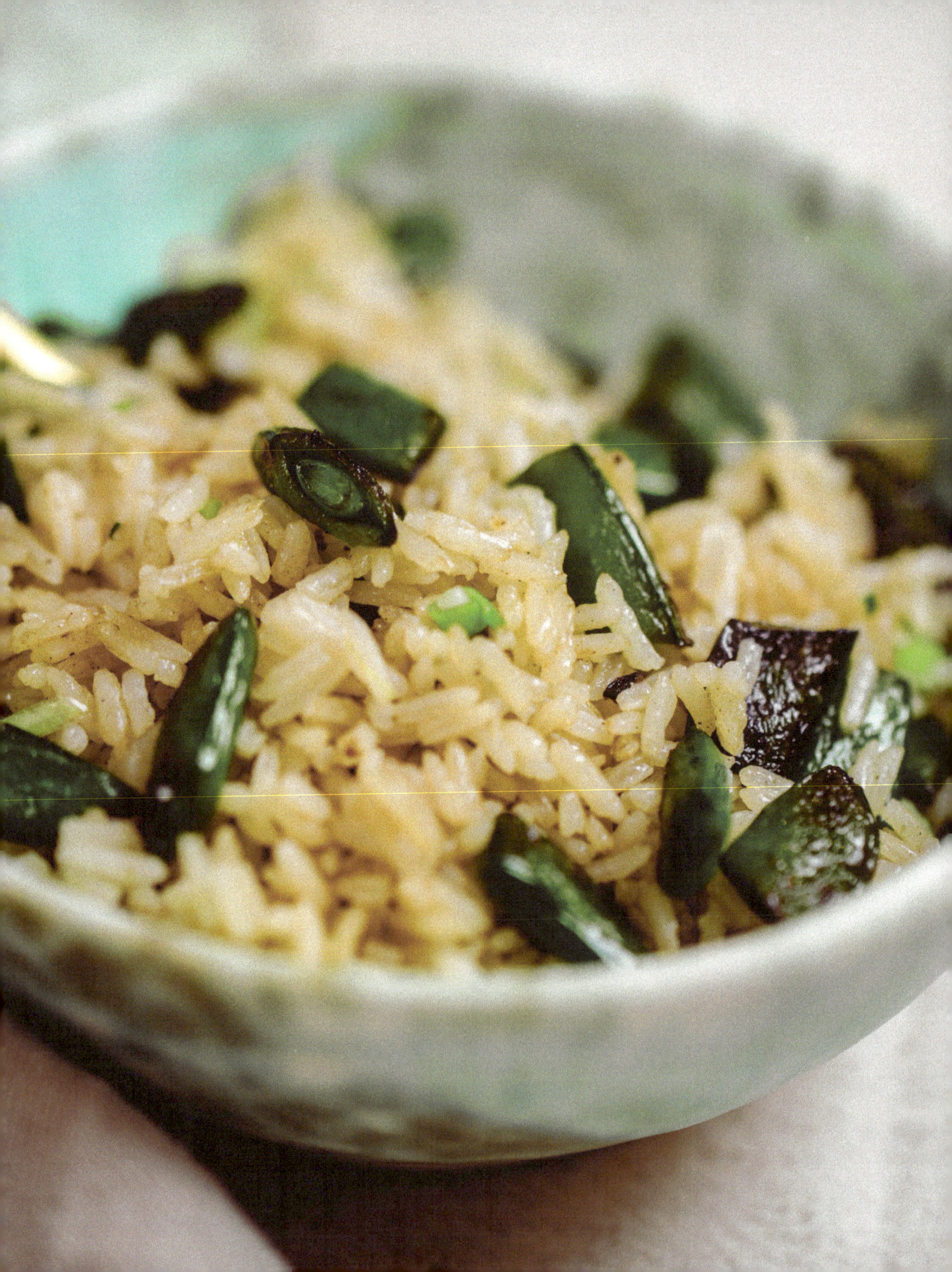

Snap Pea Brown Butter Rice

Brown rice contains more nutritious parts of the grain, including the bran, compared to white rice. Because the bran is intact, it takes longer to cook than white rice. If you are short on time, feel free to use white rice instead, just make sure to reduce the stock amount and time, following the instructions on the package. You can also use an Instant Pot or rice cooker to reduce the time for brown rice.

YIELD: 4 SERVINGS

INGREDIENTS

1 cup brown rice

2 cups vegetable stock, preferably homemade (page 84), non-MSG stock, or water

2 tablespoons unsalted butter

1 cup sugar snap peas or snow peas, trimmed and sliced thin on the bias

2 scallions, trimmed and thinly sliced

Kosher salt and fresh ground pepper

INSTRUCTIONS

1. In a medium-sized pot, bring the rice, stock (or water), and a large pinch of salt to a boil. Once boiling, cover and turn heat to low. Cook for approximately 40 minutes.

2. Turn off heat and allow to sit, covered, for about 5 minutes. Remove the lid, fluff with a fork, and set aside.

3. Add the butter to a large skillet and allow to brown slightly. Add the peas and cook for a couple minutes, stirring occasionally. Season with salt and pepper.

4. Once the peas begin to brown, add the rice and stir to combine.

5. Stir in the scallions and turn off heat. Adjust seasoning if needed.

Roasted Broccoli

If you're like me and enjoy the small, charred broccoli bits, you can add a few minutes to the roasting time for this recipe. Make sure not to overcrowd the baking tray, or the broccoli won't brown as well.

INGREDIENTS

2 medium or 3 small heads broccoli (about 1½–2 pounds)

2 tablespoons olive oil

¼ teaspoon garlic granules (optional)

Kosher salt and freshly ground pepper

INSTRUCTIONS

1. Preheat oven to 400°F.

2. Cut broccoli into florets and place on a Silpat mat- or parchment-lined baking tray.

3. Drizzle with olive oil and season with garlic granules, salt, and pepper. Toss to evenly coat.

4. Roast for 20–25 minutes or until broccoli is brown on the edges. Remove and serve or allow to cool before storing.

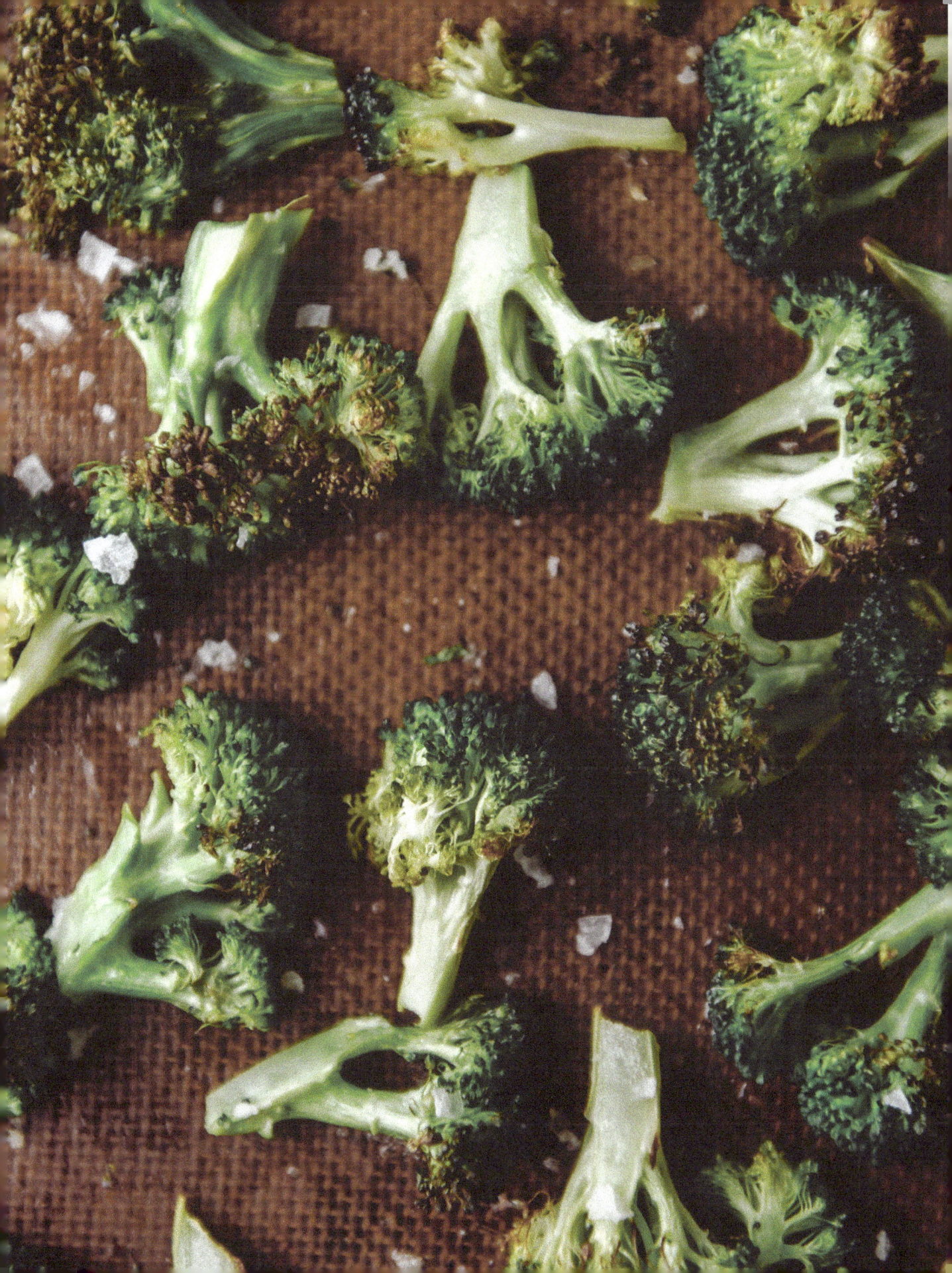

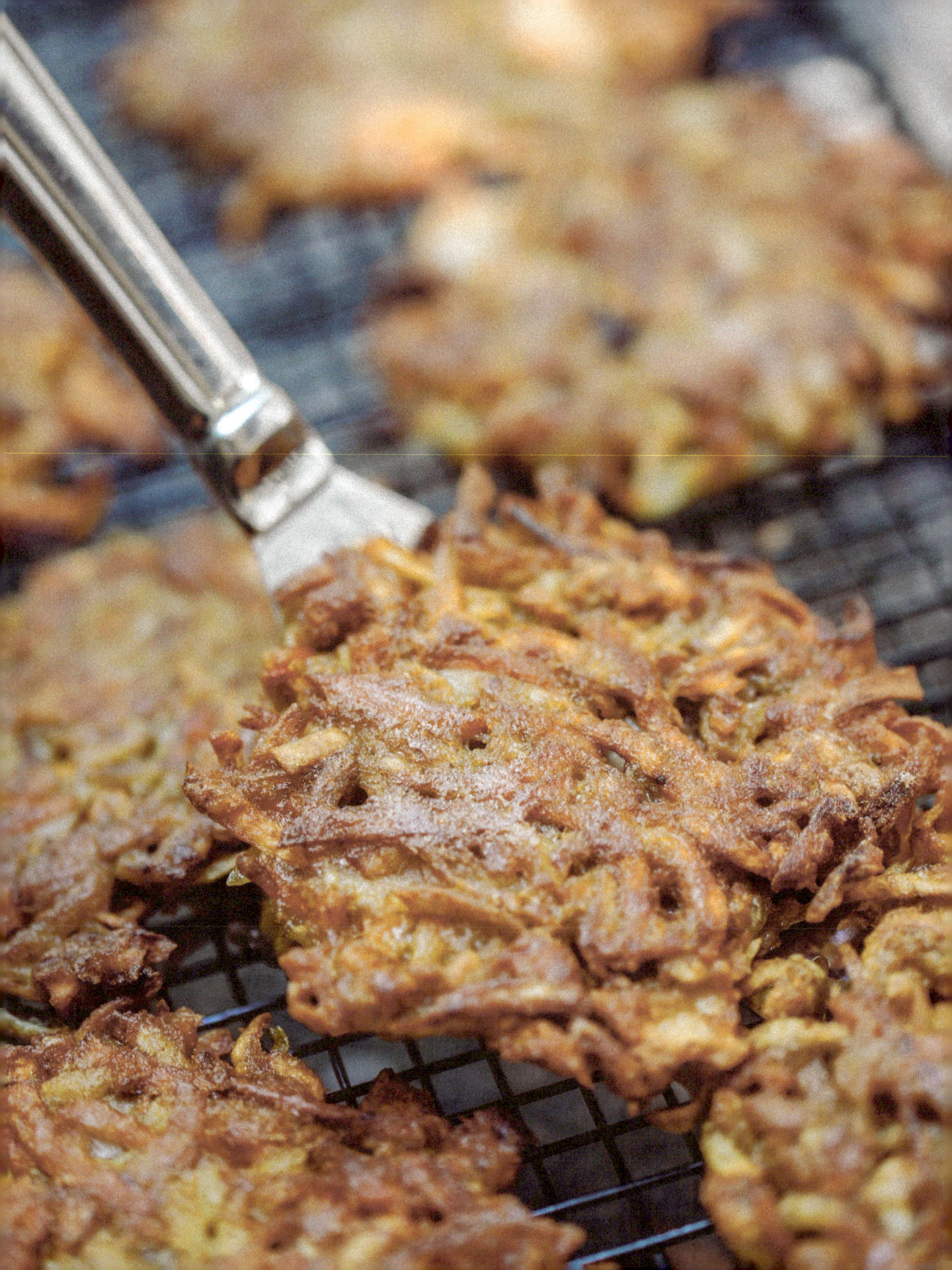

Root Vegetable Latkes

A fun twist on the standard potato latke

YIELD: 16 LATKES

INGREDIENTS

2 medium Russet potatoes

1 large carrot

1 medium sweet potato

1 parsnip

1 shallot

⅔ cup all-purpose or gluten-free flour

2 teaspoons kosher salt, plus more if needed

1 teaspoon baking powder

½ teaspoon garlic granules

1 egg

About ¼ cup high-heat oil, such as avocado oil, or ghee

Chives, for topping, sliced thin

TIP: This is great served with a salad, Herby Aioli (page 238), or even a dollop of Cinnamon Applesauce (page 62).

INSTRUCTIONS

1. Rinse the vegetables, scrubbing the potatoes if needed, and grate them with the large grater attachment to your food processor or with the coarse side of a box grater.

2. In a large bowl combine all of the grated vegetables and add the flour, salt, baking powder, garlic granules, and egg. Mix well.

3. Heat the oil in a skillet over medium-high heat. Once the oil is very hot, scoop out about ¼ cup of the latke mixture, form a ¼-inch-thick patty, and place it in the pan. Repeat a few more times, making sure you're not overcrowding the pan.

4. Brown on one side, flip over and brown on the other. Remove and allow to cool slightly on a wired rack.

5. Repeat, adding more oil if needed, until all the batter is used.

6. Top with chives and serve.

Creamy Sweet Potatoes

Unlike white potatoes, sweet potatoes can be blended without becoming gummy. I like to use these creamy sweet potatoes as a base and spoon chili on top or even Short Rib and White Bean Stew (page 99).

(page 99).

YIELD: 4–6 SERVINGS

INGREDIENTS

2 pounds sweet potatoes, peeled and cubed

½ cup milk, such as whole milk

⅛ teaspoon ground cinnamon

2 tablespoons unsalted butter, melted

Kosher salt and freshly ground pepper

INSTRUCTIONS

1. Place the sweet potatoes in a medium-sized pot and cover with water. Bring to a boil then turn heat down to simmer and cook until fork-tender. Drain and allow to cool slightly.

2. Add the potatoes, milk, cinnamon, and melted butter to a high-speed blender. Add 2 large pinches of salt and some pepper.

3. Blend just until smooth. Adjust seasoning if needed and serve.

TIP: If you prefer a more traditional mashed potato or don't have a high-speed blender, you can put the potatoes through a ricer or mash them with a pastry blender before adding the milk, cinnamon, melted butter, salt, and pepper.

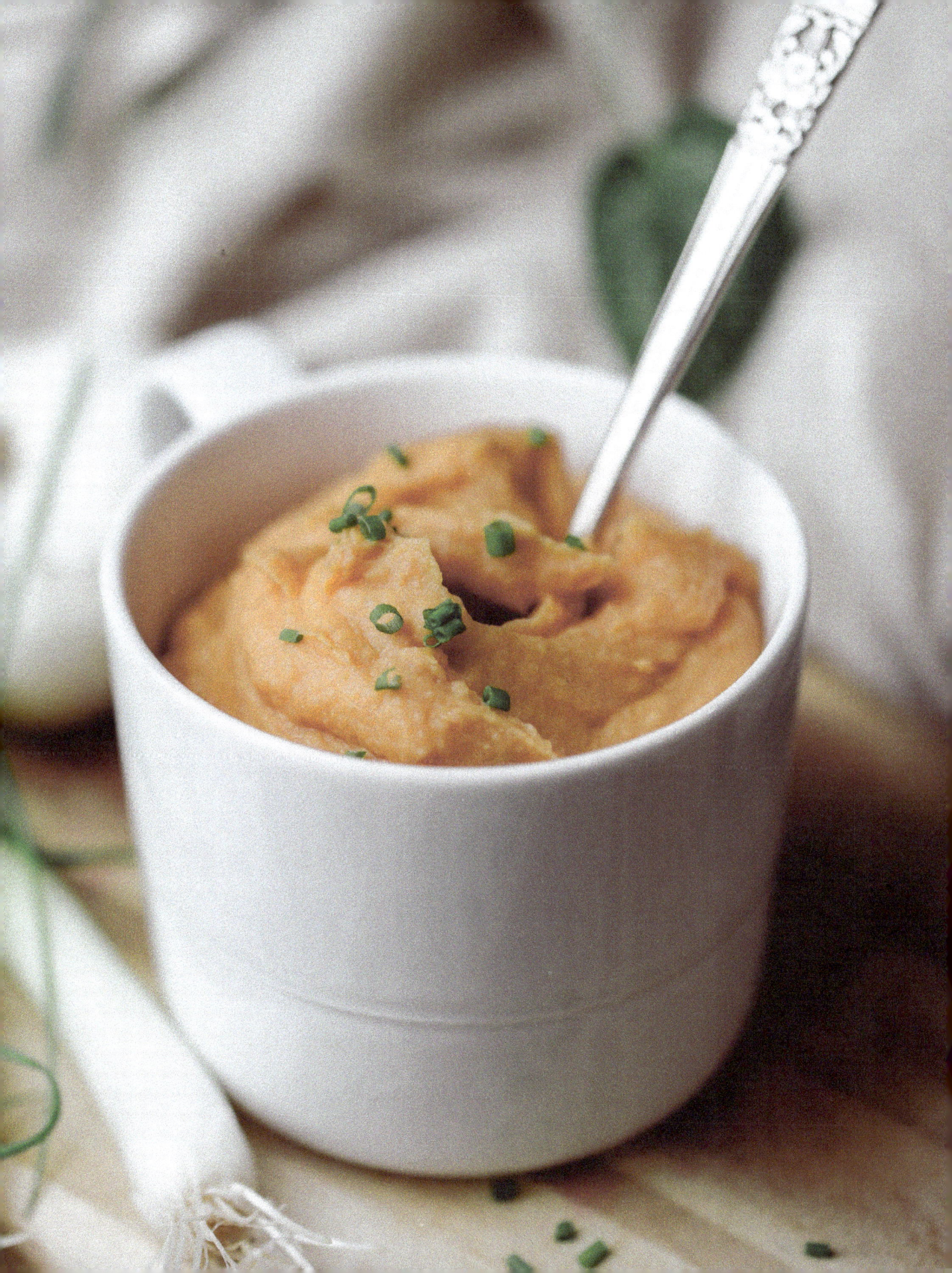

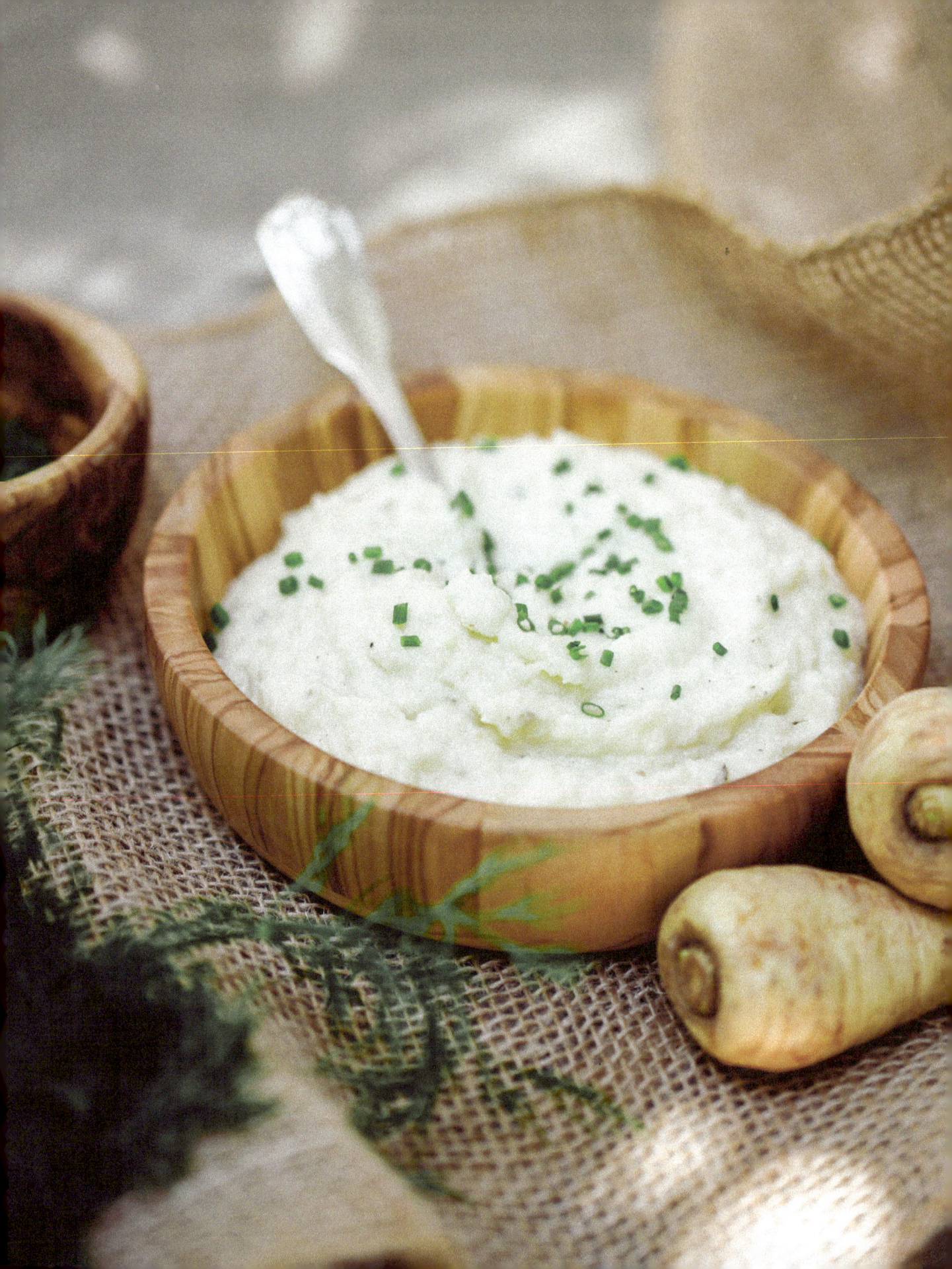

Parsnip and Turnip Purée

A delicious alternative to standard mashed potatoes

INGREDIENTS

1 medium turnip, peeled and diced, approximately ¾ pound

1 large parsnip or 2 small (you want more parsnip than turnip), peeled and diced, approximately 1 pound

1 apple, such as Granny Smith, peeled, cored, and chopped

2 tablespoons unsalted butter

½–⅔ cup vegetable or chicken stock, preferably homemade (pages 84, 86) or non-MSG stock, can substitute whole milk for a creamier texture

⅛ teaspoon dry sage

¼ teaspoon thyme

Kosher salt and freshly ground pepper

INSTRUCTIONS

1. Place the turnip and parsnip in a large pot of water and bring to a boil. Turn down to a gentle boil for about 10 minutes. Add the chopped apple and cook another 5 minutes or until the vegetables are fork-tender.

2. Drain and cool slightly.

3. Add the vegetables along with the rest of the ingredients to a food processor or high-speed blender. Season with some salt and pepper and blend until almost smooth. Adjust seasoning if needed.

Crispy Smashed Potatoes

These crispy potatoes are one of my favorite side dishes, especially drizzled with one of the Herby Aiolis (page 238).

(page 238)

YIELD: 4 SERVINGS

INGREDIENTS

6–8 medium red potatoes, unpeeled (about 2 pounds)

About 2 tablespoons olive oil

½ teaspoon garlic granules

Kosher salt and freshly ground pepper

INSTRUCTIONS

1. Line a large baking tray with a Silpat mat or parchment paper.
2. Scrub the potatoes if needed and rinse them with water. Cut the potatoes in half.
3. Place the potatoes in a medium-sized pot and cover with water, allowing 1 inch of water above the potatoes. Bring to a light boil and continue cooking until almost fork-tender. You should be able to pierce them with a fork easily but without them falling apart.
4. Preheat oven to 425°F.
5. Drain the potatoes, but do not rinse. Allow them to cool slightly. Once the potatoes are cool enough to handle, place them skin side up on the baking tray so they are evenly spread out.
6. Using a flat-bottomed bowl or similar, smash each piece so they are flattened a little more than halfway.
7. Brush them with olive oil and top with the garlic granules. Sprinkle them generously with salt and pepper.
8. Bake for 25–30 minutes until the potato skins start to brown and crisp.
9. Remove them from the oven and allow to cool slightly.

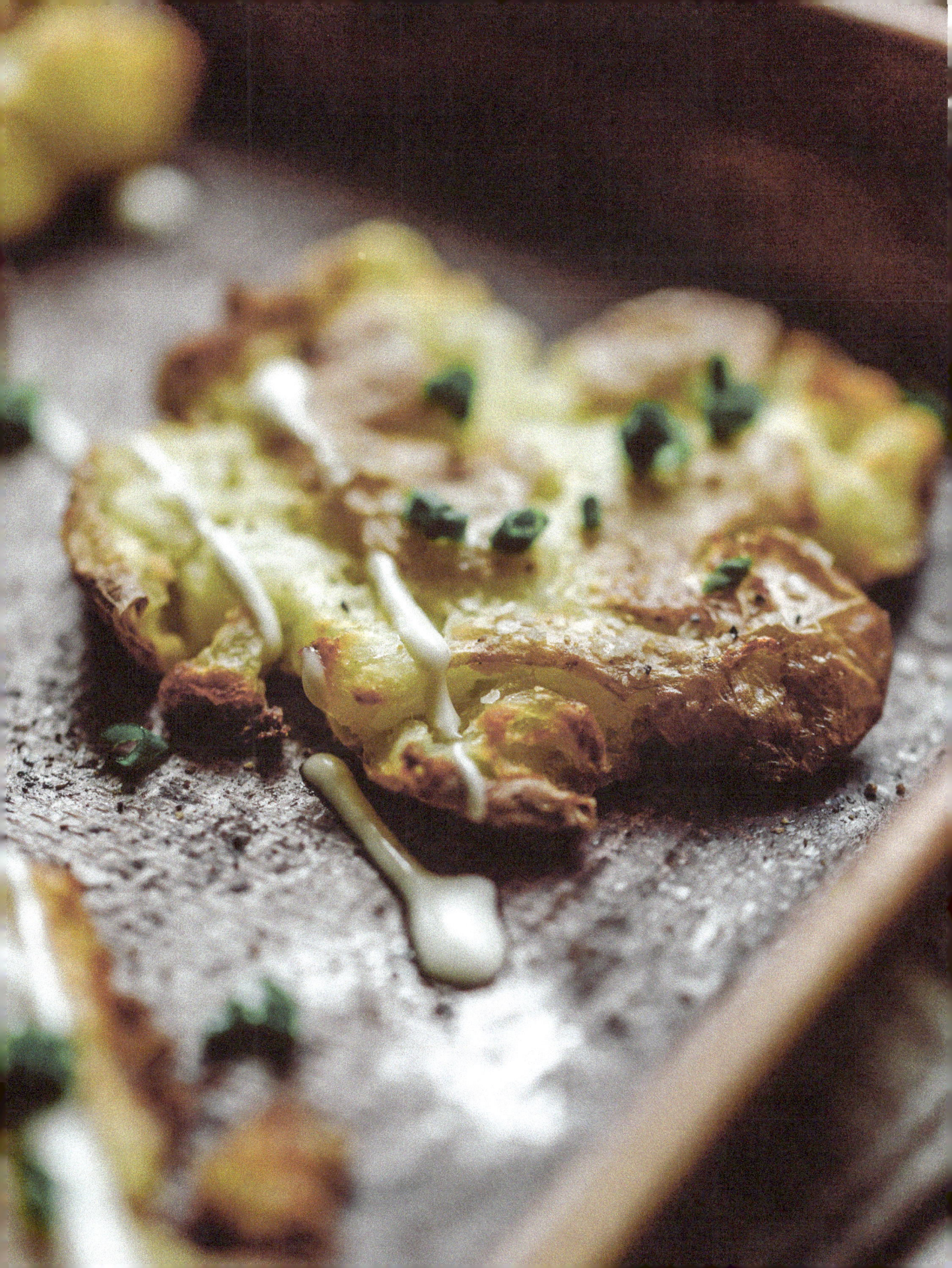

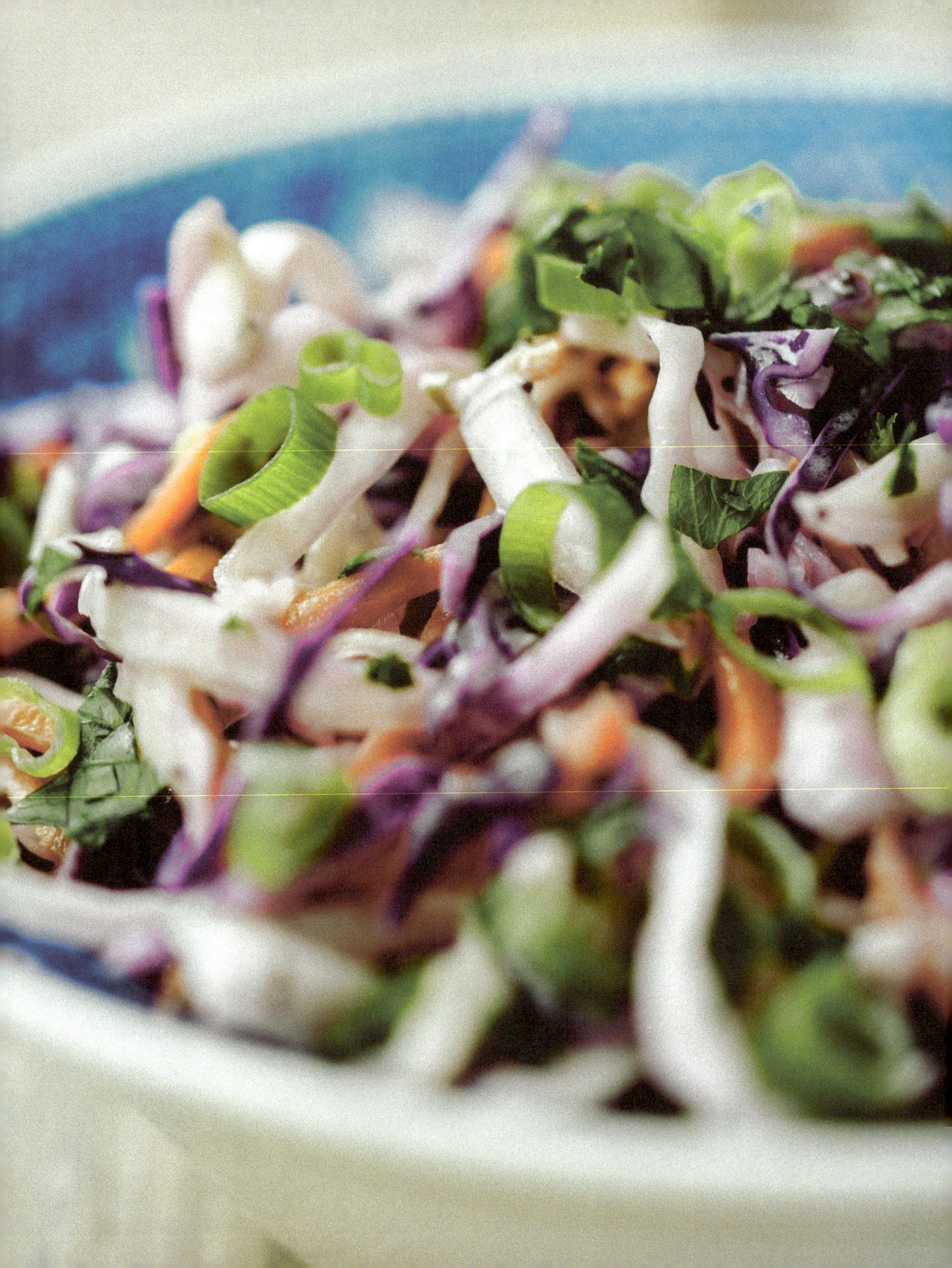

Rainbow Slaw

Store-bought slaw can be loaded with unnecessary amounts of sugar and mayonnaise. This version is still creamy but much lighter than your average Southern coleslaw.

YIELD: 6 SERVINGS

INGREDIENTS

2 cups purple cabbage, thinly sliced

2 cups green cabbage, thinly sliced

1 cup shredded carrots

2 scallions, trimmed and thinly sliced

¼ cup parsley, finely chopped

1 recipe Creamy Poppy Seed Dressing (page 235) (optional to leave out the poppy seeds)

Salt and freshly ground pepper

TIP: Other fun add-ins include chopped cilantro, diced jalapeños, ground cumin, or a little cayenne.

INSTRUCTIONS

1. Add all the ingredients into a large bowl and stir.

2. Season to taste with salt and pepper.

Twice-Baked Cheese and Chive Potatoes

For the "meat and potato" people out there

YIELD: 8 HALVES

INGREDIENTS

5 Russet potatoes

¾ cup whole milk

1 (5.3 oz) package Boursin cheese

½ cup chives, thinly sliced

½ teaspoon garlic granules

Kosher salt and freshly ground pepper

INSTRUCTIONS

1. Preheat oven to 400°F.
2. Bake the potatoes for about 1 hour 15 minutes or until fork-tender. Remove and allow to cool slightly.
3. Cut the potatoes in half lengthwise and scoop out the inside, leaving a little around the edges to create a shell.
4. Rice or mash the potato and mix in the milk, cheese, chives, and garlic granules. Season with salt and pepper to taste.
5. Place 8 halves in a 9" x 13" baking dish or similar. The other 2 halves can be composted or cooked until brown in a pan with a little olive oil (a great alternative to traditional croutons).
6. Divide the mixture among the 8 potato halves and bake for 20 minutes. Remove and serve.

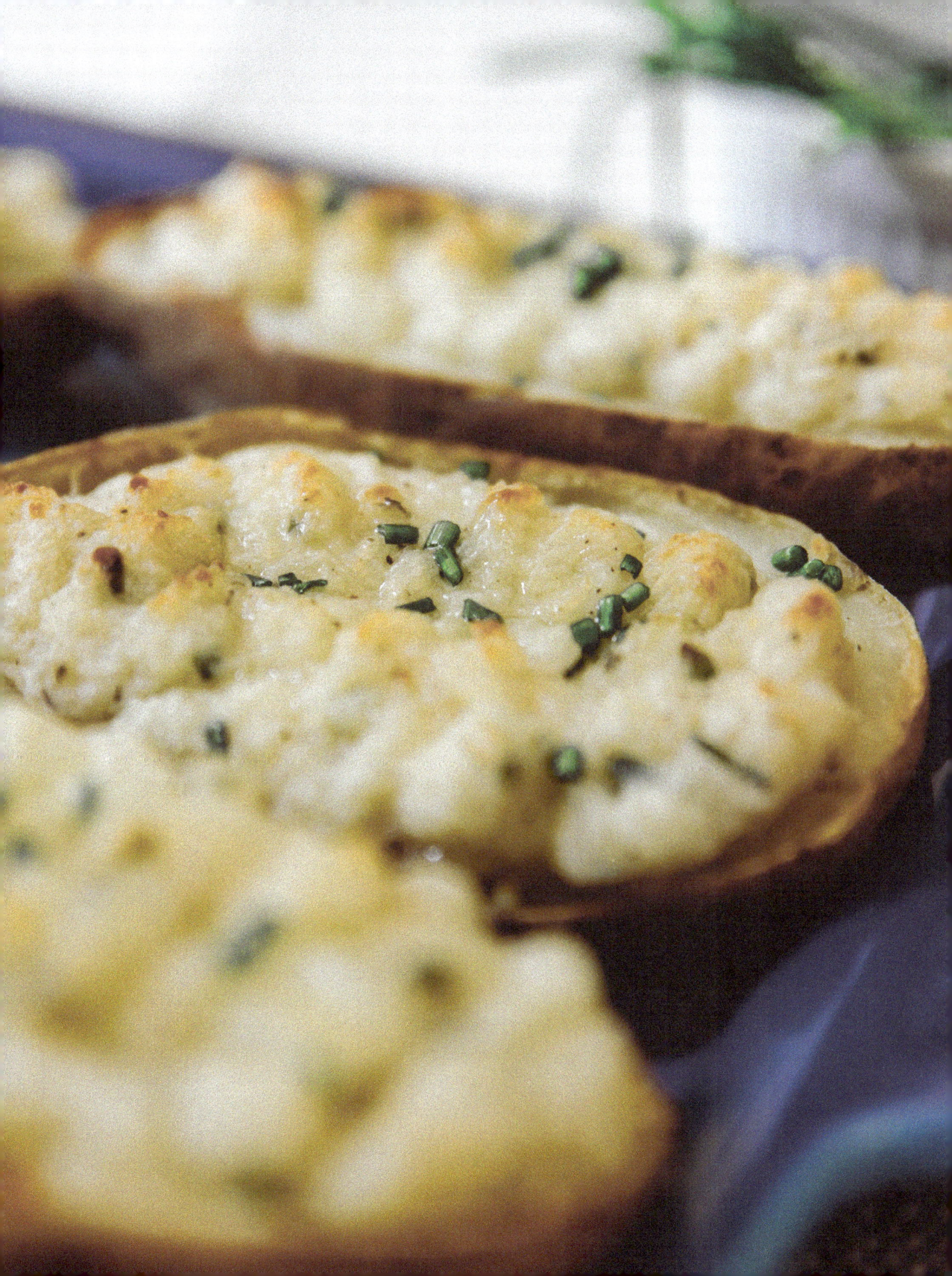

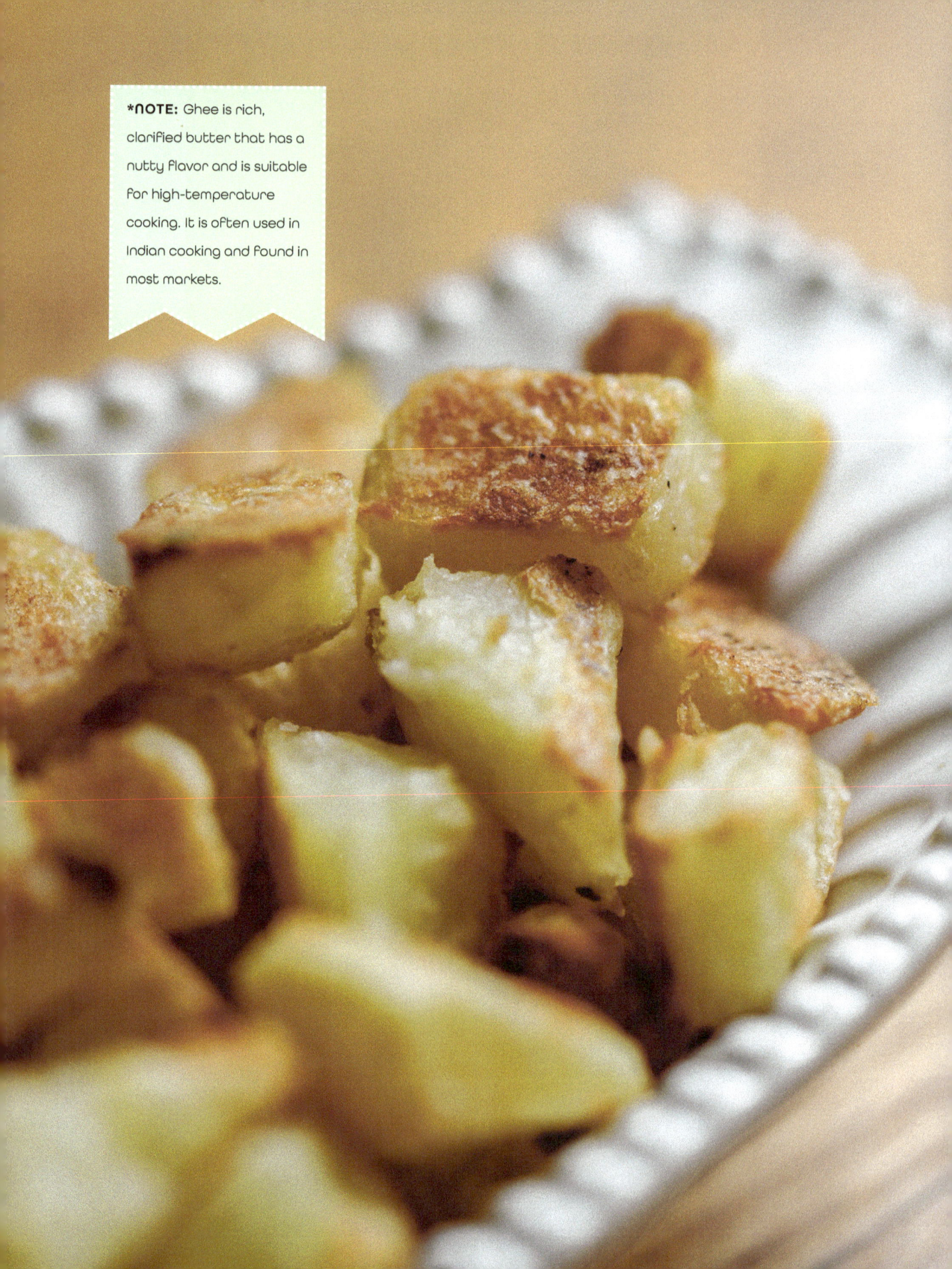

*NOTE: Ghee is rich, clarified butter that has a nutty flavor and is suitable for high-temperature cooking. It is often used in Indian cooking and found in most markets.

Roasted Garlic Potatoes

INGREDIENTS

2 pounds potatoes such as Russets or red potatoes (optional to peel), cut into 1½ -inch cubes (about 4 cups)

2 teaspoons arrowroot or cornstarch

½ teaspoon garlic granules

Kosher salt and freshly ground pepper

2 tablespoons ghee*, melted, or olive oil

INSTRUCTIONS

1. Preheat oven to 450°F and line a sheet tray with parchment paper.

2. In a large bowl, toss the potatoes with the arrowroot, garlic, salt, pepper, and melted ghee.

3. Spread out the potatoes on the parchment paper and roast until golden-brown, about 20 minutes, turning them halfway through.

Skillet Green Beans

For a side dish that's ready in about 5 minutes

YIELD: 4 SERVINGS

INGREDIENTS

1 tablespoon olive oil

1 pound green beans, trimmed

½ teaspoon garlic granules

Kosher salt and freshly ground
pepper

INSTRUCTIONS

1. Heat a large skillet over medium-high heat. Once hot, add the olive oil.

2. When the oil is hot and starts to shimmer, add the green beans. Coat in the oil and cook for a few minutes, stirring occasionally. Add a big pinch of salt. After a few minutes, the beans should start to blister and brown slightly.

3. Add the garlic granules, some pepper, and toss to coat the beans. Turn off heat and adjust seasoning if needed.

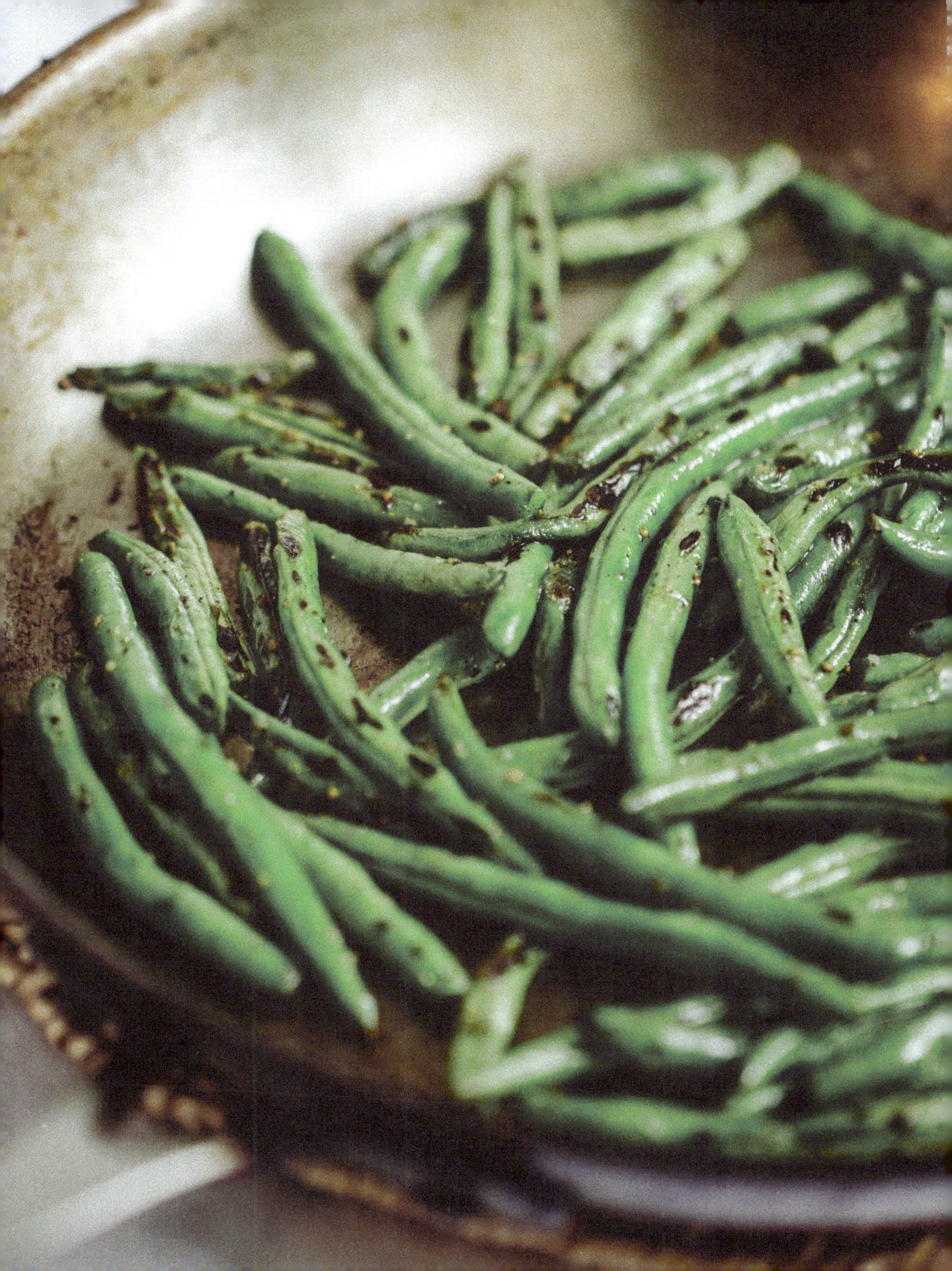

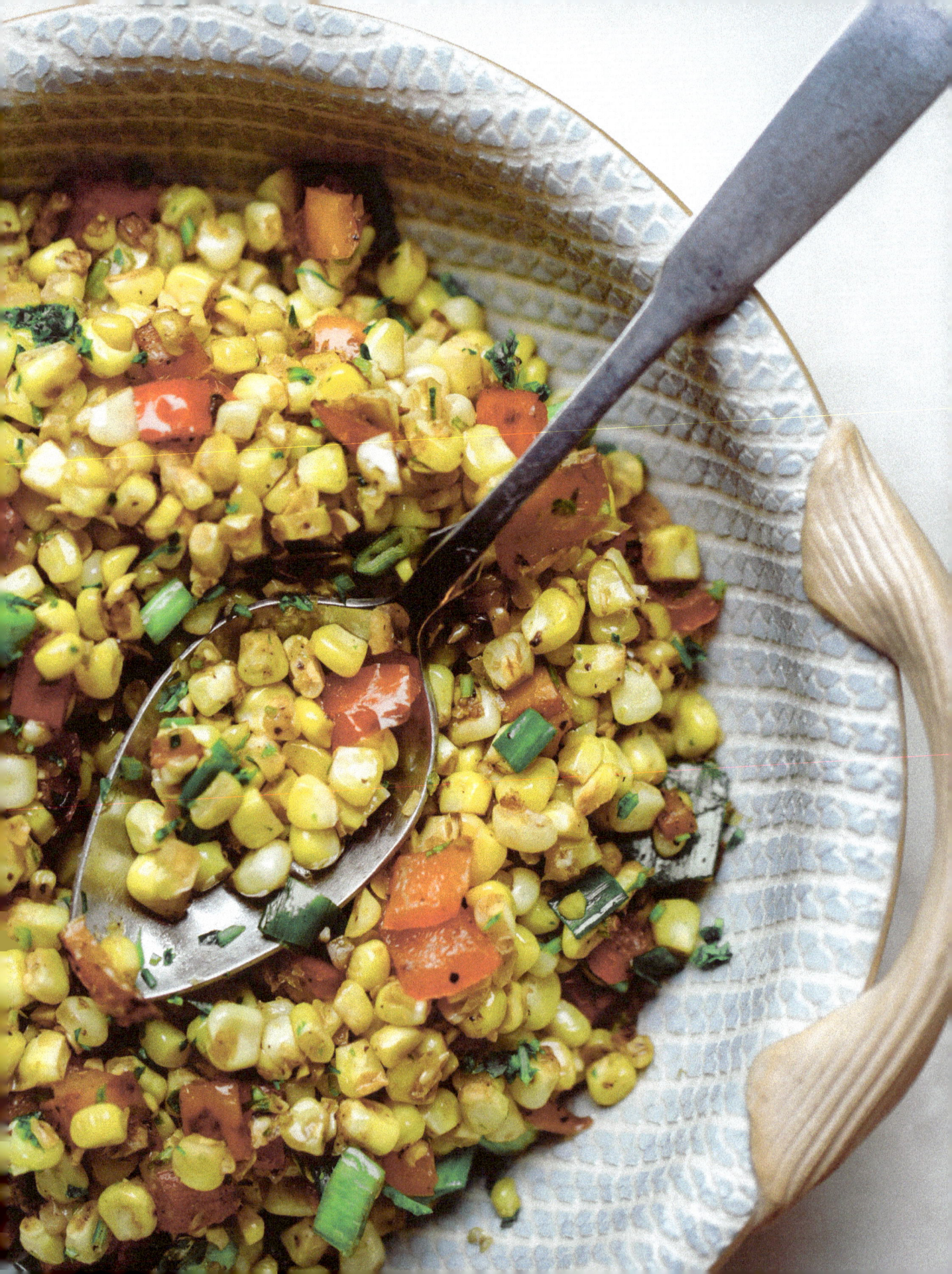

Summer Corn Sauté

This colorful dish can be a base for an animal protein, or you can bulk it up with the addition of some beans or grains.

YIELD: 4 SERVINGS

INGREDIENTS

1 tablespoon olive oil

1 red bell pepper, seeded and diced

2 cloves garlic, peeled and minced

3 scallions, thinly sliced

Kosher salt and freshly ground pepper

3 ears sweet corn, kernels cut from the cobs (about 2½ cups)

¼ cup fresh herbs such as parsley, basil, or cilantro, chopped

1 tablespoon unsalted butter

INSTRUCTIONS

1. Heat the olive oil in a skillet over medium-high heat. When the oil is hot add the bell pepper and sauté about 5 minutes.

2. Stir in the garlic and scallions along with a big pinch of salt and some pepper.

3. Add the corn and sauté for another 5 minutes, stirring occasionally.

4. Turn off heat and stir in the herbs and the butter until it is melted. Adjust seasoning if needed.

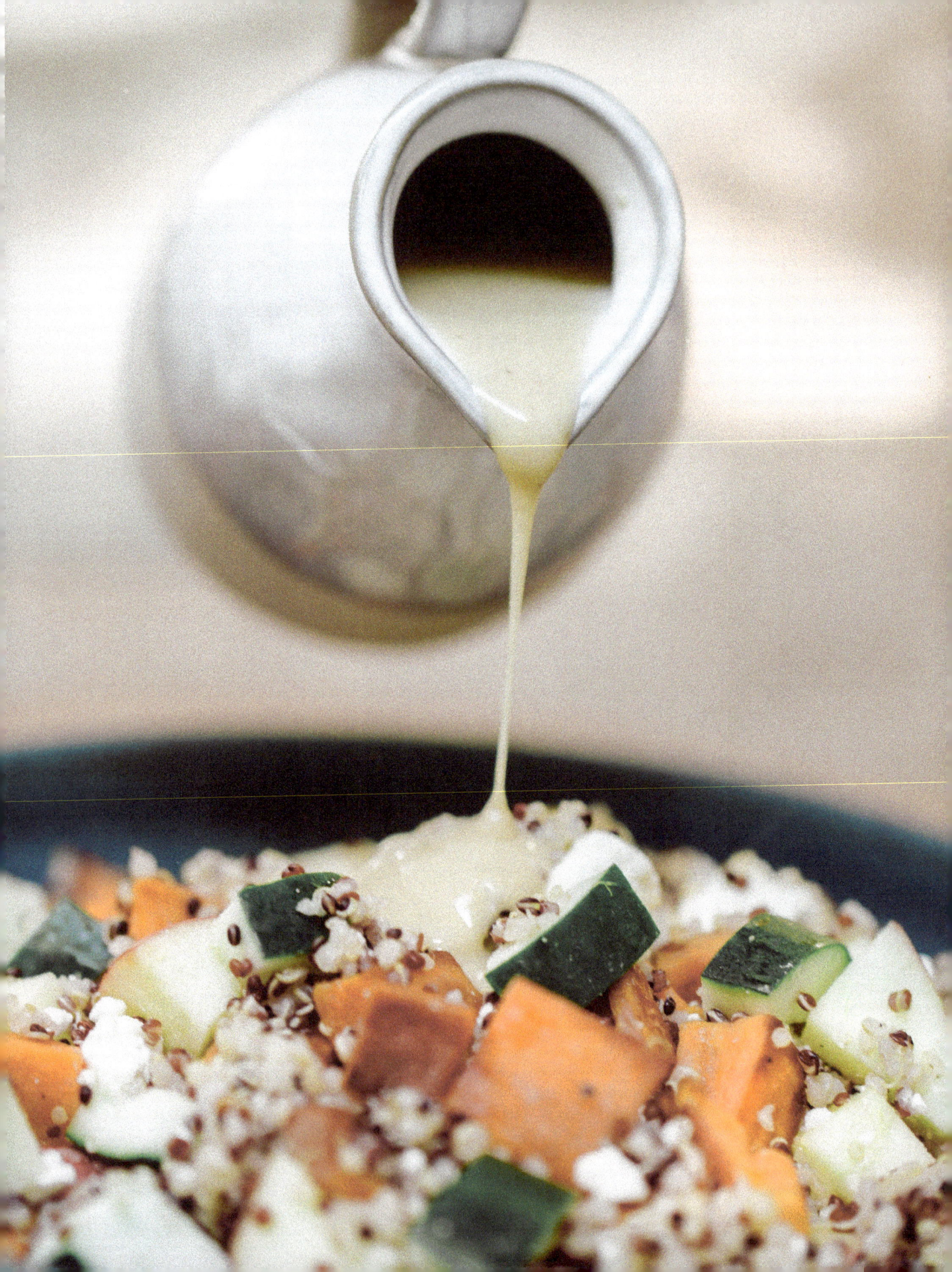

Sauces and Dips

Instant Pot Marinara 224

Mascarpone Herb Sauce 226

Tarragon Basil Sauce.. 227

Basil Sunflower Seed Pesto 228

Beet Tahini Dip.. 229

Sage Sausage Gravy 230

Holiday Gravy 231

Lemon Dijon Vinaigrette 233

Ginger Glaze 233

Honey Mustard Dressing... 234

Creamy Poppy Seed Dressing 235

Roasted Poblano and Tomatillo Salsa 236

Herby Aioli Two Ways 238

Taco Seasoning.. 239

Roasted Red Pepper Vodka Sauce 241

Super Seed Mix 242

Thai "Peanut" Sauce 243

Cauliflower Cream.. 244

Instant Pot Marinara

For a quick sauce that tastes like it has been simmering all day.

INGREDIENTS

2 tablespoons olive oil

2 large shallots, peeled and diced

3 garlic cloves, peeled and minced or grated

7–8 cups fresh tomatoes, chopped (about 3½ pounds) or if out of season use 2 (28 oz) cans whole tomatoes

½ cup stock, such as vegetable, preferably homemade (page 84), or non-MSG

1 tablespoon coconut aminos

1 tablespoon Italian seasoning

1 teaspoon dried basil

1 teaspoon dried oregano

1 bay leaf

¼ teaspoon red pepper flakes (or more if desired)

1–2 teaspoons sugar or coconut sugar (optional)

2 teaspoons kosher salt, or to taste

Freshly ground pepper

1 (6 oz) can tomato paste

INSTRUCTIONS

1. Turn the Instant Pot to sauté and pour in the olive oil. Once the oil is hot, add the shallots. Once the shallots begin to soften, add the garlic.

2. Turn off the sauté setting and add the tomatoes, stock, coconut aminos, dried herbs, bay leaf, red pepper flakes, sugar, salt, and some pepper. If you are using canned tomatoes, smash them a bit when you add them. Stir to combine.

3. Spoon the tomato paste on top but do not mix in. This will help the mixture not burn while pressurizing.

4. Close the lid and set the Instant Pot to manual (or pressure cook) for 25 minutes.

5. Once done, allow the steam to release and remove the lid.

6. Using an immersion blender, blend the marinara until desired consistency. I prefer mine to be almost smooth. If you do not have an immersion blender, you can allow the mixture to cool slightly then add it (in batches if necessary) to a high-speed blender and blend.

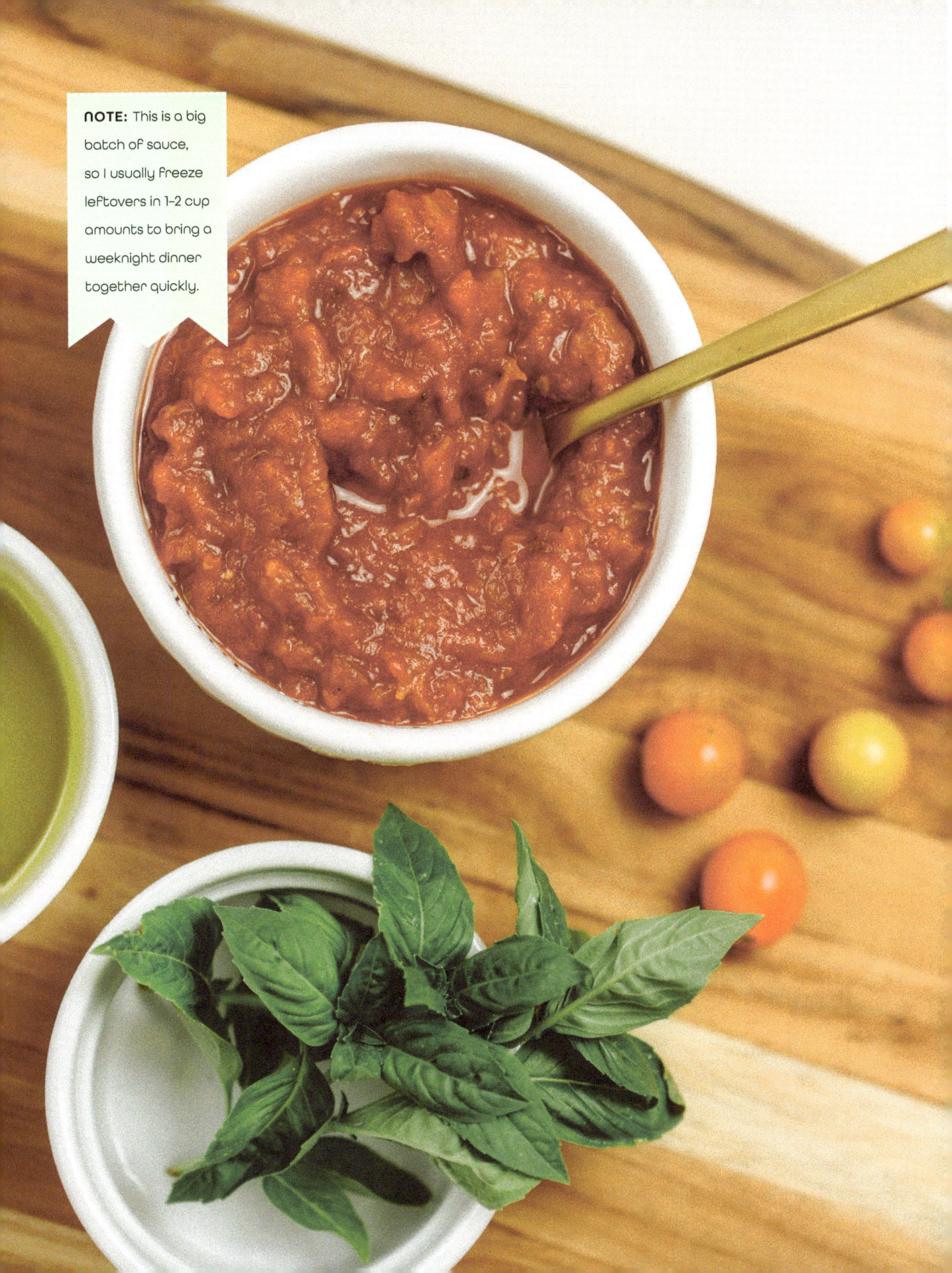

NOTE: This is a big batch of sauce, so I usually freeze leftovers in 1–2 cup amounts to bring a weeknight dinner together quickly.

Mascarpone Herb Sauce

Due to my deep love for tiramisu, I have grown very familiar with mascarpone over the years. It is a delicious, creamy cheese, originated in Italy, that can be used in many savory dishes as well.

INGREDIENTS

1 tablespoon olive oil or unsalted butter

2 shallots, peeled and diced

3 garlic cloves, peeled and grated or minced

½ cup vegetable stock, preferably homemade (page 84), or other non-MSG stock

1 (8 oz) container mascarpone cheese

½ cup chopped herbs such as mint, chives, or basil

½ lemon, juiced (optional)

Kosher salt and freshly ground pepper

Cooked pasta of choice

¼ cup sunflower seeds, toasted

INSTRUCTIONS

1. Add the olive oil or butter to a large skillet over medium heat. Once hot add the shallots and sauté for a couple minutes, then add the garlic.

2. Cook until fragrant then add the stock. Reduce slightly for a few minutes and turn off heat.

3. Add the mascarpone, herbs, and lemon juice (if using). Stir until the mascarpone is incorporated and the sauce has thickened slightly. Season to taste with salt and pepper.

4. Add the cooked pasta to the pan and toss to combine. Top with toasted sunflower seeds and serve.

This sauce is also great with chicken and vegetables.

Tarragon Basil Sauce

This was one of the few recipes I only had to test once. It's great served over Delicious Roasted Chicken (page 150) or fish.

INGREDIENTS

1 tablespoon olive oil

2 shallots, peeled and diced

2 cloves garlic, peeled and grated or minced

1 cup canned coconut milk, full fat

½ cup vegetable or chicken stock, preferably homemade (pages 84, 86), or non-MSG stock

Kosher salt and freshly ground pepper

¼ cup fresh tarragon, stemmed and chopped

¼ cup fresh basil, stemmed and chopped

Juice from ½ lemon

TIP: If not serving right away, hold off on cutting and adding the herbs. Just before serving, reheat the sauce on the stovetop and once it's hot, turn off the heat. Chop and add the herbs and stir to combine.

INSTRUCTIONS

1. In a pan add the olive oil over medium heat and once hot, sauté the shallots for a few minutes.

2. Add the garlic and cook until fragrant, about 1 minute.

3. Add the coconut milk, stock, and some salt and pepper. Simmer for about 5 minutes or until the mixture has thickened a bit.

4. Turn off heat, then add the herbs and lemon juice. Adjust seasoning if needed.

Basil Sunflower Seed Pesto

Looking for a nut- and dairy-free pesto? This recipe has you covered! Sunflower seeds are substituted here for pine nuts, and you won't even miss the Parmesan. This pesto is great over pasta, with meatballs, or used as a spread on a sandwich.

YIELD: ABOUT ½ CUP

INGREDIENTS

2 cups basil leaves

1 cup parsley

¼ cup sunflower seeds, raw

1 garlic clove, peeled

½ cup extra virgin olive oil

Squeeze of lemon (optional)

Kosher salt and freshly ground pepper

NOTE: This pesto is best used within a day or 2, or you can freeze for 2–3 months.

INSTRUCTIONS

1. Add the first 4 ingredients into a food processor and pulse a few times until the herbs are minced fine.

2. While the machine is running, slowly add the olive oil and lemon if using. Season to taste with salt and pepper.

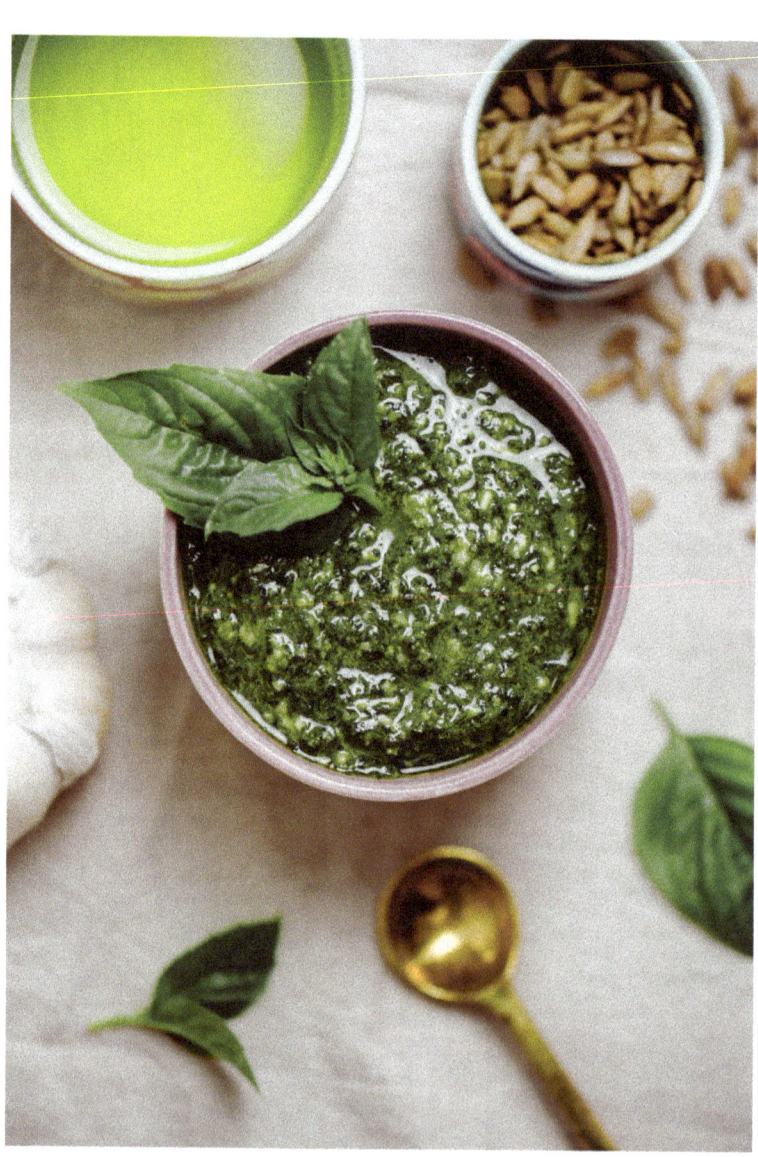

Beet Tahini Dip

This recipe started out as a dip when trying to create a beet hummus recipe. It also works great as a salad dressing if you thin it out a bit.

YIELD: ABOUT 1 CUP

INGREDIENTS

1 cooked and peeled medium beet*

1 garlic clove, peeled

Juice from ½ lemon

2 tablespoons tahini

1 teaspoon honey, or more to taste

¼ cup extra virgin olive oil

Kosher salt and freshly ground pepper

*NOTE: To cook beets, preheat oven to 400°F. Rinse beets and place in a baking dish or loaf pan along with ½ cup water. Cover with foil and bake for 45 minutes–1 hour 15 minutes depending on their size. Once you can pierce them easily with a fork, remove and allow them to cool before peeling.

INSTRUCTIONS

1. Place all ingredients into a high-speed blender and add 1–2 tablespoons water (or my favorite—beet juice from cooking) and a big pinch of salt and pepper.

2. Blend until combined and taste for seasoning.

TIP: For more of a dressing, add 1–2 tablespoons extra water or beet juice.

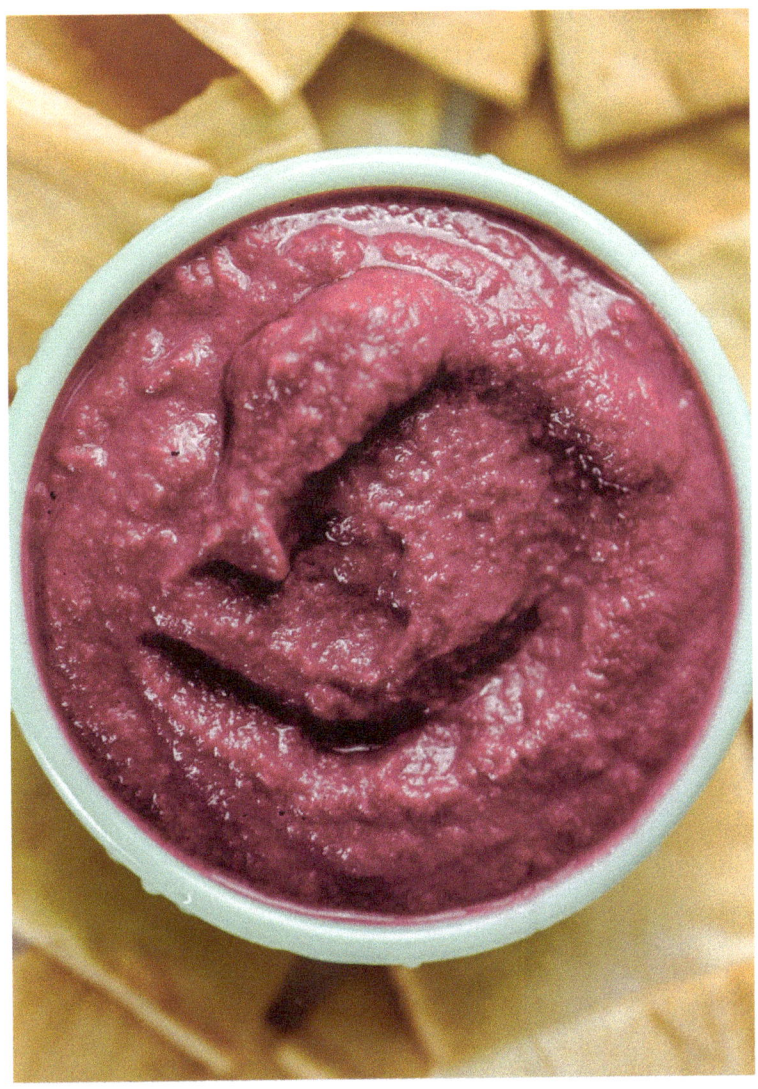

Sage Sausage Gravy

For a hearty addition to smother over Southern Biscuits (page 58)

(page 58)

YIELD: 6 SERVINGS

INGREDIENTS

1 pound Make Your Own Sausage, uncooked (page 53)

1 tablespoon chopped fresh sage leaves

2 tablespoons unsalted butter

2 tablespoons all-purpose flour or gluten-free flour

2½ cups whole milk

¼–½ teaspoon red pepper flakes (optional)

¼ teaspoon garlic granules

Salt and freshly ground pepper

INSTRUCTIONS

1. In a large skillet, cook the sausage, breaking it up as you go. After a few minutes, when the sausage is almost cooked, add the sage. Finish cooking and remove with a slotted spoon, leaving in any drippings from sausage.

2. In the same pan over medium heat, add the butter and let melt. Whisk in the flour until it is incorporated into the butter.

3. Continue to whisk until the roux turns a golden-brown, about 4–5 minutes.

4. Slowly whisk in the milk as well as the red pepper flakes (if using), garlic granules, and a pinch of salt and pepper. Add the sausage back in.

5. Cook for about 5–10 minutes over medium-low heat, until the mixture starts to thicken.

6. Adjust seasoning with salt and pepper and serve over biscuits.

Holiday Gravy

YIELD: ABOUT 1 CUP

INGREDIENTS

2 tablespoons unsalted butter

1 tablespoon all-purpose flour or gluten-free flour

About ¼ cup chicken or turkey drippings*

1 cup vegetable or chicken stock, preferably homemade (pages 84, 86), or non-MSG stock

Chopped herbs such as thyme, rosemary, or sage (optional)

Kosher salt and freshly ground pepper

*NOTE: Poultry drippings refer to the juices and fat that collect at the bottom of the pan while cooking a bird such as chicken or turkey.

INSTRUCTIONS

1. Heat the butter in a medium pot over medium-high heat. Once melted whisk in the flour.
2. Continue whisking until you cannot see any bits of flour and the roux begins to turn golden-brown.
3. Turn heat down slightly and slowly whisk in the poultry drippings then the stock and any herbs you wish to include.
4. Season with salt and pepper and simmer for about 10 minutes or until the mixture begins to reduce and thicken.
5. Turn off heat and adjust seasoning if needed.

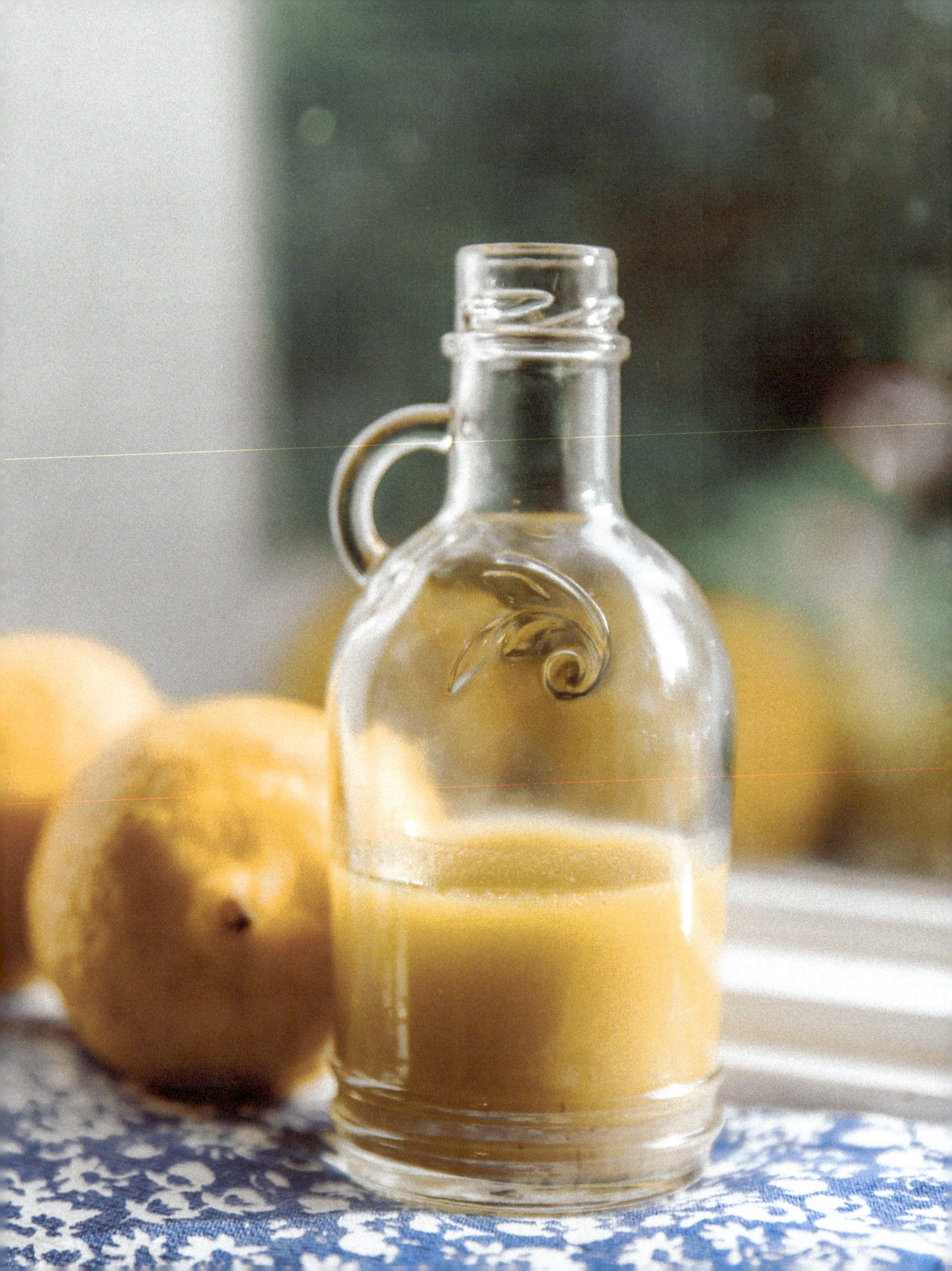

Lemon Dijon Vinaigrette

YIELD: ½ CUP

INGREDIENTS

2 tablespoons distilled white vinegar

½ lemon, juiced

1 clove garlic, peeled and grated

1 teaspoon Dijon mustard

1 tablespoon honey

¼ cup extra virgin olive oil

Kosher salt and freshly ground pepper

INSTRUCTIONS

Whisk the first 5 ingredients together in a medium-sized bowl. Slowly whisk in the olive oil. Season to taste with salt and pepper. You can also add all the ingredients to a Mason jar fitted with a lid and shake.

Ginger Glaze

This glaze might be the most used recipe in our family. I always make a double batch to keep some in the freezer. We love it on vegetable fried rice, Herby Turkey Meatballs (page 142), or as a dipping sauce for Pork Dumplings (page 162).

YIELD: ABOUT ⅔ CUP

INGREDIENTS

½ cup coconut aminos

⅓ cup water

1-inch knob fresh ginger, peeled and finely grated, about ½ teaspoon

2 tablespoons coconut sugar

1 tablespoon white distilled vinegar

1 teaspoon arrowroot starch, can substitute cornstarch

Kosher salt and freshly ground pepper

INSTRUCTIONS

1. Combine all ingredients in a small pot and whisk until you cannot see any bits of arrowroot.

2. Heat the mixture until it comes to a boil, then reduce the heat to low. Simmer for about 10 minutes, stirring occasionally until it starts to bubble and thickens slightly. Remove from heat and adjust seasoning if needed.

Honey Mustard Dressing

Homemade dressings are a quick and easy item to add to your weekly meal prep and are a fun way to get the kids involved in the kitchen. Just add everything into a Mason jar, make sure the lid is on tight, and shake.

YIELD: ABOUT ¾ CUP

INGREDIENTS

¼ cup mayonnaise

2 tablespoons Dijon mustard

2 tablespoons honey, or more to taste

1½ tablespoon distilled white vinegar

1 small clove garlic, peeled and finely grated

2 tablespoons extra virgin olive oil

Kosher salt and freshly ground pepper

INSTRUCTIONS

Add the first 5 ingredients to a bowl along with some salt and pepper. Slowly whisk in the olive oil and adjust seasoning if needed. You can also add all the ingredients to a Mason jar fitted with a lid and shake.

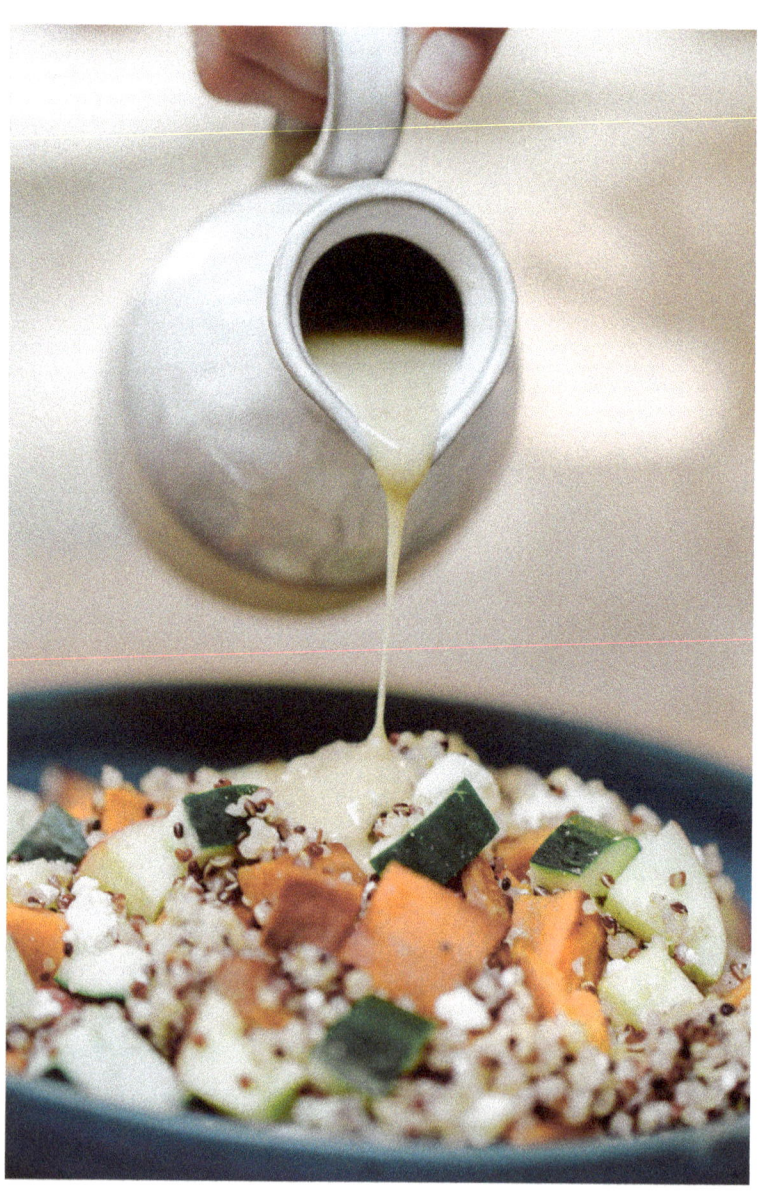

Creamy Poppy Seed Dressing

Kudos to you if you are the kind of person who goes the extra step and makes your own mayonnaise. I am not.

YIELD: ABOUT ½ CUP

INGREDIENTS

2 tablespoons extra virgin olive oil

¼ cup mayonnaise

½ teaspoon Dijon mustard

1 tablespoon honey

2 tablespoons distilled white vinegar

1 teaspoon poppy seeds

Kosher salt and freshly ground pepper

INSTRUCTIONS

Whisk the first 6 ingredients in a bowl and season to taste with salt and pepper.

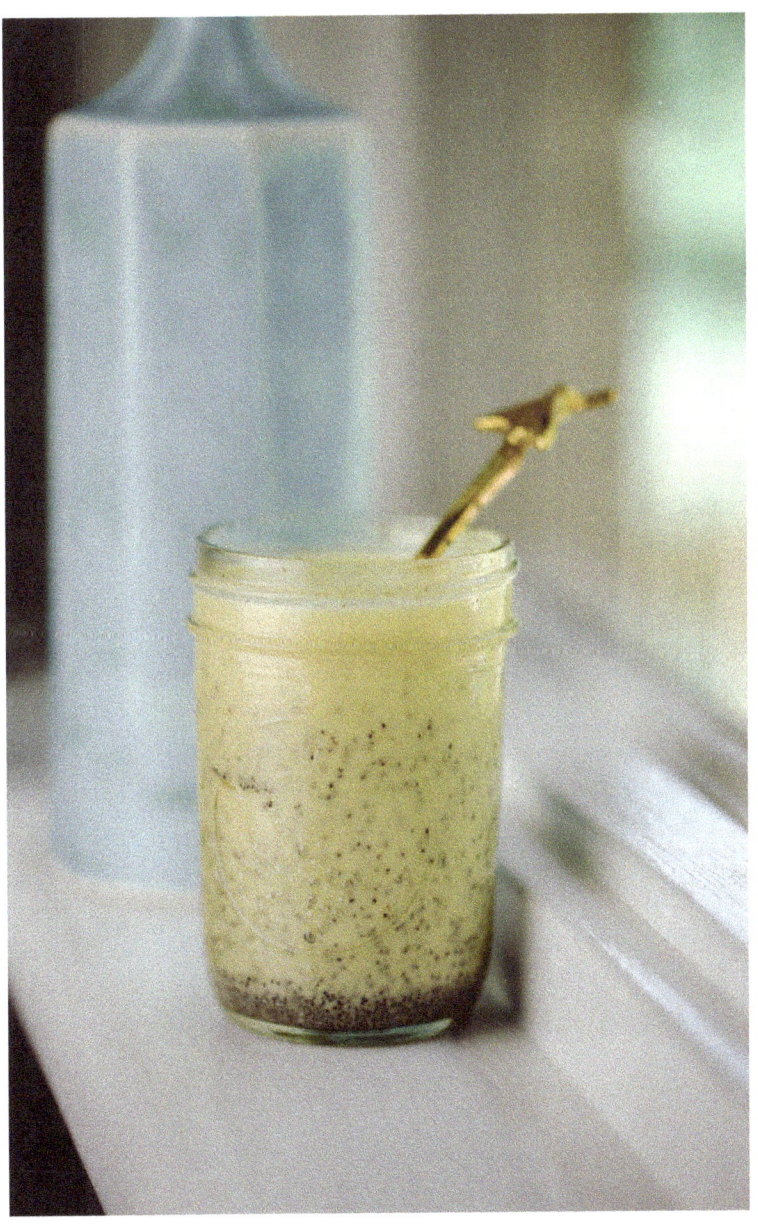

Roasted Poblano and Tomatillo Salsa

YIELD: 2 CUPS

INGREDIENTS

3 poblano peppers

1 pound tomatillos, or 4–5 medium, husks removed

Olive oil

3 scallions, trimmed and thinly sliced

1 garlic clove, peeled and grated or minced

½ teaspoon red pepper flakes (optional)

½ cup cilantro, chopped

½ cup parsley, chopped

Kosher salt and freshly ground pepper

INSTRUCTIONS

1. Preheat oven to 450°F.
2. Place the peppers and the tomatillos on a parchment-lined baking tray. Roast for 25 minutes and remove the tomatillos. Set them aside.
3. Toss the scallions with a little olive oil and add to the parchment-lined tray next to the peppers. Flip the peppers over and place back in the oven for another 5–10 minutes so that most of the peppers are blistered.
4. Remove the tray from the oven and place peppers in a bowl. Cover with plastic wrap for 15 minutes to loosen the skin. Then uncover, peel the peppers, remove the seeds and stems, and dice.
5. Add all the ingredients to a high-speed blender or food processor and season with salt and pepper. Blend until desired consistency and adjust seasoning if needed.

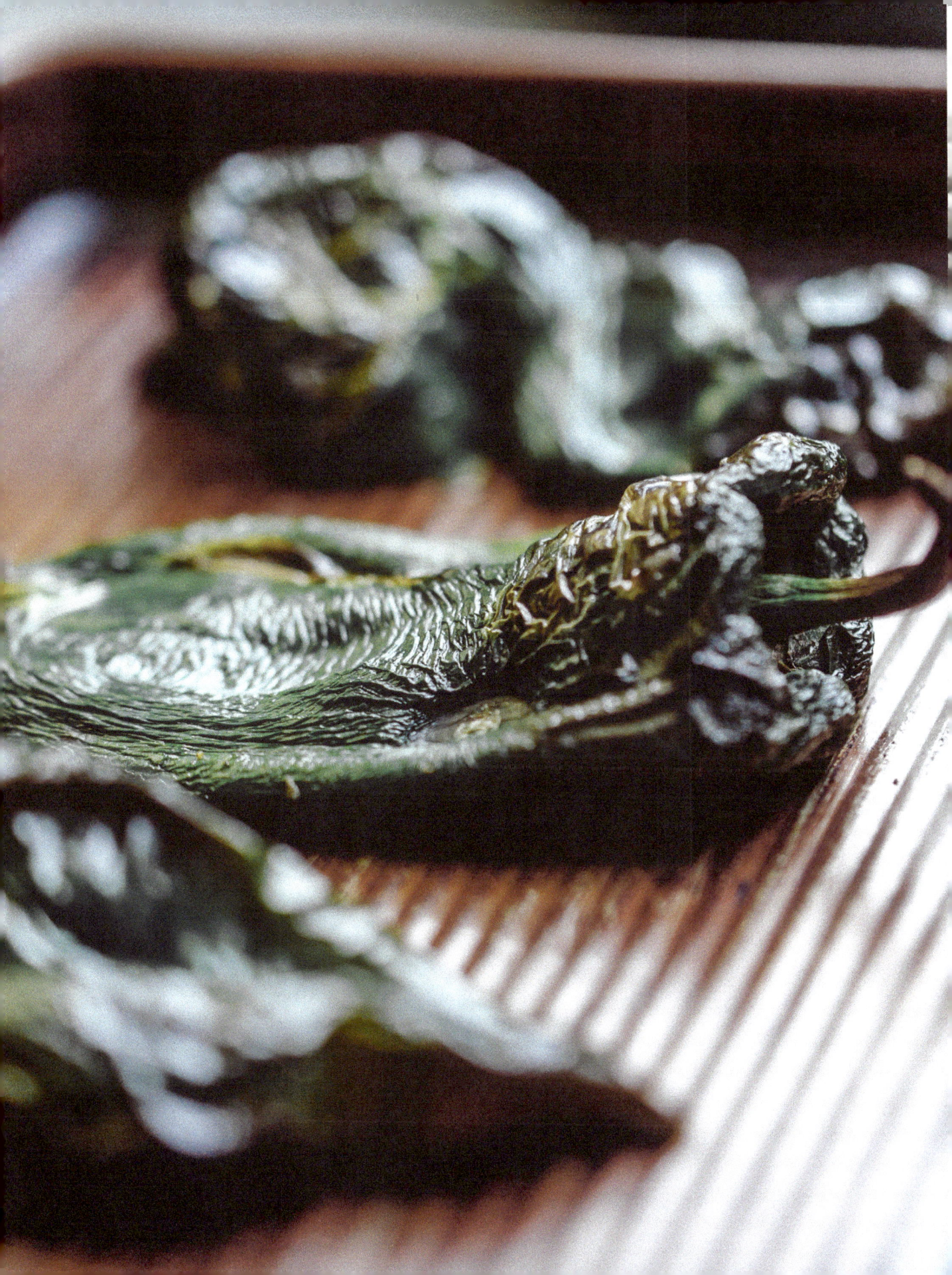

Herby Aioli Two Ways

YIELD: ABOUT ½ CUP

INGREDIENTS

Base

⅓ cup mayonnaise

3 tablespoons extra virgin olive oil

1 small clove garlic

Several fresh chives or green part of 1 scallion

Kosher salt and freshly ground pepper

Parsley Lemon

2 teaspoons lemon juice

½ cup fresh parsley (some stems OK)

Cilantro Lime

2 teaspoons lime juice

½ cup fresh cilantro (some stems OK)

INSTRUCTIONS

1. Place all the base ingredients into a high-speed blender and add herb and citrus of choice. Blend until smooth. Adjust seasoning if needed. You can also chop the herbs by hand and mix together in a bowl.

2. If the aioli is going to be used as more of a dressing, you can add a tablespoon of water to thin the mixture.

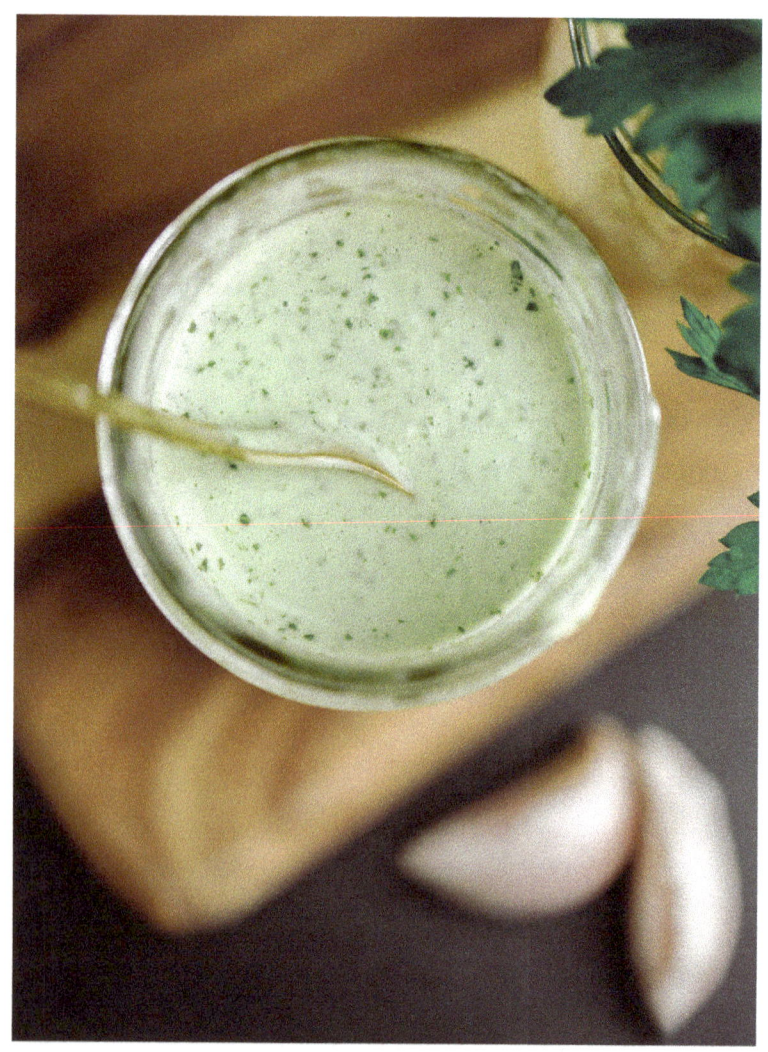

Taco Seasoning

Because it's hard to find taco seasoning without the onion granules

YIELD: ABOUT ¼ CUP

INGREDIENTS

1 tablespoon chili powder

1 tablespoon ground cumin

1 tablespoon garlic granules

1 teaspoon paprika

1 teaspoon oregano

½ teaspoon coconut sugar

INSTRUCTIONS

Mix all ingredients in a bowl.

Can store at room temperature for several months.

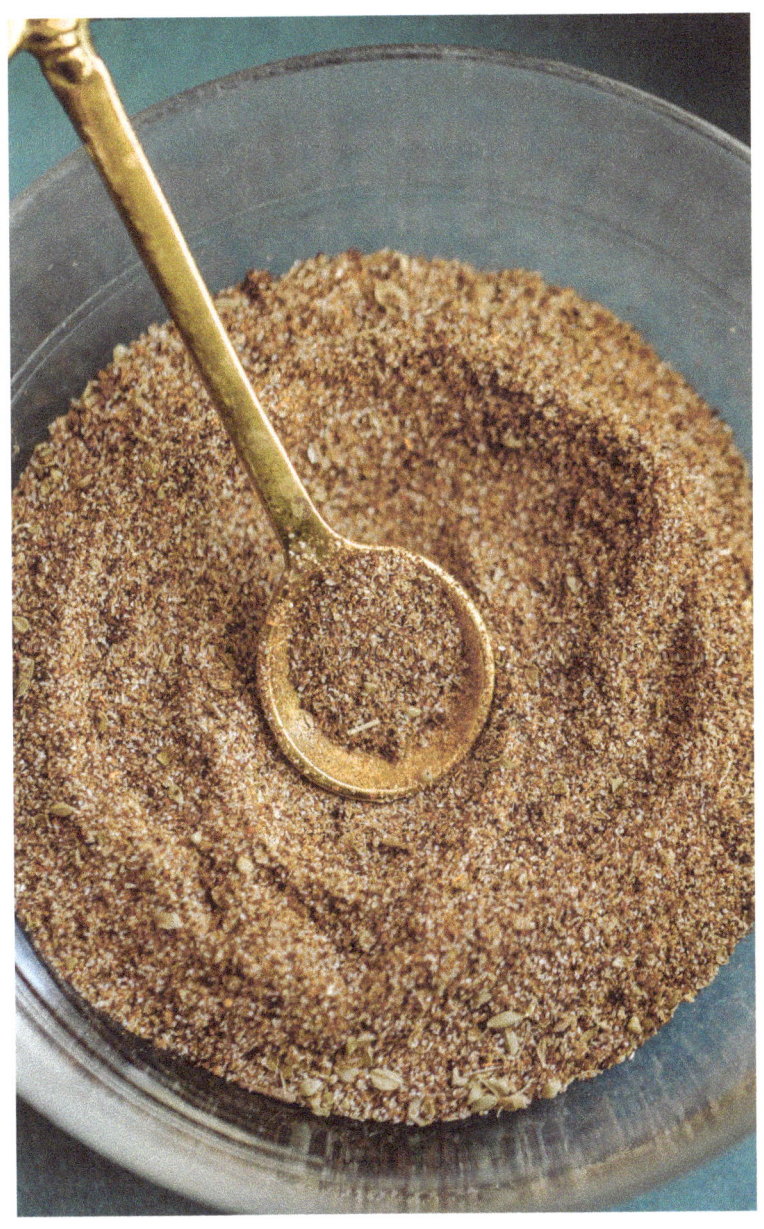

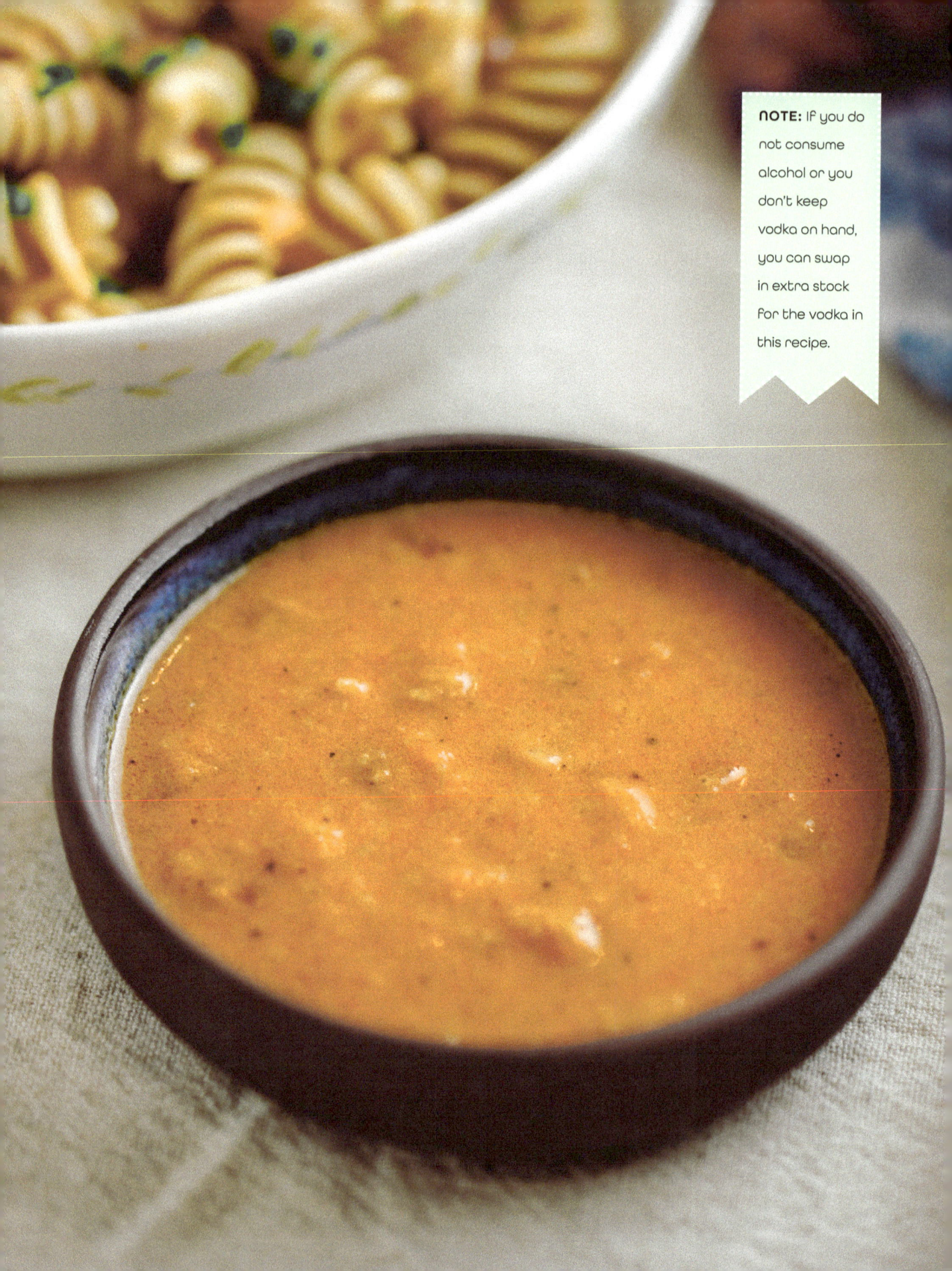

NOTE: If you do not consume alcohol or you don't keep vodka on hand, you can swap in extra stock for the vodka in this recipe.

Roasted Red Pepper Vodka Sauce

YIELD: 1½ CUPS

INGREDIENTS

1 cup jarred roasted red peppers, drained

½ cup canned coconut milk, plus more if needed

½ cup stock such as vegetable or chicken, preferably homemade (pages 84, 86), or non-MSG stock

¼ cup plain hummus

1 tablespoon olive oil

1 shallot, finely chopped

2 garlic cloves, peeled and minced or grated

¼ cup vodka

Pinch of red pepper flakes

Fresh basil to top (optional)

Kosher salt and freshly ground pepper

TIP: This sauce is great tossed with pasta and Banzo Balls (page 112).

INSTRUCTIONS

1. In a high-speed blender, add the roasted red peppers, coconut milk, stock, and hummus along with some salt and pepper. Blend until smooth and set aside.

2. Heat a skillet or pot over medium-high heat and add the olive oil. Once the oil is hot, add the shallot to the pan and stir to coat in the oil. Allow to cook for a couple of minutes until it barely starts to brown. Then add the garlic and a large pinch of salt and pepper.

3. After about a minute carefully add the vodka. Reduce by about half, then add the red pepper mixture from the blender.

4. Bring to a light boil then turn heat down and simmer for about 10 minutes. The mixture should begin to thicken slightly.

5. Add the red pepper flakes and turn off heat. Check for seasoning and adjust if needed. I like to add another splash of coconut milk here, then top with fresh basil, if using.

Super Seed Mix

This mix was adapted from a Trader Joe's product that was discontinued many years ago. It gives a nice crunch to the Super Seed Granola (page 37). I also like to add a tablespoon of it to the pot when I am cooking grains for added nutrients.

YIELD: ⅓ CUP

INGREDIENTS

3 tablespoons hemp hearts

2 tablespoons chia seeds

1½ tablespoons flax seeds

1½ tablespoons poppy seeds

INSTRUCTIONS

Mix all the ingredients together and store in a tightly sealed container at room temperature.

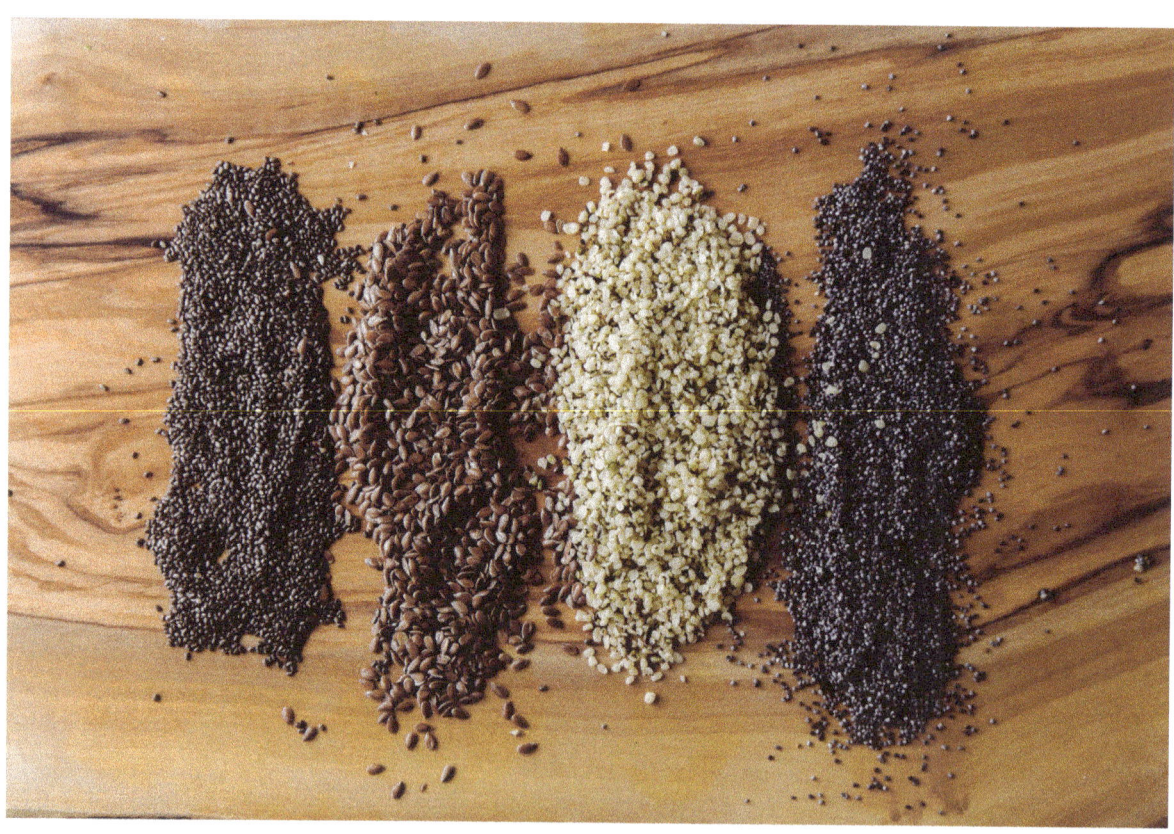

Thai "Peanut" Sauce

A nut-free Thai sauce that goes with everything from grilled vegetables to grains and noodles

YIELD: ABOUT 1 CUP

INGREDIENTS

1-inch knob ginger, peeled

1 garlic clove, peeled

1 scallion, trimmed

¼ cup sunflower seed butter

¼ cup coconut aminos

¼–½ teaspoon red pepper flakes

Juice of ½ lime

1 teaspoon honey, only if sunflower seed butter is not sweetened

Kosher salt and freshly ground pepper

INSTRUCTIONS

1. Add all the ingredients into a high-speed blender or food processor along with 2–3 tablespoons water and blend until smooth. You can add more or less water depending on how thick you'd like the sauce, but it does thicken over time.

2. Season to taste with salt and pepper.

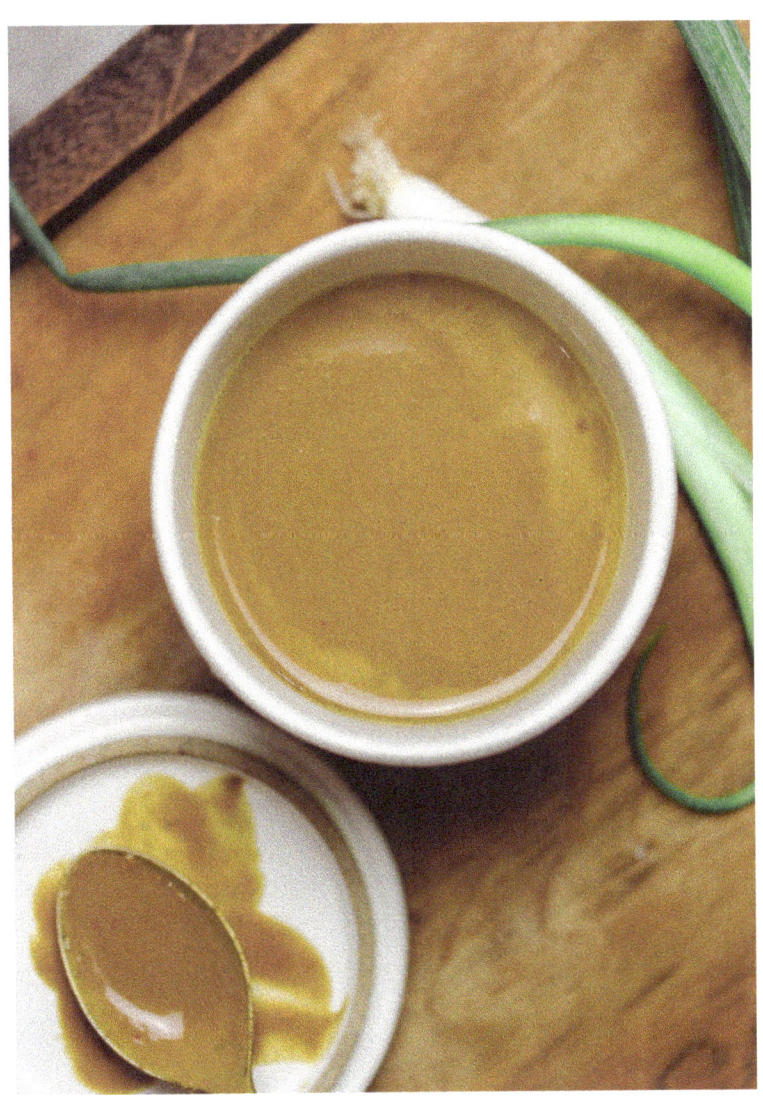

Cauliflower Cream

This is a great replacement for the canned cream of mushroom or cream of chicken products you see at the grocery store that are usually filled with unwanted, processed ingredients.

YIELD: 2½ CUPS

INGREDIENTS

1 head cauliflower, cut into florets (about 16 oz)

½ cup vegetable or chicken stock, preferably homemade (pages 84, 86), or non-MSG stock

¼ teaspoon garlic granules

½ teaspoon Italian seasoning

1 tablespoon unsalted butter, melted

Kosher salt and freshly ground pepper

INSTRUCTIONS

1. Bring a medium-sized pot of water to a boil and add the cauliflower. Turn heat down to medium-low and lightly boil until the cauliflower is tender, about 8–10 minutes. Drain and cool slightly.

2. Place cauliflower in a high-speed blender with the rest of the ingredients and some salt and pepper. Blend until smooth. Adjust seasoning if needed.

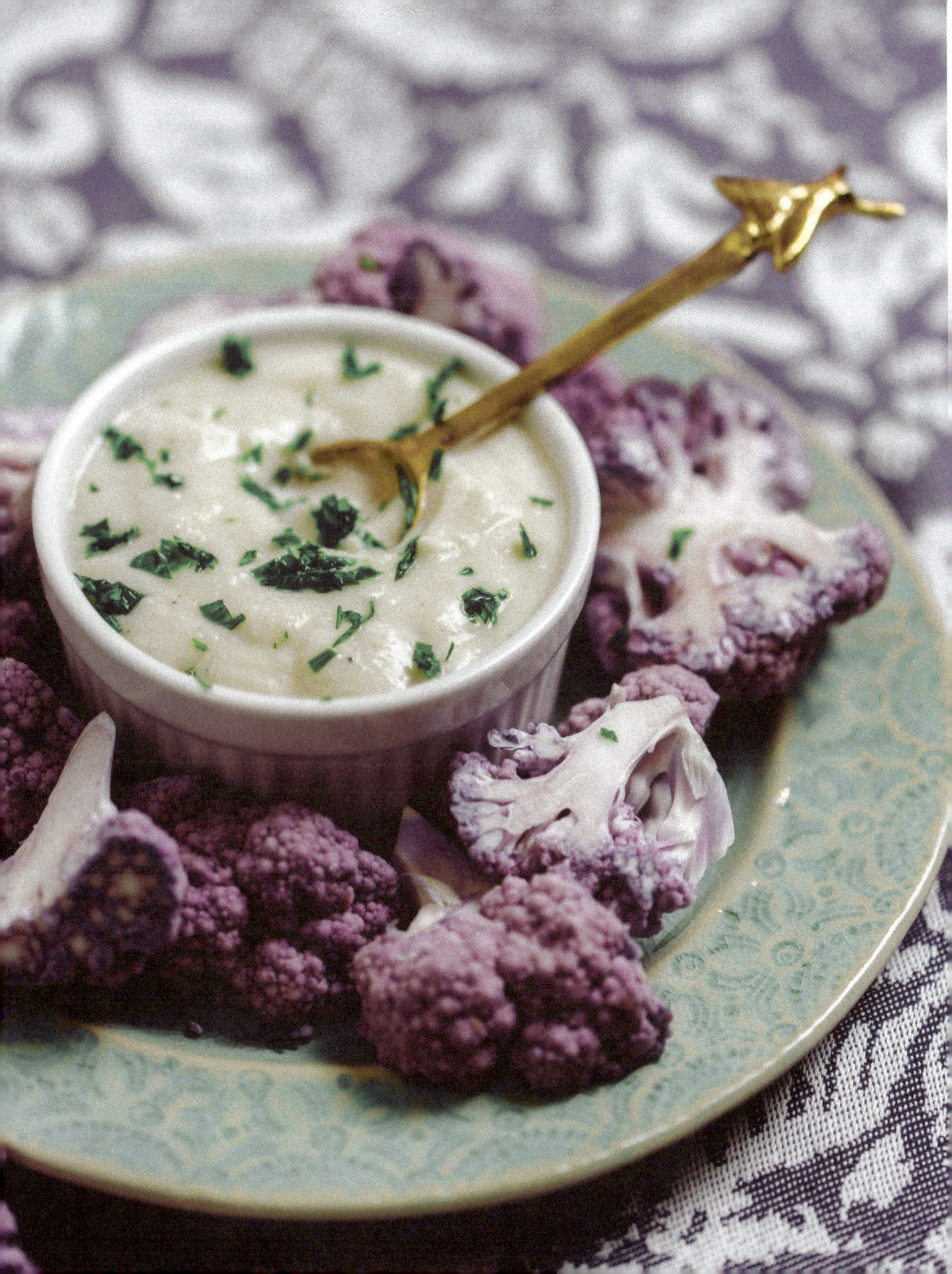

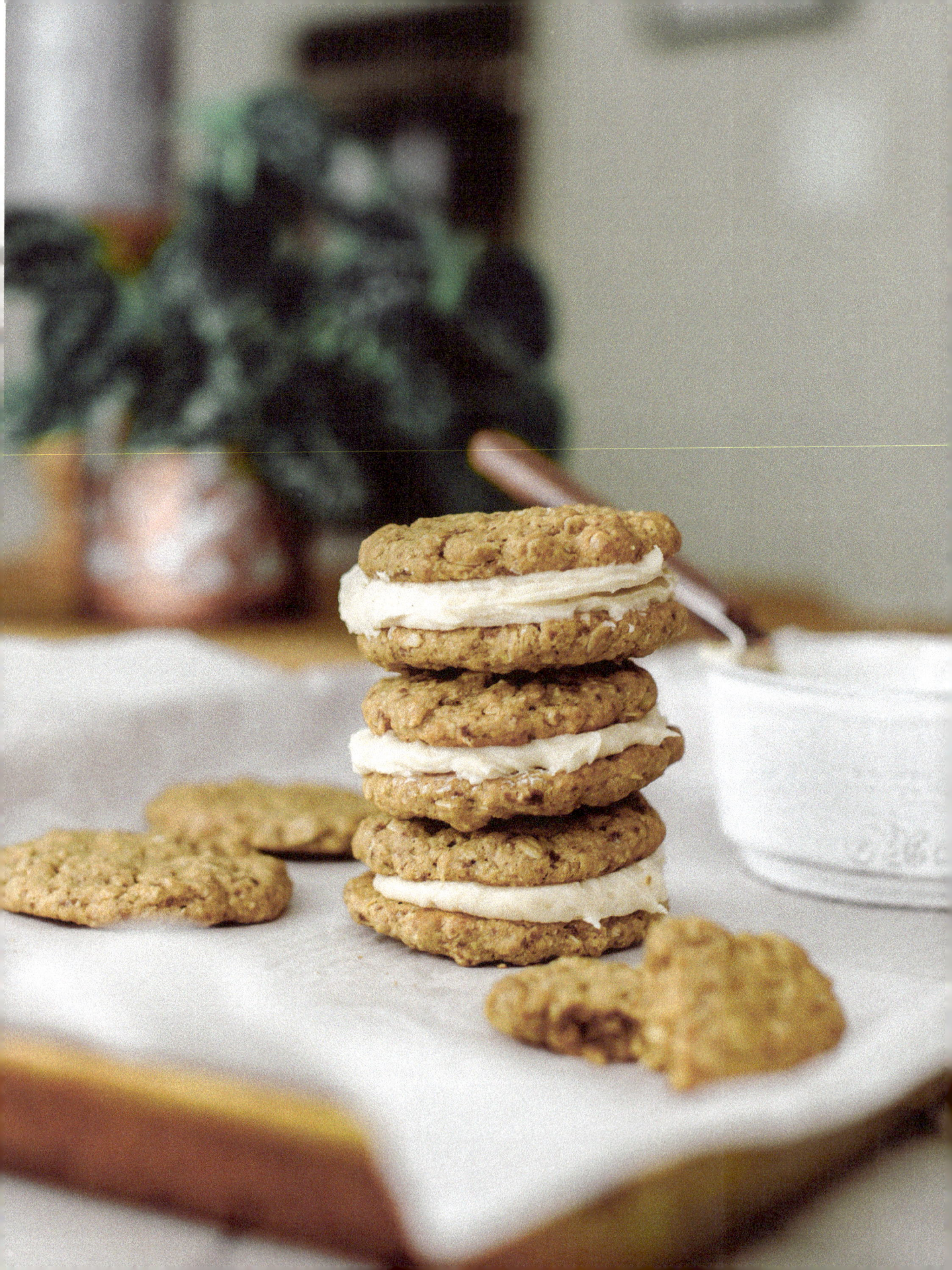

Sweets

Mixed Berry Jam 248

Oatmeal Cookie Cream Pies 250

Berry Crumble Bars 252

Grandma's Peach and Blueberry Cobbler 255

Strawberry Rhubarb Crisp 256

Coconut Whipped Cream 259

Coconut Caramel Sauce 259

Go-To Pie Crust 260

Caramel Pear Tartlets 263

Cinnamon Apple Galette 264

Mixed Berry Jam

Every year as the weather starts to warm up, I look forward to all the delicious fruit available at the farmers market. At least once a year I make a large batch of jam and store it in small Mason jars to pull out throughout the fall and winter. This jam is great mixed into oatmeal, yogurt, or spooned over pancakes and waffles.

YIELD: ABOUT 2 CUPS

INGREDIENTS

2 pounds berries such as blueberries, strawberries, and blackberries, washed (quarter the strawberries if large)

About ⅔ cup sugar, or more if berries are out of season, can substitute coconut sugar

¼ teaspoon kosher salt, or more to taste

Juice of ½ lemon

INSTRUCTIONS

1. In a medium-sized pot mix the fruit with the sugar and allow to sit for about 15 minutes until the berries have released some of their juices. Bring the mixture to a boil and then reduce to a simmer. Add the salt.

2. Cook, stirring occasionally, for 30 minutes or until the mixture thickens. If you like your jam thicker, simmer for another 10–15 minutes.

3. Add the lemon juice and turn off heat. At this point you can leave the jam chunky or blend with an immersion blender until desired consistency. Alternatively, allow the jam to cool slightly then place in a high-speed blender and blend.

4. Place the jam in the refrigerator and cool completely. It will keep for 2–3 weeks covered in the fridge.

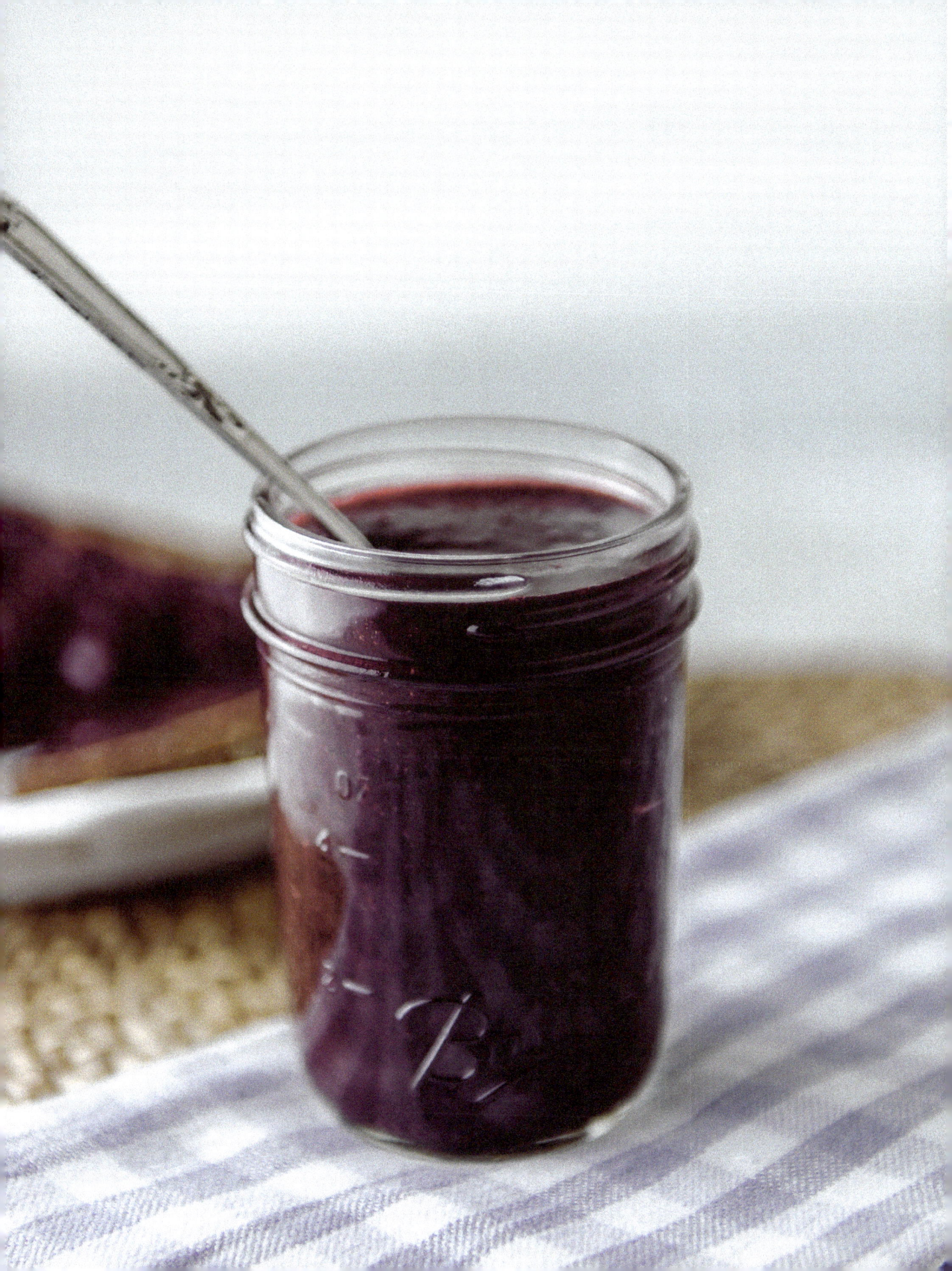

Oatmeal Cookie Cream Pies

This is my attempt to create a less-processed version of the Little Debbie Oatmeal Creme Pies I loved as a child. The cookies are great by themselves or made into cream pies. I love to keep them in the freezer and when I am craving one, I let it sit out at room temperature for about 10 minutes before enjoying.

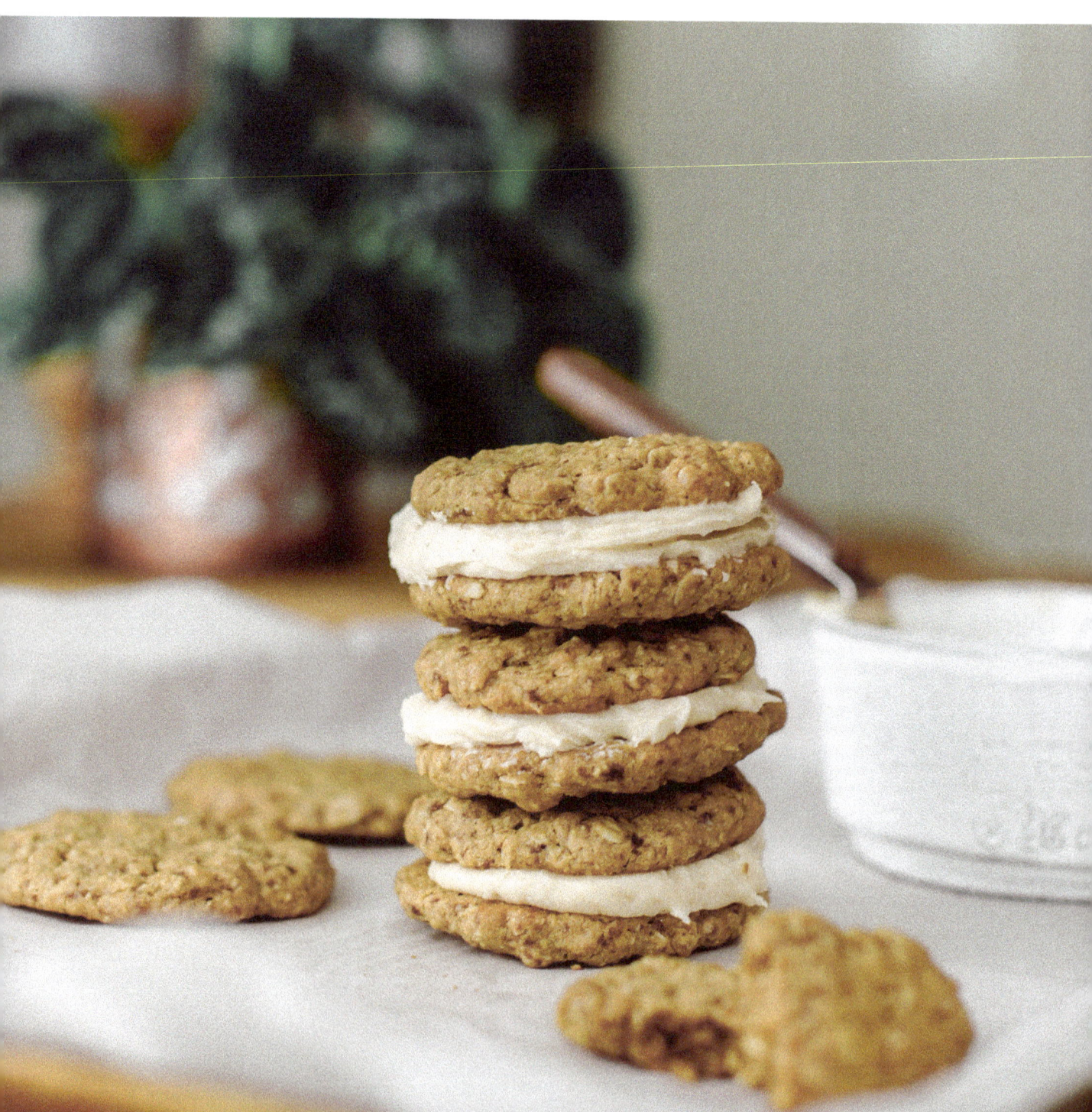

INGREDIENTS

Cookies

¼ cup unsalted butter, room temperature

¼ cup coconut oil (or another ¼ cup unsalted softened butter)

1 cup dark brown sugar

1 egg

1 teaspoon pure vanilla extract

½ cup oat flour (page 13)

¾ cup all-purpose or gluten-free flour such as Bob's Red Mill

1 cup rolled oats

1 teaspoon baking powder

¼ teaspoon baking soda

¾ teaspoon ground cinnamon

½ teaspoon salt

Filling

4 tablespoons unsalted butter, room temperature

⅓ cup cream cheese, room temperature

½ teaspoon pure vanilla extract or vanilla bean paste

¼ teaspoon ground cinnamon

⅛ teaspoon kosher salt

1⅓ cups powdered sugar

INSTRUCTIONS

Cookies

1. Preheat oven to 375°F.
2. In a stand mixer beat the butter and coconut oil (or additional butter) together with a paddle attachment.
3. Once combined add the dark brown sugar and continue mixing, scraping down the sides when needed.
4. Add the egg and vanilla extract. Mix until combined.
5. In a bowl add the oat flour, all-purpose flour, oats, baking powder, baking soda, cinnamon, and salt. Mix until the ingredients are evenly distributed.
6. Then add the dry ingredients in 3 batches into the mixer and mix only until combined. Don't overmix.
7. Scoop the dough out into 18 portions (about golf-ball size) and press down each cookie about halfway.
8. Bake for 8–10 minutes or until the edges begin to turn golden-brown. Remove and set aside to cool.

Filling

1. In a stand mixer with a whisk attachment add the butter and cream cheese.
2. Whisk until combined and smooth. Then add the vanilla, cinnamon, and salt.
3. Whisk until smooth and add the powdered sugar in 2–3 batches until mixture is smooth.
4. To assemble, once cooled, flip 9 of the cookies over.
5. Divide filling evenly in the cookie centers. Then top with remaining cookies. Press down lightly.

I prefer to store them in the fridge or even freezer until just before serving. If you keep them in the freezer, allow them to sit at room temperature for about 10 minutes before serving.

Berry Crumble Bars

YIELD: 16 SMALL SQUARES

INGREDIENTS

12 tablespoons unsalted butter, room temperature

¾ cup cane sugar or coconut sugar

1 teaspoon pure vanilla extract

1½ cups all-purpose or gluten-free flour

¾ cup oat flour (page 13)

½ teaspoon kosher salt

1 cup Mixed Berry Jam (page 248 or other migraine-friendly jam)

1 cup Super Seed Granola (page 37)

INSTRUCTIONS

1. Preheat oven to 350°F.
2. Line an 8" x 8" dish with parchment paper, leaving extra to hang over the sides.
3. Using a stand mixer fitted with the paddle attachment or hand beaters, beat the butter until it is soft and light in color. Then add the sugar and vanilla. Mix until combined.
4. In a separate bowl, whisk together the flour, oat flour, and salt.
5. While the mixer is on low-speed, slowly add the dry ingredients. Mix just until incorporated, scraping down the sides if needed as you go.
6. Place ⅔ of the dough in the parchment-lined dish and press down so it covers the bottom evenly. Then spread the jam on top of the dough.
7. Combine the granola with remaining dough and evenly spread out on top of the jam. Press down and bake for about 45 minutes or until the top begins to lightly brown.
8. Remove from the oven and allow to cool before slicing and removing from the pan.

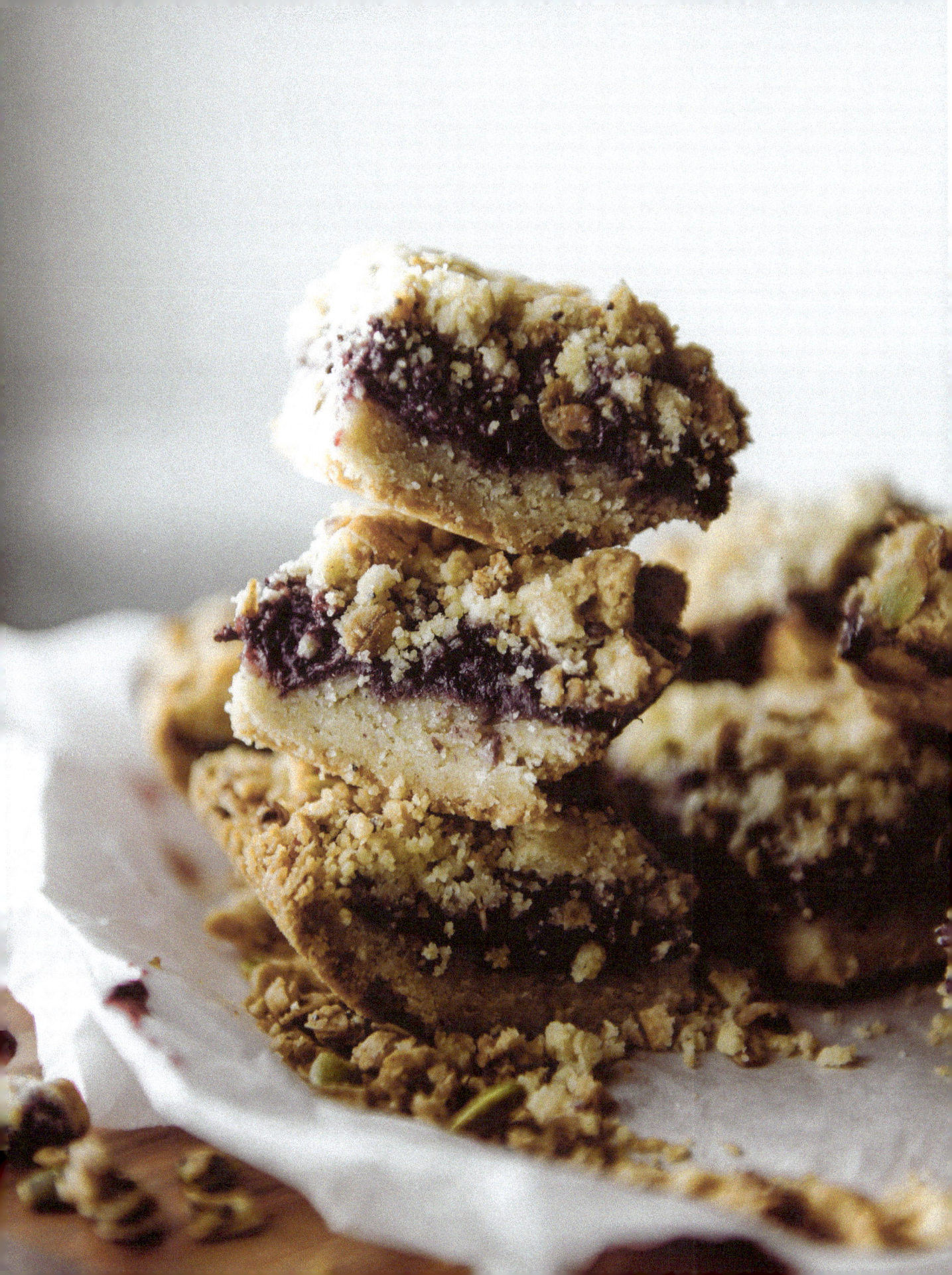

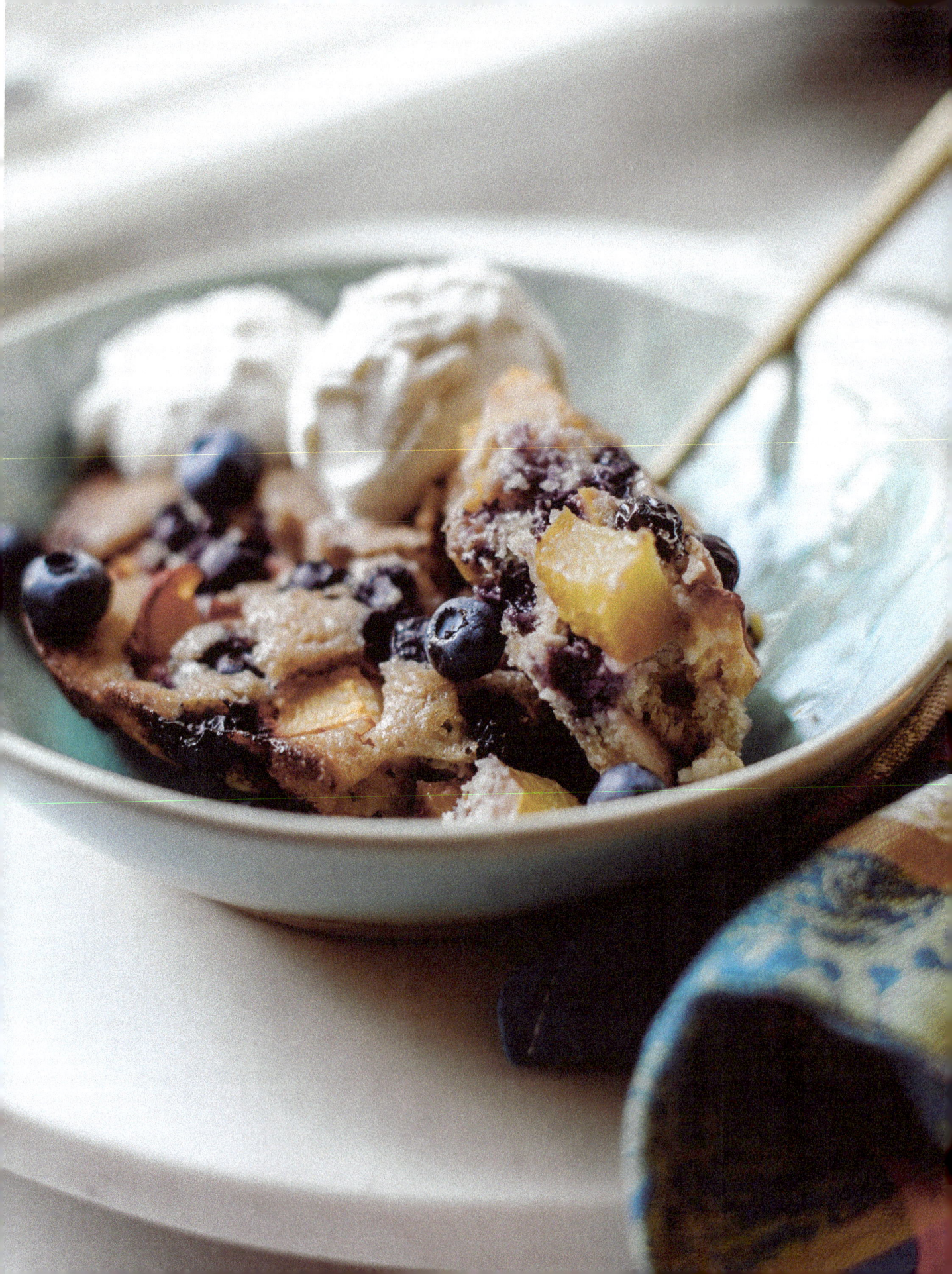

Grandma's Peach and Blueberry Cobbler

This is another recipe inspired by my grandma. I was around 8 years old the first time I watched her make this dessert at my grandparents' mountain house in Boone, North Carolina. She made it look so easy, and I remember counting the minutes until we all finished dinner and I was able to try some. She served it with a big scoop of ice cream right on top, and I couldn't get enough. I managed to devour a second serving almost as quickly as the first.

YIELD: 8 SERVINGS

INGREDIENTS

4 tablespoons unsalted butter

1 cup self-rising flour

⅔ cup light brown sugar or coconut sugar

1 teaspoon ground cinnamon

¼ teaspoon kosher salt

1 cup whole milk

Juice of ½ lemon

3 cups fresh, ripe peaches, pitted and diced, about 3 peaches

1½ cups fresh blueberries

Ice cream or whipped cream, to serve. Delicious with Coconut Whipped Cream (page 259) on top

INSTRUCTIONS

1. Preheat oven to 425°F.
2. Melt butter in an 11" x 8" casserole dish or comparably sized cast-iron pan in the oven as it preheats for about 10 minutes. The butter should begin to brown slightly. Remove from the oven.
3. Meanwhile, mix together the flour, sugar, cinnamon, and salt.
4. Add the milk and lemon juice and stir to combine.
5. Pour the batter over the melted butter.
6. Evenly distribute the fruit over the batter and place back in preheated oven.
7. Bake for about 25 minutes or until golden-brown on top. Allow it to cool slightly before serving.

Strawberry Rhubarb Crisp

I love to make this crisp when I am entertaining. It's not too heavy and can be made earlier in the day. You can add a big dollop of Coconut Whipped Cream (page 259) or ice cream on top.

INGREDIENTS

Filling

3 heaping cups sliced rhubarb, ½-inch slices

3 heaping cups strawberries, halved or quartered depending on their size

½ cup coconut sugar or cane sugar

⅛ teaspoon ground cinnamon

¼ teaspoon kosher salt

1½ tablespoons arrowroot, can substitute cornstarch

Juice of 1 lemon

Topping

¼ cup coconut sugar

1 cup old-fashioned oats

½ cup all-purpose flour or gluten-free flour

¼ teaspoon salt

6 tablespoons cold unsalted butter

INSTRUCTIONS

1. Preheat oven to 400°F.

2. In a large bowl, add the rhubarb, strawberries, sugar, cinnamon, salt, arrowroot, and lemon juice. Mix until thoroughly combined.

3. Pour the mixture into a cast-iron pan or an 8" x 8" size dish or similar.

4. For the topping, mix the coconut sugar, oats, flour, and salt in a bowl. You can use the same bowl as the filling to mix, just make sure you scraped out most of the filling. Cut the butter into chunks then using a pastry blender cut the butter into the dry ingredients. The butter should be about the size of a small bean when finished.

5. Once well combined, evenly distribute the topping over the filling and place in the oven.

6. Bake for 30–40 minutes or until the edges are golden-brown. Remove and allow to cool.

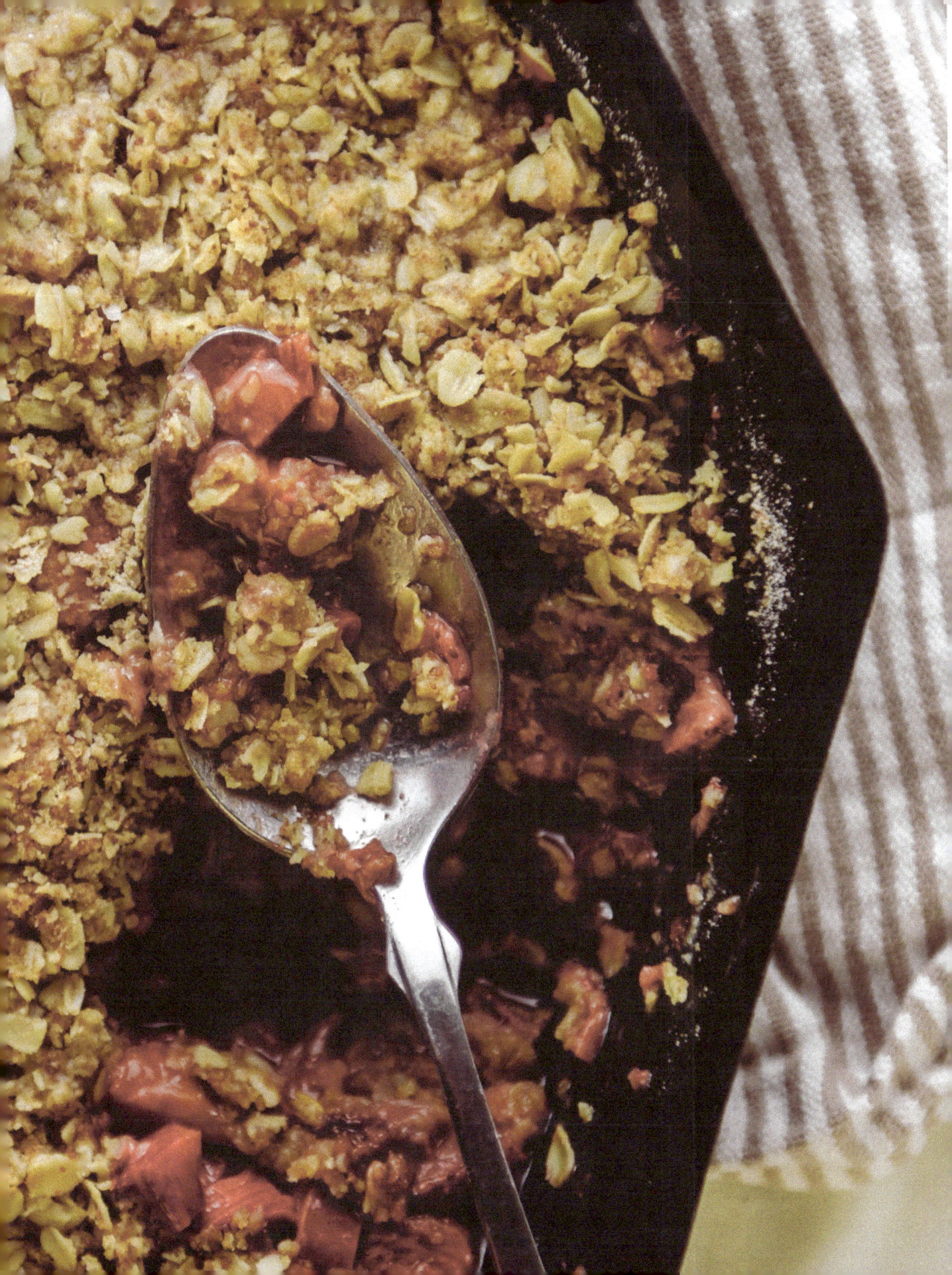

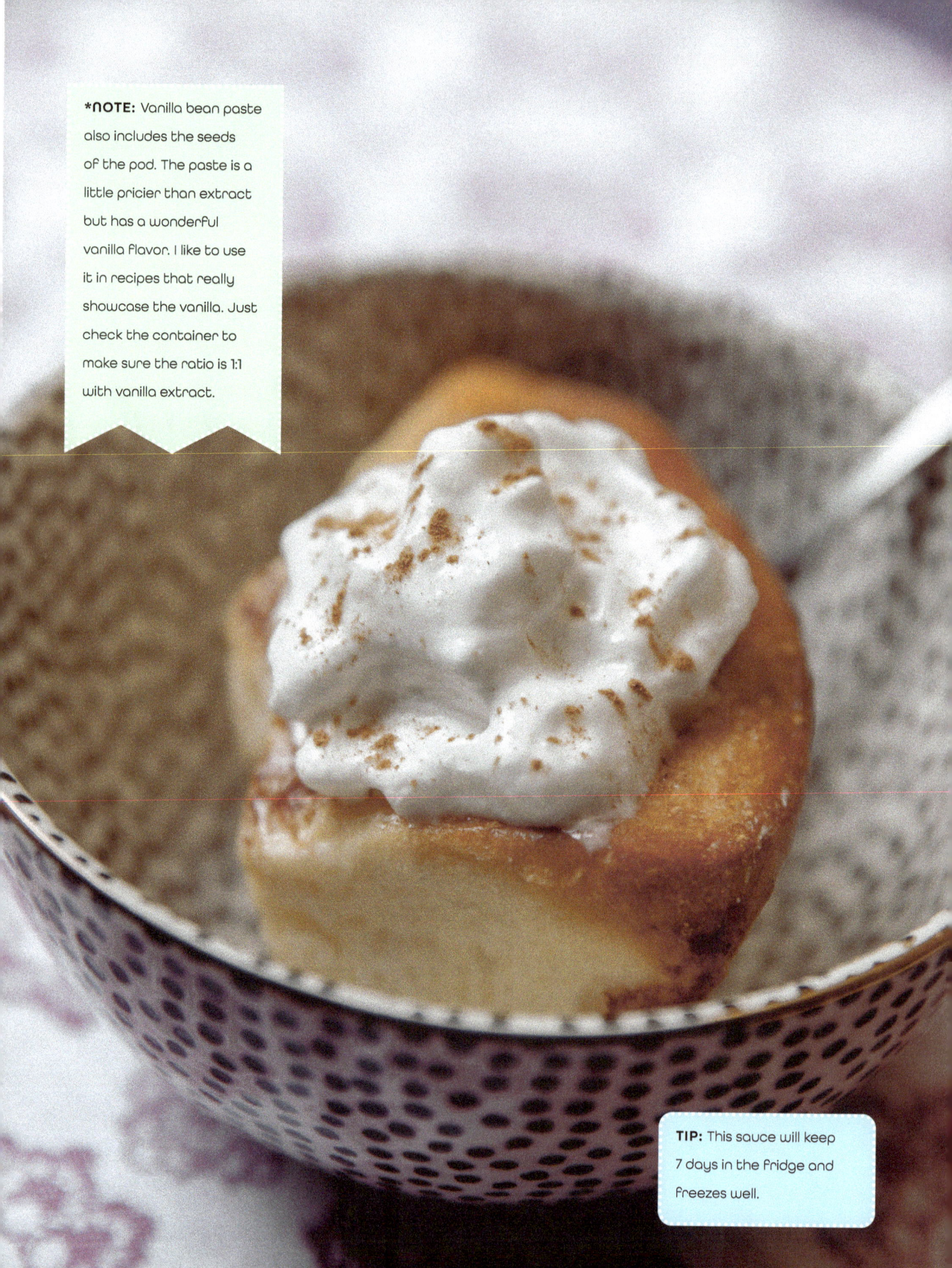

*NOTE: Vanilla bean paste also includes the seeds of the pod. The paste is a little pricier than extract but has a wonderful vanilla flavor. I like to use it in recipes that really showcase the vanilla. Just check the container to make sure the ratio is 1:1 with vanilla extract.

TIP: This sauce will keep 7 days in the fridge and freezes well.

Coconut Whipped Cream

This whipped cream is a nice dairy-free alternative. Be sure to chill the coconut before beginning. You can use canned coconut cream, or if you have full-fat coconut milk, the cream (fat) will separate, and you can carefully extract it from the can. The leftover liquid can be used in smoothies or sauces. Thai Kitchen coconut milk and Whole Foods 365 coconut milk work best in this recipe.

YIELD: ABOUT 2 CUPS

INGREDIENTS

1 cup coconut cream, chilled for 12–24 hours in the fridge

1½ tablespoons powdered sugar, or more to taste

1 teaspoon pure vanilla extract or vanilla bean paste*

Kosher salt

INSTRUCTIONS

1. Place the coconut cream in a stand mixer fitted with a paddle attachment. Beat on medium high for a few minutes until the mixture looks light and fluffy and has almost doubled in size.

2. Add the powdered sugar, vanilla (or vanilla bean paste), and a small pinch of salt.

Coconut Caramel Sauce

For a dairy-free caramel sauce that's great on desserts like the Cinnamon Apple Galette (page 264) or Caramel Pear Tartlets (page 263), or you can drizzle it on ice cream

YIELD: ¾–1 CUP

INGREDIENTS

2 tablespoons coconut oil or unsalted butter

¾ cup coconut sugar or light brown sugar

1 cup full-fat coconut milk

¼ teaspoon kosher salt

1 teaspoon pure vanilla extract or vanilla bean paste (see Note)

INSTRUCTIONS

1. Add the oil or butter and the sugar to a small sauce pot.

2. Melt over medium heat.

3. Stir in the coconut milk and salt.

4. Turn heat to low and with a heavy simmer going, reduce mixture by about half, for about 15 minutes.

5. Turn off heat and stir in the vanilla. Allow it to cool. The mixture will continue to thicken as it cools.

Go-To Pie Crust

This has been my go-to pie crust recipe ever since I can remember. Feel free to substitute gluten-free flour if gluten is a trigger for you. I have made many gluten-free pie crusts and learned that they are more delicate, so be extra careful when rolling it out and remember you can patch any holes. It doesn't have to look perfect.

YIELD: 1 PIE CRUST

INGREDIENTS

1¼ cups all-purpose flour or gluten-free flour

¼ teaspoon kosher salt

2 teaspoons sugar

½ cup or 1 stick unsalted butter, cold and cut into chunks

About ½ cup cold water

INSTRUCTIONS

1. Combine the flour, salt, and sugar in a medium-sized bowl.
2. Using a pastry blender, cut in the cold butter until the pieces are the size of peas.
3. Starting with ⅓ cup, add the water and stir. You should have a few crumbs at the bottom of the bowl. If it looks too dry, add the rest of the water and stir.
4. Place the dough onto a clean, lightly floured surface and pat the dough into a thick square.
5. For the cut and stack method, cut the dough in half from the top using a bench scraper. Stack one half on the other, adding any crumbs on top. Press down lightly and repeat 5–7 times. This is what is going to give you all those flaky layers.
6. Wrap the dough in plastic wrap and place in the fridge until you are ready to roll out the dough. It will keep in the fridge for 24 hours, or you can freeze it.
7. To roll out the dough, place it on a lightly floured surface and sprinkle a little flour on top so it does not stick to the rolling pin.
8. Starting in the center of the dough, roll out in each direction to form a circle. It helps to turn the dough slightly as you work, making sure there is enough flour on the counter so the dough does not stick as you roll it out.
9. Continue rolling until the circle of dough is about an inch wider than the pie dish. Using the rolling pin to help transport the dough, carefully place the dough over the pie dish and press lightly on the bottom and sides. Crimp the top edges of the dish.

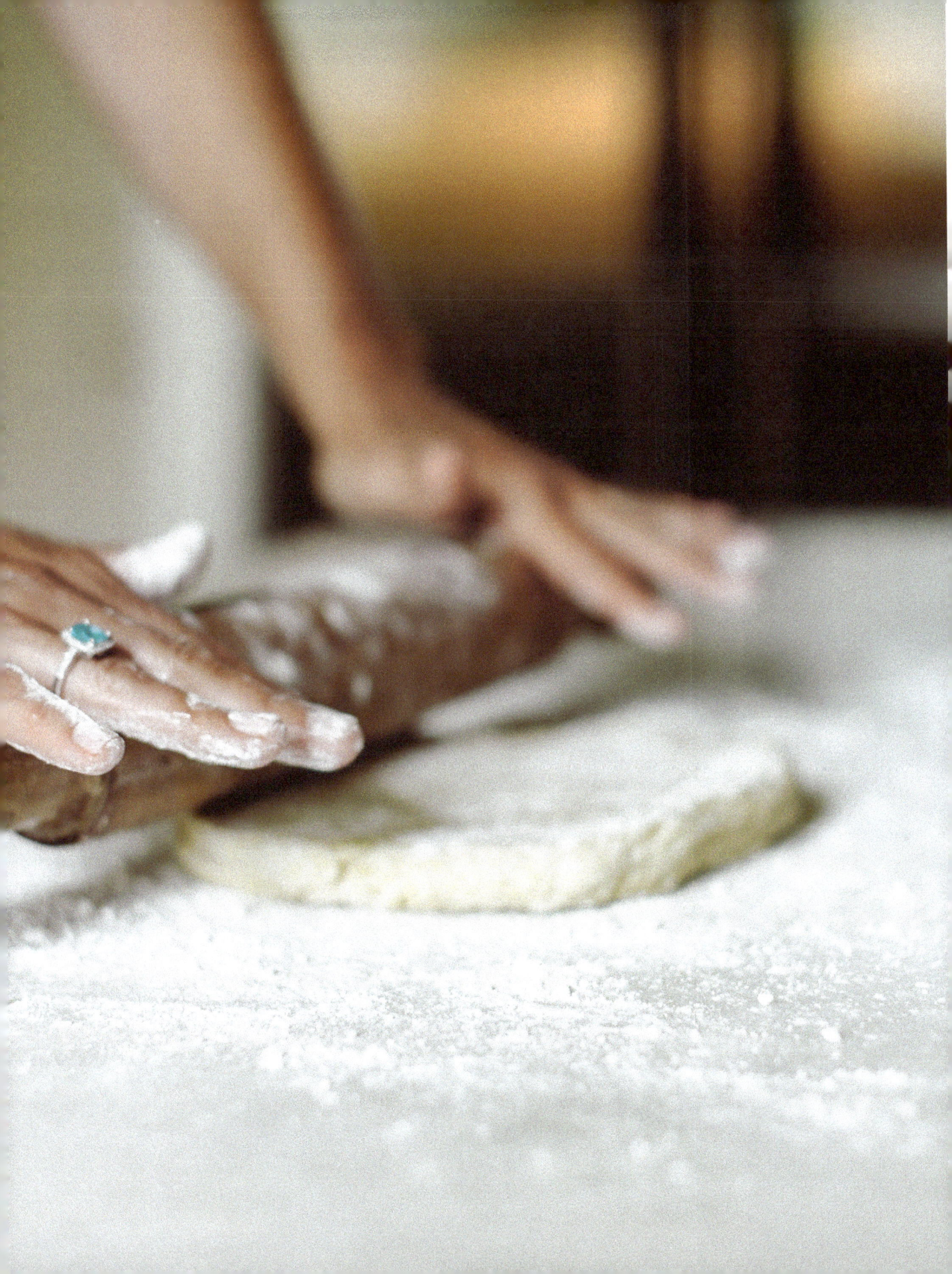

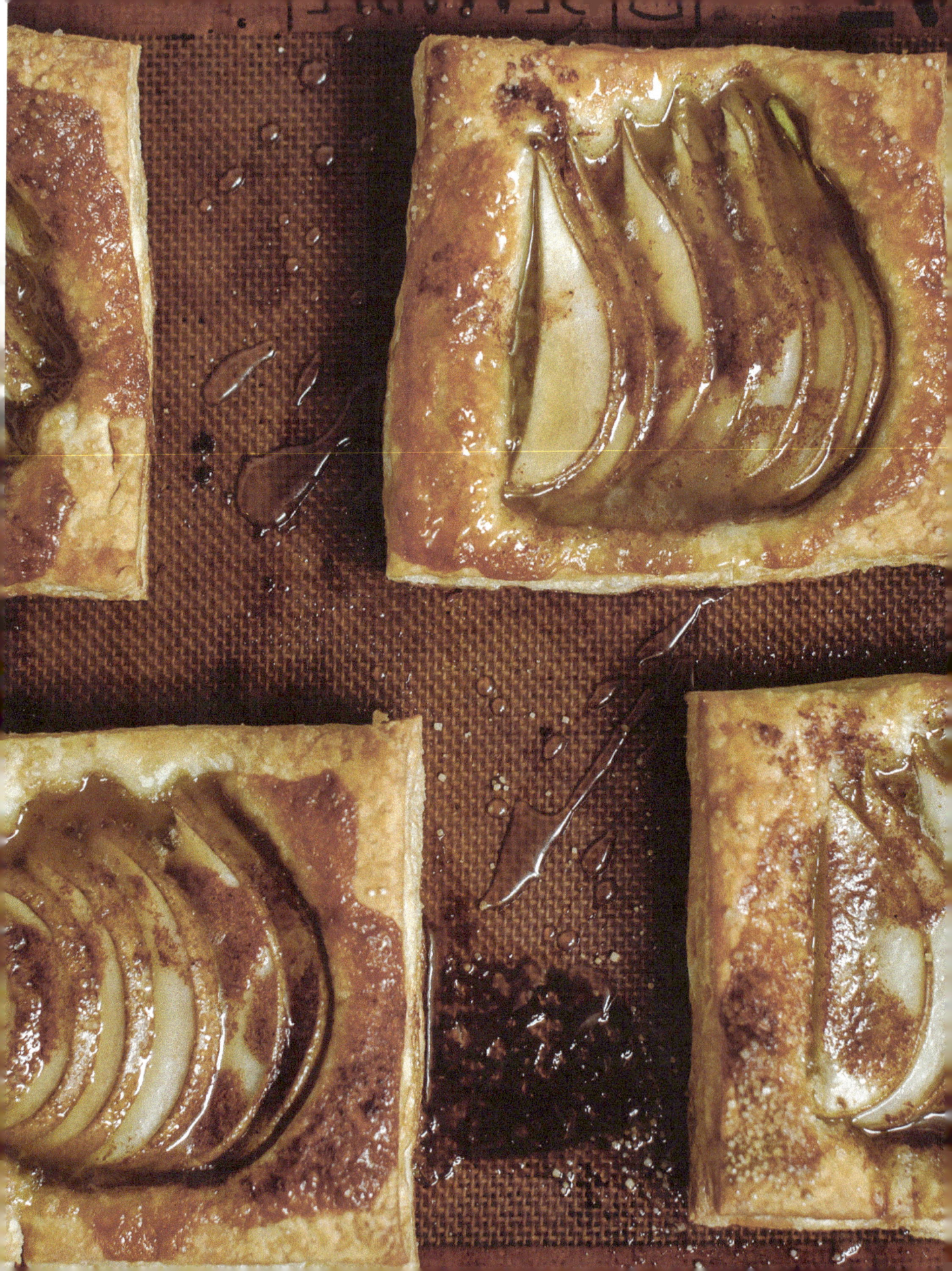

Caramel Pear Tartlets

I don't use many processed ingredients, but once in a while ready-made puff pastry is a nice shortcut. Once the pastry has defrosted, this dessert comes together rather quickly and is always a festive dessert for a fall gathering.

YIELD: 8 TARTLETS

INGREDIENTS

2 sheets frozen puff pastry (approximately 400 grams)

1 recipe Coconut Caramel Sauce (page 259)

4 tablespoons unsalted butter, room temperature

½ teaspoon ground cinnamon

⅛ teaspoon ground nutmeg

Kosher salt

3 pears such as Bosc, Bartlett, or Anjou

2 tablespoons turbinado sugar

INSTRUCTIONS

1. Preheat oven to 400°F and line 2 sheet trays with Silpat mats or parchment paper.
2. While the puff pastry is defrosting at room temperature, make the Coconut Caramel Sauce. Once the sauce is made, set it off to the side and allow it to cool completely.
3. Combine the butter, cinnamon, nutmeg, and a small pinch of salt in a small bowl and stir together. Set aside.
4. Core the pears by cutting off all 4 sides. Discard (or compost!) the core and slice the pears into ⅛-inch slices.
5. To cut and assemble the tartlets, cut each piece of puff pastry into 4 even squares or rectangles, creating 8 total.
6. Using about ⅔ of the caramel sauce, divide it among each square of puff pastry, spooning a little in the center of each and gently spreading it almost to the edges, leaving about ½ inch around the edges without sauce. It's OK if some of the sauce drips off the side of the puff pastry.
7. Divide the pear slices on top of the caramel sauce, fanning them out in a line down the center of each tartlet.
8. Divide the butter mixture on top of each so that there are a few small dollops of butter on top of the pears.
9. Sprinkle with turbinado sugar and bake for 20–30 minutes. Remove and allow to cool slightly.
10. Drizzle with the remaining caramel sauce and serve.

Cinnamon Apple Galette

A galette, to me, is a beautiful, more rustic (read: easier) version of a pie. They can be sweet or savory, and you can change up the ingredients based on the time of year.

YIELD: 8 SERVINGS

INGREDIENTS

4 apples such as Golden Delicious, peeled and sliced

1 teaspoon ground cinnamon

¼ cup light brown sugar (can substitute coconut sugar)

1 tablespoon arrowroot or cornstarch

Juice of ½ lemon

⅛ teaspoon ground ginger

¼ teaspoon kosher salt

1 teaspoon pure vanilla extract

1 recipe Go-To Pie Crust (page 260)

1 egg, lightly beaten

1 tablespoon turbinado sugar

Coconut Caramel Sauce, about ½ recipe (page 259)

INSTRUCTIONS

1. Preheat oven to 400°F and line a baking sheet with a Silpat mat or parchment paper.

2. Place the sliced apples in a large bowl with the cinnamon, light brown sugar, arrowroot, lemon juice, ginger, salt, and vanilla. Mix so all the apples are evenly coated. Set it aside.

3. Roll out your pie crust on a clean surface and carefully transfer it to the baking sheet.

4. Place the apples in the middle of the pie crust, leaving about 2 inches around the outside. If there is a little liquid at the bottom of the bowl, you can pour that over the apples after you have placed them on the pie crust.

5. Fold the edges of the pie crust up over the apples, leaving the apples in the center exposed.

6. Brush the crust with the egg and sprinkle with turbinado sugar.

7. Bake for about 35 minutes or until the crust starts to brown.

8. Allow to cool slightly before slicing and drizzle with Coconut Caramel Sauce. Also great with vanilla ice cream.

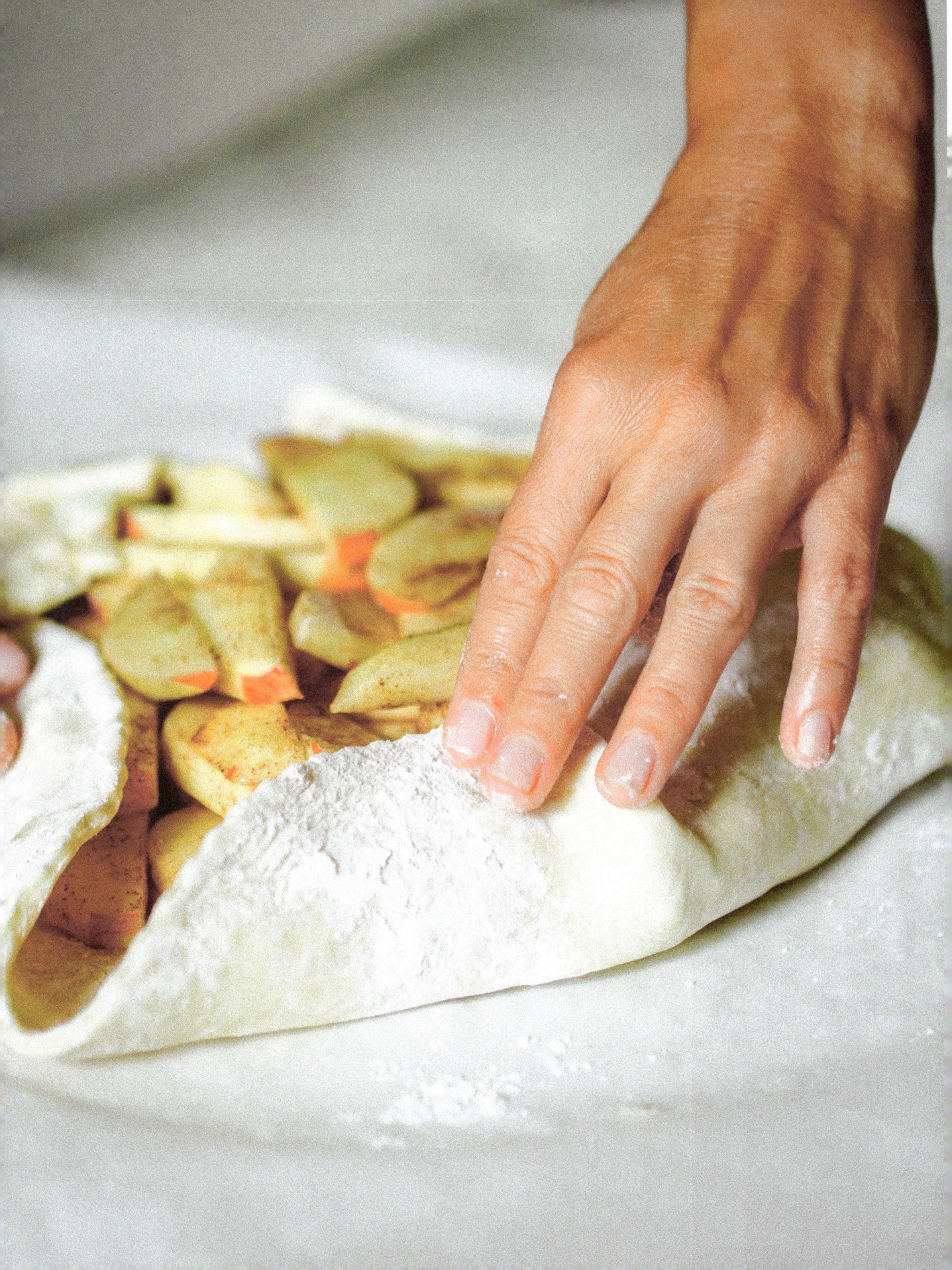

Index

A

Açaí Berry Bowl — 31, 37

Acorn Squash, Sausage and Apple Stuffed — 154

Aioli, Cilantro and Lime — 115, 238

Aioli, Parsley Lemon — 238

Alfredo, Butternut Squash Fettuccine — 178

Aminos, Coconut — 77, 116, 124, 127, 130, 133, 146, 162, 198, 224, 233, 243

Apple — 21, 25, 34, 34, 42, 45, 49, 62, 87, 154, 209, 264

Apple Cider Soup — 87

Apple Galette, Cinnamon — 264

Apple Pancakes with Sage Leaves — 34

Applesauce, Cinnamon — 34, 41, 42, 45, 62, 205

Arrowroot Starch — 116, 217, 233, 256, 264

Arugula — 100, 103, 104, 107

Asparagus — 186, 193, 194

Autumn Squash and Apple Cider Soup — 87

Avocado — 9

Avocado Oil — 13, 99, 116, 189, 205

B

Baba Ghanoush — 65

Bamboo Shoots — 153

Bananas — 9

Banzo Balls — 112, 241

Basic Pasta Dough — 166, 167

Basil — 78, 92, 112, 141, 149, 158, 181, 182, 221, 226, 227, 228, 241

Basil Hummus — 78

Basil Sunflower Seed Pesto — 141, 158, 228

Beans — 9, 14, 74, 78, 92, 96, 99, 115, 120, 157, 218

Beans and Greens Turkey Stew — 96

Beef — 9, 15, 99, 130, 141, 157, 169

Beef Meatballs, Classic Italian — 141

Beet Pasta, Creamy — 177

Beet Tahini Dip — 103, 104, 229

Bell Peppers, Southwestern Stuffed — 157

Bench Scraper — 11, 170, 174, 260

Berry and Beet Smoothie — 24

Berry Crumble Bars — 252

Berry Jam, Mixed — 248, 252

Biscuits, Southern — 58

Black Bean Burgers — 120

Black Bean Grain Bowl — 115

Blender — 11, 13, 17–28, 62, 65, 74, 77, 78, 88, 91, 92, 146, 177, 178, 209, 224, 229, 236, 238, 241, 243, 244, 248

Blueberry — 23, 28, 31, 38, 50, 66, 248, 252, 255

Blueberry Bites — 66

Blueberry Cobbler, Grandma's Peach — 255

Blueberry Coffee Cake — 37, 38

Blueberry Smoothie — 23

Bolognese Sauce — 11, 169

Breakfast — 33–58

Breakfast Bake — 49

Breakfast Hash — 54

Broccoli, Roasted — 186, 202

Burgers, Black Bean — 120

Burgers, Mediterranean Turkey — 149

Burgers, Ultimate Salmon — 190

Butternut Squash Alfredo Fettuccine — 178

C

Cabbage — 130, 153, 162, 213

Caramel — 259, 263, 264

Caramel Pear Tartlets — 259, 263

Caramel Sauce, Coconut — 259

Carrot — 42, 49, 86, 87, 91, 92, 120, 123, 127, 130, 137, 150, 153, 169, 173, 177, 198, 205, 213

Cauliflower — 27, 28, 103, 116, 124, 133, 137, 198, 244

Cauliflower Bites, Cornmeal-Crusted — 124

Cauliflower Cream Sauce — 133, 137, 244

Cauliflower Fried Rice — 198

Cauliflower, General Tso's — 116

Cauliflower, Roasted Chickpea, Salad, — 103

Cheese — 9, 46, 57, 100, 107, 119, 123, 138, 149, 154, 157, 158, 177, 178, 181, 182, 214, 251

Chicken — 53, 86, 92, 95, 96, 99, 108, 133, 134, 136, 137, 138, 145, 146, 150, 161, 169, 178, 209, 226, 227, 231, 241, 244

Chicken Empanadas with Zucchini and Corn — 138

Chicken, Ginger with Lemongrass — 146

Chicken Lettuce Wraps — 134

Chicken, Mama's Wild Rice Casserole — 136, 137

Chicken Orzo Soup with Ginger — 92

Chicken, Roasted with Herb Butter — 150

Chicken Salad with Grapes — 108

Chicken, Shredded Taco — 161

Chicken Stock — 86, 91, 95, 96, 137, 178, 209, 227, 231, 241, 244

Chicken Sweet Potato Meatballs — 145

Chickpea — 14, 65, 77, 103, 112

Chickpea and Cauliflower Salad — 103

Classic Italian Beef Meatballs — 141

Cinnamon — 20, 34, 37, 38, 41, 42, 49, 62, 81, 87, 206, 251, 255, 256, 259, 263, 264

Cinnamon Apple Galette — 259, 264

Cinnamon Applesauce — 34, 41, 42, 45, 62, 205

Cobbler, Grandma's Peach and Blueberry — 255

Coconut — 11, 14, 15, 18, 19, 20, 21, 22, 23, 25, 26, 28, 31, 34, 37, 38, 41, 42, 45, 49, 50, 53, 58, 66, 69, 77, 81, 87, 88, 91, 116, 124, 127, 130, 133, 138, 141, 145, 146, 162, 189, 198, 221, 224, 227, 233, 239, 241, 243, 248, 251, 252, 255, 256, 259, 260, 263, 264

Coconut Bites — 69

Coconut Caramel Sauce — 14, 259, 263, 264

Coconut-Crusted Fish Tacos with Mango Salsa — 189

Coconut Whipped Cream — 31, 255, 256, 259

Coffee Cake, Power Blueberry — 37, 38

Cookie, Oatmeal, Cream Pies — 250

Corn — 13, 81, 119, 124, 138, 157, 182, 189, 193, 221

Corn Ravioli, Sweet — 182

Corn Sauté — 221

Cornmeal-Crusted Cauliflower Bites — 124

Cream Pies, Oatmeal Cookie — 250

Creamy Beet Pasta — 177

Creamy Gnocchi with Peas and Carrots — 173

Creamy Pasta Skillet, Grown-Up — 133

Creamy Poppy Seed Dressing — 235

Creamy Sweet Potatoes — 206

Crisp, Strawberry Rhubarb — 256

Crispy Smashed Potatoes — 210

Curry, Thai Vegetable with Ramen — 127

D

Delicious Roasted Chicken with Herb Butter — 150

Dietary Triggers — 8, 9

Dip, Beet Tahini — 103, 104, 229

Dips — 73, 74, 77, 78, 103, 124, 229, 233

Dressing, Honey Mustard — 104, 234

Dressing, Lemon Dijon Vinaigrette — 100–101, 194, 233

Dressing, Poppy Seed — 108, 213, 235

Dressings — 15, 100, 103, 104, 107, 108, 229, 233, 234, 235, 238

Duck Gumbo — 95

Dumplings, Pork — 162, 233

E

Egg Frittata Muffins — 46

Empanadas, Chicken with Zucchini and Corn — 138

F

Fettuccine Alfredo, Butternut Squash — 178

Fettuccine Noodles — 167

Fish — 9, 12, 15, 185, 186, 189, 190, 193, 194, 227

Fish en Papillote — 193

Fish Tacos, Coconut-Crusted with Mango Salsa — 189

Food Processor — 11, 42, 49, 58, 62, 66, 69, 74, 112, 120, 137, 138, 146, 169, 181, 182, 205, 209, 228, 236, 243

Freezer Staples — 15

Fridge Staples — 15

Frittata, Migraine-Friendly — 54, 57

Fruit — 9, 15, 62, 66, 69, 70, 87, 100, 104, 107, 108, 154, 248, 250, 252, 255, 256, 263, 264

Fully Loaded Sweet Potatoes — 158

G

Galette, Apple Cinnamon — 259, 264

Garlic — 9, 46, 53, 54, 57, 65, 73, 74, 77, 78, 81, 84, 86, 87, 91, 92, 95, 96, 99, 103, 112, 115, 116, 119, 120, 124, 127, 133, 134, 137, 138, 141, 142, 145, 146, 149, 150, 153, 154, 157, 162, 169, 173, 190, 193, 198, 202, 205, 210, 214, 217, 218, 221, 224, 226–230, 233, 234, 236, 238, 239, 241, 243, 244

Garlic, Herb-Roasted — 73

Garlic Potatoes, Roasted — 217

Garlic, Roasted, White Bean Dip — 73, 74

General Tso's Cauliflower — 116

Ghanoush — 65

Ginger — 18, 24, 28, 37, 92, 116, 134, 142, 146, 153, 162, 186, 198, 233, 243, 264

Ginger Chicken with Lemongrass — 146

Ginger Glaze — 116, 134, 142, 153, 186, 233

Glazed Salmon Quinoa Bowl — 186

Gnocchi — 11, 165, 170, 173, 174

Gnocchi, Peas and Carrots — 173

Gnocchi with Sage Brown Butter Sauce, Pumpkin — 174

Go-To Pie Crust — 123, 260, 264

Grain Bowl, Black Bean — 115

Grandma Parker's Pasta Bolognese — 169

Grandma's Peach and Blueberry Cobbler — 255

Granola, Super Seed — 31, 37, 38, 242, 252

Grape — 25, 100, 108

Grape and Radicchio Salad — 100

Gravy — 9, 58, 230, 231

Gravy, Holiday — 231

Gravy, Sage Sausage — 58, 230

Green Beans, Skillet — 218

Greens — 96, 100, 103, 104, 107, 189, 190

Grilled Shrimp and Asparagus Salad — 194

Grown-Up Creamy Pasta Skillet — 133

Gumbo, Duck — 95

H

Harvest Vegetable Pie — 123

Hash, Saturday Morning — 54

Herb Butter, Delicious Roasted Chicken — 150

Herb-Roasted Garlic — 73

Herb Sauce, Mascarpone — 226

Herby Aioli Two Ways — 120, 124, 205, 210, 238

Herby Glow Smoothie — 21

Herby Turkey Meatballs — 142, 233

Hidden Veggie Smoothie — 27

Holiday Gravy — 231

Honey Mustard Dressing — 104, 234

Hummus, Roasted Red Pepper — 77

Hummus, Sweet Pea and Basil — 78

I

Instant Pot — 12, 95, 99, 112, 141, 146, 161, 169, 201, 224

Instant Pot Marinara — 224

Italian Meatballs, Beef — 141

J

Jam, Mixed Berry — 248, 252

Johnny's Pumpkin Muffins — 45

K

Kitchen Tools — 11, 12

L

Latkes, Root Vegetable — 205

Lemon Dijon Vinaigrette — 100–101, 194, 233

Lemongrass, Ginger Chicken — 146

Lettuce Wraps, Chicken — 134

M

Make Your Own Sausage — 49, 53, 54, 57, 95, 137, 154, 158, 169, 230

Mama's Chicken and Wild Rice Casserole — 136, 137

Mango — 18, 21, 25, 27, 50, 189

Mango Salsa, Coconut-Crusted Fish Tacos with — 189

Maple — 15, 20, 28, 31, 34, 37, 38, 42, 45, 49, 50, 62, 69, 70, 81, 90, 107, 123

Maple Chili Pumpkin Seeds — 70, 90, 107

Maple Curry Pumpkin Seeds — 70

Marinara Sauce — 112, 141, 146, 224

Mascarpone Herb Sauce — 226

Meat — 9, 12, 15, 53, 95, 99, 108, 130–162, 169, 170, 214

Meatballs — 141, 142, 145, 228, 233

Meatballs, Chicken Sweet Potato — 145

Meatballs, Classic Italian Beef — 141

Meatballs, Herby Turkey — 142, 233

Meaty Mains — 7, 129–162

Mediterranean Turkey Burgers — 149

Migraine-Free Morning Glory Muffins — 42

Migraine-Friendly Frittata — 54, 57

Migraine Triggers — 8, 9

Mint — 18, 19, 226

Minty Mango Kale Smoothie — 18

Mixed Berry and Beet Smoothie — 24

Mixed Berry Jam — 248

Mixed Greens and Quinoa Salad — 104

Moo Shu Bowl — 153

Muffins — 13, 41, 42, 45, 46, 62, 174

Mustard Dressing, Honey — 104, 234

N

Noodles, Fettuccine — 167

O

Oat Flour — 13, 34, 38, 42, 45, 49, 112, 120, 141, 142, 145, 251, 252

Oatmeal Cookie Cream Pies — 250

Oats — 13, 20, 37, 38, 41, 42, 50, 66, 69, 112, 120, 141, 142, 145, 248, 250, 251, 252, 256

Orzo Soup, Chicken — 92

Overnight Oats Three Ways — 50

P

Pancakes — 34, 248

Pantry Staples — 13, 14

Papillote, Fish en — 193

Parsnip and Turnip Purée — 209

Pasta — 11, 65, 73, 133, 150, 165–182, 226, 228, 241

Pasta, Bolognese, Grandma Parker's — 169

Pasta, Butternut Squash Fettuccine Alfredo — 178

Pasta, Creamy Beet — 177

Pasta Dough — 166, 167, 181, 182

Pasta Skillet, Grown-Up Creamy — 133

Pastry Blender — 11, 41, 154, 206, 256, 260

Pea Brown Butter Rice, Snap — 201

Pea Hummus — 78

Pea Ravioli, Spring — 181

Peach — 18, 28, 31, 255

Peach and Blueberry Cobbler, Grandma's — 255

Peach Pie Smoothie (or Bowl) — 28

"Peanut" Sauce, Thai — 130, 243

Pear — 26, 50, 263

Pear Tartlets, Caramel — 262

Peas and Carrots, Creamy Gnocchi with — 173

Peppers, Southwestern Stuffed Bell — 157

Pesto, Basil Sunflower Seed — 141, 158, 228

Pie Crust — 11, 123, 260, 264

Pie, Harvest Vegetable — 123

Pie, Savory Root Vegetable — 123

Pink Dragon Smoothie — 26

Popcorn Toppings, Sweet and Savory — 81

Poppy Seed Dressing — 108, 213, 235

Pork — 15, 53, 54, 130, 153, 162, 233

Pork Dumplings — 162, 233

Potato — 11, 54, 57, 84, 86, 91, 112, 123, 170, 174, 205, 210, 214, 217

Potato Meatballs, Chicken Sweet — 145

Potatoes, Creamy Sweet — 206

Potatoes, Crispy Smashed — 210

Potatoes, Roasted Garlic — 54, 57, 217

Potatoes, Twice-Baked Cheese and Chive — 214

Power Blueberry Coffee Cake — 37, 38

Pumpkin — 20, 37, 45, 50, 70, 87, 107, 174

Pumpkin Gnocchi with Sage Brown Butter Sauce — 174

Pumpkin Muffins — 45

Pumpkin Seeds Two Ways — 70

Purée, Parsnip and Turnip — 209

Q

Quick Moo Shu Bowl — 153

Quinoa — 14, 104, 119, 153, 186

Quinoa Bowl, Glazed Salmon — 186

Quinoa and Mixed Greens Salad — 104

Quinoa Taco Filling — 119

R

Radicchio — 100

Rainbow Slaw — 213

Ramen, Thai Vegetable Curry — 127

Ravioli, Spring Pea — 181

Ravioli, Sweet Corn — 182

Red Pepper Hummus — 77

Rhubarb — 22, 256

Rhubarb Crisp, Strawberry — 256

Rice, Cauliflower Fried — 198

Rice Casserole, Mama's Chicken and Wild — 136, 137

Ricer — 11, 170, 174, 206

Roasted Blueberry Smoothie — 23

Roasted Broccoli — 186, 202

Roasted Chicken with Herb Butter — 150

Roasted Chickpea and Cauliflower Salad — 103

Roasted Garlic — 73, 74

Roasted Garlic Potatoes — 54, 57, 217

Roasted Garlic White Bean Dip — 73, 74

Roasted Grape and Radicchio Salad — 100

Roasted Poblano and Tomatillo Salsa — 236

Roasted Red Pepper Hummus — 77

Roasted Red Pepper Vodka Sauce — 112, 141, 241

Root Vegetable Latkes — 205

Root Vegetable Soup — 91

S

Sage — 34, 53, 58, 99, 123, 150, 154, 158, 169, 174, 178, 182, 185, 209, 230, 231

Sage Brown Butter Sauce — 174, 182

Sage Sausage Gravy — 230

Salad — 7, 13, 83, 100, 103, 104, 107, 108, 119, 120, 194, 229

Salad, Chicken, with Grapes — 108

Salad, Grilled Shrimp and Asparagus — 194

Salad, Roasted Chickpea and Cauliflower — 103

Salmon Burgers — 190

Salmon, Glazed, Quinoa Bowl — 186

Salsa, Roasted Poblano and Tomatillo — 236

Saturday Morning Breakfast Hash — 54

Sauce, Coconut Caramel — 259

Sauce, Mascarpone Herb — 182, 226

Sauce, Roasted Red Pepper Vodka — 241

Sauce, Tarragon Basil — 227

Sauce, Thai "Peanut" — 243

Sauces — 7, 9, 11, 14, 15, 65, 130, 141, 146, 167, 169, 170, 173, 174, 178, 181, 182, 223–244, 259, 263, 264

Sausage — 9, 49, 53, 54, 57, 58, 95, 137, 154, 158, 169, 230

Sausage and Apple Stuffed Acorn Squash — 154

Sausage Gravy, Sage — 58, 230

SB&J Smoothie — 25

Seafood — 7, 185–194

Seasonal Quinoa and Mixed Greens Salad — 104

Seed Mix — 37, 242

Seeds — 9, 13, 14, 15, 19, 20, 25, 27, 28, 31, 37, 38, 50, 53, 66, 69, 70, 87, 96, 100, 107, 108, 116, 124, 130, 134, 141, 146, 158, 186, 213, 226, 228, 235, 242, 243, 252

Short Rib and White Bean Stew — 99, 206

Shredded Taco Chicken — 161

Shrimp — 194

Shrimp and Asparagus Salad, Grilled — 194

Sides — 7, 197–221

Silpat — 12, 22, 37, 41, 42, 45, 46, 58, 65, 70, 100, 123, 124, 138, 141, 142, 154, 202, 210, 252, 263, 264

Skillet Green Beans — 218

Slaw, Rainbow — 213

Smoothies — 7, 11, 15, 17–28, 174, 259

Snacks — 7, 9, 19, 45, 61–81, 174

Snap Pea Brown Butter Rice — 201

Snickerdoodle Muffins with Streusel Topping — 41, 45

Soups — 83, 87, 91, 92

Southern Biscuits — 58, 230

Southwestern Stuffed Bell Peppers — 157

Spring Pea Ravioli — 181

Spring Strawberry and Arugula Salad — 107

Squash — 87, 104, 112, 154, 178, 193

Squash, Butternut Fettuccine Alfredo — 178

Squash, Sausage and Apple Stuffed Acorn — 154

Stew — 7, 11, 12, 83, 95, 96, 99, 206

Stew, Beans and Greens Turkey — 96

Stew, Short Rib and White Bean — 99, 206

Stir-Fried Udon — 130

Stocks — 83, 84, 86, 87

Strawberry — 19, 22, 26, 28, 31, 50, 69, 107, 248, 256

Strawberry and Arugula Salad — 107

Strawberry Coconut Bites — 11, 69

Strawberry Mint Refresher — 19

Strawberry Rhubarb Crisp — 256

Strawberry Rhubarb Smoothie — 22

Stocks, Soups, Stews, and Salads — 7, 83–108, 206

Stuffed Bell Peppers — 157

Summer Corn Sauté — 221

Super Seed Granola — 31, 37, 38, 242, 252

Super Seed Mix — 37, 242

Sweet Corn Ravioli — 182

Sweet Pea and Basil Hummus — 78

Sweet Potato — 20, 49, 91, 104, 123, 145, 158, 205, 206

Sweet Potato Apple Breakfast Bake — 49

Sweet Potato Meatballs, Chicken — 145

Sweet Potato Pie Smoothie — 20

Sweet Potatoes, Creamy — 206

Sweet Potatoes, Fully Loaded — 158

Sweet and Savory Popcorn Toppings — 81

Sweets — 247–264

T

Taco Chicken, Shredded — 161

Tacos, Coconut-Crusted Fish with Mango Salsa — 189

Taco Filling, Quinoa — 119

Taco Seasoning — 119, 145, 157, 161, 239

Tahini — 15, 65, 77, 78, 103, 104, 229

Tahini, Beet, Dip — 103, 104, 229

Tahini Dressing — 103, 104, 229

Tarragon Basil Sauce — 227

Tartlets, Caramel Pear — 259, 263

Thai "Peanut" Sauce — 130, 243

Thai Vegetable Curry with Ramen — 127

Tomatillo Salsa, Roasted Poblano — 236

Turkey — 15, 53, 96, 130, 133, 142, 145, 149, 169, 231

Turkey Burgers, Mediterranean — 149

Turkey Meatballs, Herby — 142, 233

Turkey Stew — 96

Turnip — 84, 86, 91, 209

Turnip Purée, Parsnip — 209

Twice-Baked Cheese and Chive Potatoes — 214

U

Udon, Stir-Fried — 130

Ultimate Salmon Burgers — 190

V

Vanilla — 14, 20, 28, 34, 37, 38, 41, 42, 45, 49, 50, 251, 252, 259, 264

Vegetable — 9, 11, 13, 15, 27, 46, 57, 83, 84, 86, 87, 91, 92, 96, 99, 103, 104, 111, 123, 127, 137, 138, 145, 158, 169, 170, 177, 178, 186, 193, 201, 205, 209, 224, 226, 227, 231, 241, 243, 244

Vegetable Curry with Ramen, Thai — 127

Vegetable Latkes, Root — 205

Vegetable Harvest, Pie — 123

Vegetable Soup — 91

Vegetable Stock — 15, 84, 87, 91, 92, 96, 119, 127, 137, 178, 201, 209, 224, 226, 227, 231, 241, 244

Vegetarian Mains — 7, 111–127

Veggie Smoothie — 27

Vinaigrette, Lemon Dijon — 100–101, 194, 233

Vinegar — 9, 87, 116, 138, 233, 234, 235

Vodka Sauce, Roasted Red Pepper — 112, 141, 241

W

Whipped Cream, Coconut — 31, 255, 256, 259

White Bean Dip — 73, 74

White Bean Stew — 99, 206

Wild Rice, Chicken Casserole — 136, 137

Wraps, Chicken Lettuce — 134

Y

Yeast — 9

Z

Zucchini — 138

Zucchini and Corn, Chicken Empanadas — 138

About the Authors

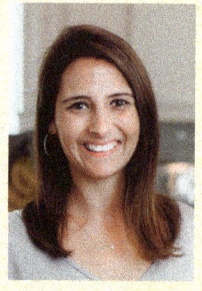

CAT BROWNE is a personal chef, nutrition educator, and healthy lifestyle advocate. Cat graduated from the College of Charleston and quickly realized while working in the industry that cooking was her calling. She soon enrolled in The Culinary Institute of America at Greystone, in Napa Valley, California. She earned the Culinary Achievement Award and helped to start the school's first farm to table program following graduation. In 2015 Cat returned to her hometown of Raleigh, North Carolina, to start her personal chef company, Culinary Solutions. Cat provides meal prep services to families, teaches cooking classes, and caters to many allergies and dietary restrictions. With over 15 years' experience, Cat is passionate about helping people discover a whole foods lifestyle through healthy, flavorful meals that focus on fresh ingredients. Cat lives in Raleigh with her two young children.

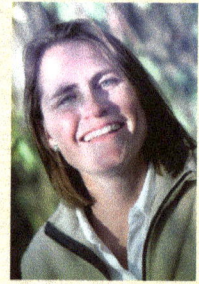

LAURIE HARTFORD, MS, RD, has a BA in biology with a concentration in nutrition from Cornell University and an MS in nutrition from Boston University. She is a registered dietician. She previously worked as a dietician in pediatrics for Dartmouth Hitchcock Medical Center and for the Cystic Fibrosis team at the University of Kentucky. Laurie is currently in private practice in the Bay Area.

Cat and Laurie connected through Cat's father and Laurie's husband, who have worked together in the health-care industry.

www.ingramcontent.com/pod-product-compliance
Lightning Source LLC
Chambersburg PA
CBHW041532120626
46551CB00018B/2663

9 7 9 8 9 9 9 0 6 7 2 1 0